theclinics.com

PEDIATRIC CLINICS OF NORTH AMERICA

International Adoption: Medical and Developmental Issues

GUEST EDITORS
Lisa H. Albers, MD, MPH
Elizabeth D. Barnett, MD
Jerri Ann Jenista, MD
Dana E. Johnson, MD, PhD

October 2005 • Volume 52 • Number 5

SAUNDERS

An Imprint of Elsevier, Inc.
PHILADELPHIA   LONDON   TORONTO   MONTREAL   SYDNEY   TOKYO

W.B. SAUNDERS COMPANY
A Division of Elsevier Inc.

1600 John F. Kennedy Boulevard • Suite 1800 • Philadelphia, Pennsylvania 19103

http://www.theclinics.com

THE PEDIATRIC CLINICS OF NORTH AMERICA	Volume 52, Number 5
October 2005	ISSN 0031-3955
Editor: Carin Davis	ISBN 1-4160-2751-3

The ideas and opinions expressed in *The Pediatric Clinics of North America* do not necessarily reflect those of the Publisher. The Publisher does not assume any responsibility for any injury and/or damage to persons or property arising out of or related to any use of the material contained in this periodical. The reader is advised to check the appropriate medical literature and the product information currently provided by the manufacturer of each drug to be administered to verify the dosage, the method and duration of administration, or contraindications. It is the responsibility of the treating physician or other health care professional, relying on independent experience and knowledge of the patient, to determine drug dosages and the best treatment for the patient. Mention of any product in this issue should not be construed as endorsement by the contributors, editors, or the Publisher of the product or manufacturers' claims.

The Pediatric Clinics of North America (ISSN 0031-3955) is published bi-monthly by W.B. Saunders Company, Corporate and Editorial offices: 1600 JFK Boulevard, Suite 1800, Philadelphia, PA 19103-2822. Accounting and Circulation offices: 6277 Sea Harbor Drive, Orlando, FL 32887-4800. Periodicals postage paid at Orlando, FL 32862, and additional mailing offices. Subscription prices are $135.00 per year (US individuals), $246.00 per year (US institutions), $177.00 per year (Canadian individuals), $320.00 per year (Canadian institutions), $200.00 per year (international individuals), $320.00 per year (international institutions), $68.00 per year (US students), $100.00 per year (Canadian students), and $100.00 per year (foreign students). To receive student/resident rate, orders must be accompanied by name of affiliated institution, date of term, and the signature of program/residency coordinator on institution letterhead. Orders will be billed at individual rate until proof of status is received. Foreign air speed delivery is included in all Clinics subscription prices. All prices are subject to change without notice. POSTMASTER: Send address changes to *The Pediatric Clinics of North America*, W.B. Saunders Company, Periodicals Fulfillment, Orlando, FL 32887-4800. **Customer Service: 1-800-654-2452 (US). From outside of the US, call 1-407-345-4000.** E-mail: hhspcs@harcourt.com.

The Pediatric Clinics of North America is also published in Spanish by McGraw-Hill Inter-americana Editores S.A., Mexico City, Mexico; in Portuguese by Reichmann and Affonso Editores, Rua Comandante Coelho 1085, CEP 21250, Rio de Janeiro, Brazil; and in Greek by Althayia SA, Athens, Greece.

The Pediatric Clinics of North America is covered in *Index Medicus, Excerpta Medica, Current Contents, Current Contents/Clinical Medicine, Science Citation Index, ASCA, ISI/BIOMED,* and *BIOSIS.*

Printed in the United States of America.

GUEST EDITORS

LISA ALBERS, MD, MPH, Adoption Program, Developmental Medicine Center, Children's Hospital Boston, Boston, Massachusetts

ELIZABETH D. BARNETT, MD, Associate Professor of Pediatrics, Boston University School of Medicine; and Maxwell Finland Laboratory for Infectious Diseases, Boston Medical Center, Boston, Massachusetts

JERRI ANN JENISTA, MD, Pediatrician, Department of Pediatrics and Emergency Medicine, St. Joseph Mercy Hospital, Ann Arbor, Michigan

DANA E. JOHNSON, MD, PhD, Department of Pediatrics, University of Minnesota, International Adoption Clinic, University of Minnesota Children's Hospital, Minneapolis, Minnesota

CONTRIBUTORS

LISA ALBERS, MD, MPH, Adoption Program, Developmental Medicine Center, Children's Hospital Boston, Boston, Massachusetts

ELIZABETH D. BARNETT, MD, Associate Professor of Pediatrics, Boston University School of Medicine; and Maxwell Finland Laboratory for Infectious Diseases, Boston Medical Center, Boston, Massachusetts

JULIA M. BLEDSOE, MD, Clinical Associate Professor of Pediatrics, Division of General Pediatrics, University of Washington School of Medicine; Co-Director, Center for Adoption Medicine; Staff Pediatrician, FAS Diagnostic and Prevention Network, University of Washington, Seattle, Washington

JENNIFER CHAMBERS, MD, MPH & TM, Assistant Professor, Department of Pediatrics, University of Alabama; Director, International Adoption Clinic, Birmingham, Alabama

LIN H. CHEN, MD, Director of the Travel Medicine Center, Division of Infectious Diseases, Mount Auburn Hospital; Assistant Clinical Professor of Medicine, Harvard Medical School, Cambridge, Massachusetts

EILEEN COSTELLO, MD, Assistant Clinical Professor of Pediatrics, Boston University Medical School, Boston; Southern Jamaica Plain Health Center, Jamaica Plain, Massachusetts

SUSAN SOON-KEUM COX, Vice President, Holt International Children's Services, Eugene, Oregon

JULIAN K. DAVIES, MD, Clinical Assistant Professor of Pediatrics, Division of General Pediatrics, University of Washington School of Medicine; Co-Director, Center for Adoption Medicine; Staff Pediatrician, FAS Diagnostic and Prevention Network, University of Washington, Seattle, Washington

KATHRYN N. DOLE, MS, OTR/L, International Adoption Clinic, Fairview–University Medical Center, University of Minnesota; Department of Special Education, Minneapolis Public Schools, Minneapolis, Minnesota

JERRI ANN JENISTA, MD, Pediatrician, Department of Pediatrics and Emergency Medicine, St. Joseph Mercy Hospital, Ann Arbor, Michigan

DANA E. JOHNSON, MD, PhD, Department of Pediatrics, University of Minnesota, International Adoption Clinic, University of Minnesota Children's Hospital, Minneapolis, Minnesota

JUDITH ECKERLE KANG, MD, Department of Pediatrics, New York Presbyterian Hospital, Weill Cornell Medical Center, New York, New York

JOY LIEBERTHAL, LMSW, President, Also-Known-As, New York, New York

PATRICK MASON, MD, PhD, International Adoption Center, Inova Fairfax Hospital for Children; Northern Virginia Endocrinologists, Fairfax, Virginia

LAURIE C. MILLER, MD, Associate Professor of Pediatrics; Director, International Adoption Clinic, Tufts University School of Medicine, The Floating Hospital for Children–New England Medical Center, Boston, Massachusetts

LISA NALVEN, MD, MA, FAAP, Director, Developmental Pediatrics–Adoption Screening and Evaluation Program, Valley Center for Child Development, Ridgewood, New Jersey; Clinical Assistant Professor, Department of Pediatrics, Columbia University College of Physicians and Surgeons, New York, New York

CHRISTINE NARAD, APRN, BC, International Adoption Center, Inova Fairfax Hospital for Children, Fairfax, Virginia

ELAINE E. SCHULTE, MD, MPH, Associate Professor of Pediatrics, Medical Director, International Adoption Program, Department of Pediatrics, Albany Medical College, Albany, New York

KAY SELIGSOHN, PhD, Adoption Program, Children's Hospital Boston, Boston, Massachusetts

SARAH H. SPRINGER, MD, Chair, American Academy of Pediatrics Section on Adoption and Foster Care; Medical Director, International Adoption Health Services of Western Pennsylvania, Pediatric Alliance, PC, Pittsburgh, Pennsylvania

CAROL WEITZMAN, MD, Department of Pediatrics, Yale University School of Medicine, New Haven, Connecticut

CONTENTS

Despite the popularity of international adoption in North America
and Western Europe as a means to build a family, the knowledge
of health care professionals is often limited regarding the historical
context of this phenomenon as well as the motivations and process
experienced by adoptive parents. Although international adoption
is viewed as an acceptable if not admirable method of forming
kinships in accepting countries, opinions in the international community are mixed. Whether international adoptions increase or are
drastically curtailed depends on addressing the misgivings that
many countries have about placing their children abroad. Concerns
center in two broad areas: sensitivity toward preservation of family
and culture and whether the process has sufficient integrity to act
in the best interests of children and birth parents.

International adoption pairs the most vulnerable and high-risk
pediatric population with the lowest risk parent group. International adoption also presents unique and rewarding challenges
for primary care pediatricians. After receiving information from
the medical reviewer, a parent must determine whether or not
this child is "their child." The position of the medical reviewer is to
provide the family with as much information as possible about
the health status of the child by explaining the terminology in the
report and assessing the photograph or videotape. It is also the

reviewer's job to guide the parent's expectations of the adoption by explaining the inherent differences in the development of children in institutions. In the preadoption phase, we must remember that our ultimate goal is to aid in the permanent placement of a child with a family that has realistic expectations and is well prepared to aid that child to reach his or her fullest potential.

Pretravel consultation before international adoption must encompass standard advice for those who travel, advice for those who are exposed to the newly adopted child, and information about caring for a new child during travel. Children who travel to meet siblings may need special accommodations before and during travel. Data on the health of internationally adopted children illustrate the risk of exposing family members and close contacts to some infectious diseases during or after international adoption. Parents, family members, and close contacts of the newly adopted child should be given advice to reduce their own and their child's risk. Targeted preadoption counseling, close attention to hygiene and safety advice, and prompt identification and treatment of infections lead to the safest and most trouble-free adoption travel experience.

Health care professionals play a critical role in providing age-appropriate immunizations and assessing newly arrived internationally adopted children for infectious diseases. A systematic approach to screening for infectious diseases combined with assessment of signs and symptoms that could be related to diseases prevalent in the child's country of origin supports children's long-term health and that of their new families.

The arrival of a newly adopted child into the family is usually a joyous time. Behavioral concerns arise in many internationally adopted children, most of whom are infants or toddlers at the time of placement with their adoptive families. Problems with feeding, sleeping, and other daily activities are often prominent in the first few weeks after the adoption. Some children display emotional distress and developmental delays; however, most recover rapidly. Anticipatory guidance from the pediatrician can assist families and children with this major life transition.

After international adoption, routine screenings for infectious and nutritional diseases, lead exposure, and vision and hearing difficulties are early priorities for children's postadoptive health care. Specific health concerns raised before adoption should also be reviewed after children arrive home with their families. Once appropriate postadoptive screenings and immunizations have been initiated, the challenge for the primary care provider is to determine the intervals and content of future follow-up visits. Clinical decision making is influenced by a specific child's age, acute medical needs, and developmental assessments.

Growth delay is one of the most common and persistent findings in children who have been adopted from abroad. Although the cause is not clearly understood, it may be related to the observed phenomenon of psychosocial short stature described in children from abusive and neglectful settings in western countries. Fortunately, adopted children generally experience significant improvement in growth after joining their new family, but this may put girls at risk for early and rapidly progressing puberty. This review should help the health care team to understand these issues and work better with the adoptive parents to ensure a child's smooth transition into family life.

Prenatal alcohol and drug exposures are a significant concern in many domestic and international adoptions. This article addresses the following substance exposures for children: alcohol, opiates, tobacco, marijuana, cocaine, and methamphetamines. For each substance, we review the teratogenicity of the exposure and identify the spectrum of neurodevelopmental issues that can present in children exposed to this substance. Diagnosis of the spectrum of fetal alcohol outcomes is also discussed. When possible, we provide country-specific statistics on exposure risks for adopted children.

Children adopted internationally and their families are a heterogeneous group. Internationally-adopted children have been reported to have a range of developmental and behavioral difficulties. The authors describe the current evidence documenting developmental outcomes for children and common behavioral and mental health concerns including attachment difficulties that may impact children and their families after international adoption. Pediatricians must be thoughtful to individualize the care of adoptive children and not make assumptions shortly after adoption. It is critical to avoid using "standard" parenting advice that may not apply to children who have experienced loss, deprivation, separation, and instability in their early lives. By listening to families, carefully evaluating children, and monitoring progress over time, pediatricians can avoid the pitfall of oversimplifying and underestimating the complexity and challenges that these families face. Instead, pediatric primary care providers can play a key role in maximizing the potential of an internationally adopted child and his or her family.

As a result of their preadoptive histories and experiences, internationally adopted children, especially those with a history of institutionalization, can present with a complex profile of developmental and behavioral issues. Although many children demonstrate significant recovery and resilience after joining their adoptive homes, others go on to have mild or sometimes more severe developmental and behavioral issues. This high-risk population requires comprehensive evaluation, monitoring, and interventions by professionals with expertise in child development and knowledge of the impact of institutionalized care to support optimal developmental and behavioral outcomes for children and their families. This article focuses on strategies for evaluation and management of long-term developmental and/or behavioral difficulties exhibited by postinstitutionalized children.

Families who adopt internationally often need assistance in determining which factors they need to consider when making educational decisions for their child, and they frequently seek guidance from their physician. Understanding how the educational system functions, how it differs from the medical system, and how children who have been adopted internationally can succeed in school is important for health care providers, because this information helps parents in making proactive decisions for their children. Internationally adopted children have the best chance of maximizing their learning potential when medical and educational professionals work together to assist families as they plan for their child's education.

Children who are internationally adopted are at increased risk of developmental and behavioral concerns, including attention disorders, learning disorders, and autistic spectrum disorders. In attempting to promote their child's optimal development and well-being, parents of internationally adopted children are faced with the additional stress of having many unanswered and unanswerable questions about their child's early origins. As a result, internationally adopted children and their parents need the support and counsel of their pediatrician as they grow and develop into adulthood. A combination of traditional, complementary, and alternative therapies is the rule rather than the exception for most children with developmental challenges.

As international adoption has become more "mainstream," the issues recently addressed in domestic adoption have become more important in adoptions involving children originating in other countries. Certain groups of prospective adoptive parents, such as gay or lesbian couples, single parents, and parents with disabilities, have begun to apply to adopt in ever increasing numbers. Children who may have been considered unadoptable in the past are now routinely being offered to prospective adoptive parents. The numbers and ages of the children placed and the spacing between adoptions have come under scrutiny. The rates of adoption dissolutions and disruptions are being examined carefully by the receiving and sending countries. There is a pressing need for research into numerous social aspects of adoption.

Intercountry adoption is an extremely sensitive and emotional issue for the citizens of the sending countries as well as for those in other, often more affluent, countries who adopt these children. It must be a priority to respect the dignity of the child's birth country as well as the dignity of the child.

GOAL STATEMENT

The goal of *Pediatric Clinics of North America* is to keep practicing physicians and residents up to date with current clinical practice in pediatrics by providing timely articles reviewing the state-of-the-art in patient care.

ACCREDITATION

The *Pediatric Clinics of North America* is planned and implemented in accordance with the Essential Areas and Policies of the Accreditation Council for Continuing Medical Education (ACCME) through the joint sponsorship of the University of Virginia School of Medicine and Elsevier. The University of Virginia School of Medicine is accredited by the ACCME to provide continuing medical education for physicians.

The University of Virginia School of Medicine designates this educational activity for a maximum of 90 category 1 credits per year, 15 category 1 credits per issue, toward the AMA Physician's Recognition Award. Each physician should claim only those credits that he/she actually spent in the activity.

The American Medical Association has determined that physicians not licensed in the US who participate in this CME activity are eligible for AMA PRA category 1 credit.

Category 1 credit can be earned by reading the text material, taking the CME examination online at http://www.theclinics.com/home/cme, and completing the evaluation. After taking the test, you will be required to review any and all incorrect answers. Following completion of the test and evaluation, your credit will be awarded and you may print your certificate.

FACULTY DISCLOSURE

The University of Virginia School of Medicine, as an ACCME accredited provider, endorses and strives to comply with the Accreditation Council for Continuing Medical Education (ACCME) Standards of Commercial Support, Commonwealth of Virginia statutes, University of Virginia policies and procedures, and associated federal and private regulations and guidelines on the need for disclosure and monitoring of proprietary and financial interests that may affect the scientific integrity and balance of content delivered in continuing medical education activities under our auspices.

The University of Virginia School of Medicine requires that all CME activities accredited through this institution be developed independently and be scientifically rigorous, balanced and objective in the presentation/discussion of its content, theories and practices.

All authors/editors participating in an accredited CME activity are expected to disclose to the readers relevant financial relationships with commercial entities occurring within the past 12 months (such as grants or research support, employee, consultant, stock holder, member of speakers bureau, etc.). The University of Virginia School of Medicine will employ appropriate mechanisms to resolve potential conflicts of interest to maintain the standards of fair and balanced education to the reader. Questions about specific strategies can be directed to the Office of Continuing Medical Education, University of Virginia School of Medicine, Charlottesville, Virginia.

The authors/editors listed below have identified no financial or professional relationships for themselves, their spouse/partner: Lisa H. Albers, MD, MPH; Elizabeth D. Barnett, MD; Jennifer Chambers, MD, MPH & TM; Susan Soon-keum Cox; Carin Davis, Acquisitions Editor; Kathryn N. Dole, MS, OTR/L; Jerri Ann Jenista, MD, MS; Dana E. Johnson, MD, PhD; Judith Echerle Kang, MD; Joy Lieberthal, LMSW; Patrick W. Mason, MD, PhD; Laurie C. Miller, MD; Lisa Nalven, MD, MA, FAAP; Christine Narad, APRN, BC; Elaine E. Schulte, MD, MPH; Kay Seligsohn, PhD; Sarah H. Springer, MD; and, Carol Weitzman, MD.

The author listed below has identified the following financial or professional relationships: Lin H. Chen, MD is consultant, travel health advisor, and serves on the editorial board for American Health.

The following authors have not provided disclosure information: Julia M. Bledsoe, MD; Eileen Costello, MD; and, Julian K. Davies, MD.

Disclosure of Discussion of Non-FDA Approved Uses for Pharmaceutical and/or Medical Devices: **The University of Virginia School of Medicine, as an ACCME provider, requires that all authors identify and disclose any "off label" uses for pharmaceutical and medical device products. The University of Virginia School of Medicine recommends that each physician fully review all the available data on new products or procedures prior to clinical use.**

TO ENROLL

To enroll in the *Pediatric Clinics of North America* Continuing Medical Education program, call customer service at **1-800-654-2452** or visit us online at www.theclinics.com/home/cme. The CME program is available to subscribers for an additional fee of $205.00.

ELSEVIER
SAUNDERS

Pediatr Clin N Am 52 (2005) xiii–xv

PEDIATRIC CLINICS
OF NORTH AMERICA

Preface

International Adoption: Medical and Developmental Issues

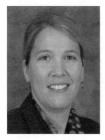 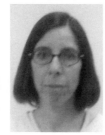 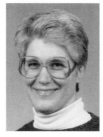 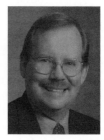

Lisa Albers, MD, MPH   Elizabeth D. Barnett, MD   Jerri Ann Jenista, MD   Dana E. Johnson, MD, PhD
Guest Editors

For more than a decade, international adoption has been increasing world-wide, with 22,884 children born abroad adopted by United States citizens in 2004. The experiences of children with a history of international adoption may be widely disparate. For example, for 50 years, families have welcomed children from orphanages or foster families in Korea into their homes and their hearts while children born in the former Soviet Union or China, residing primarily in child welfare institutions, have been joining families for only a decade. Although the children of international adoption may share some similar experiences with domestically adopted children or with immigrant or refugee children, their situation from birth to adulthood is unique from a myriad of medical, developmental and behavioral perspectives. These children often join their families after experiencing significant malnutrition, neglect and deprivation while residing in child welfare institutions. Infectious diseases and prenatal substance exposures may also negatively impact their growth and development as well. While most children thrive after joining their families, a substantial minority may continue to have chronic medical, developmental or behavioral concerns.

As discussed by Johnson, children are internationally adopted within a complex array of political and familial factors—yet appreciating any individual child's trajectory of growth and development within the context of their new family is critical to optimizing any individual child's long-term potential. While pediatric health care providers work with families and children before, during, or after international adoption, little information is provided during medical or nursing school, pediatric residency, or other graduate school training programs to prepare clinicians for this unique yet gratifying experience.

This volume aims to provide primary care and specialty providers with a framework for addressing the needs of internationally adopted children and their families from before adoption into adulthood. Progressing from preadoption consultation to identity development, we review evidence from the literature where possible and describe current clinical standards of care where available.

Articles by Chambers, Barnett, and Chen review considerations for providers when they review preadoption records, help families prepare to travel and meet their new family members and perhaps provide long-distance consultation to families while abroad. Davies and Bledsoe review implications of prenatal substance exposure worldwide, as the demographics of maternal substance use vary widely across countries but may carry long-term implications for families. Miller, Schulte, and Springer review immediate medical, developmental, and behavioral concerns that providers may need to address relatively shortly after children join their families.

While families may be most focused on medical issues before their child's adoption, chronic medical, developmental, or behavioral needs may emerge in the months to years following adoption. The articles by Mason, Weitzman and Albers discuss long-term growth and puberty concerns as well as developmental challenges children and their families may face. Dole, Nalven, and Costello discuss practical strategies for supporting families as they deal with school systems and access mainstream and complementary and or alternative developmental services to support their children's long-term development. Jenista reviews unique considerations for nontraditional adoptive families. Articles by Cox, Lieberthal, and Eckerle Kang review implications of international adoption on any individual's ultimate identity development, including the implications of international adoption for later search for and reunion with their birth families for families who become multiracial through adoption. An annotated bibliography also suggests readings specifically geared to professionals, parents, and children.

Lisa Albers, MD, MPH
Developmental Medicine Center, Pediatrics
Children's Hospital and Harvard Medical School
Adoption Program
300 Longwood Avenue, Fegan 10
Boston, MA 02118, USA
E-mail address: lisa.albers@childrens.harvard.edu

Elizabeth D. Barnett, MD
Section of Pediatric Infectious Diseases
Boston University Medical Center
Maxwell Finland Laboratory for Infectious Diseases
774 Albany Street, 5th Floor
Boston, MA 02118, USA
E-mail address: ebarnett@bu.edu

Jerri Ann Jenista, MD
Adoption Medicine
551 Second Street
Ann Arbor, MI 48103, USA
E-mail address: jajenista@aol.com

Dana E. Johnson, MD, PhD
Division of Neonatology
International Adoption Clinic
University of Minnesota
MMC 211, 420 Delaware Street SE
Minneapolis, MN 55455, USA
E-mail address: johns008@umn.edu

ELSEVIER
SAUNDERS

PEDIATRIC CLINICS

OF NORTH AMERICA

Pediatr Clin N Am 52 (2005) 1221–1246

International Adoption: What Is Fact, What Is Fiction, and What Is the Future?

Dana E. Johnson, MD, PhD

Department of Pediatrics, University of Minnesota, International Adoption Clinic,
University of Minnesota Children's Hospital, MMC 211, 420 Delaware Street SE,
Minneapolis, MN 55455, USA

As providers of primary care for children, we are highly knowledgeable about how families are created—or are we? Although most caregivers with whom we interact become parents in the old-fashioned way, in North America and Western Europe, adoption plays a significant role in the formation of kinships. Neither domestic nor international adoption is well addressed during medical training. Inspection of five major pediatrics texts revealed from none to six pages (0%–0.2% of total pages) devoted to the topic [1–5], despite the fact that among children less than 18 years of age living with families in the United States, 1 of 40 children is adopted [6].

Adoption is a broadly accepted method of building a family and is part of our shared experience in the United States. The 2002 National Adoption Attitudes Survey [7] revealed that more than 90% of Americans had "very favorable" or "somewhat favorable" opinions about adoption, and 64% of respondents reported that a family member or close friend had been adopted. Thirty-nine percent of Americans had quite seriously or somewhat seriously considered adopting at some point in their lives, and 86% believed that adoptive parents derive the same amount or more satisfaction from raising an adopted child as they derive from raising a birth child. In addition to society's approval, adoption advocates have powerful bipartisan political allies, because 160 members of the US House of Representatives and Senate (30%) belong to the Congressional Coalition on Adoption [8].

International adoption is a growing component of adoption in the United States. In 2001, the most recent period for which accurate data are available, international adoptions made up 15% of all adoptions (127,407 total adoptions)

E-mail address: johns008@umn.edu

[9]. This percentage has tripled since 1992. The 2000 US Census reported 199,136 international adoptees younger than 18 years of age living with families in the United States (12.5% of adopted children) [6]. In 2001, the rate of children who joined families through international adoption was 4.7 for every 1000 children born in the United States and 5.6 for every 1000 children born in Canada [9–12]. In some US states, Canadian provinces, and Western European countries, the rates were twice that high (Figs. 1 and 2) [9–13]. Therefore, it is virtually inevitable that providers of primary pediatric care are going to come into contact with families in their practice who are considering or who have adopted internationally.

On the surface, international adoption seems to be a win-win situation. On first encounter, you see elated parents with their newly arrived, scrubbed, well-fed, and immaculately dressed child. Parents with room for a child in their hearts matched with a needy orphan—what could be better? On closer examination, however, international adoption is a series of juxtapositions: separation and loss with dreams fulfilled, poverty with wealth, colonialism with self-determination, exploitation with altruism, religious law with secular law, and best interest of the group with best interest of the individual to mention but a few. The polar view-points of two contemporary figures in this debate illustrate this best. Mother

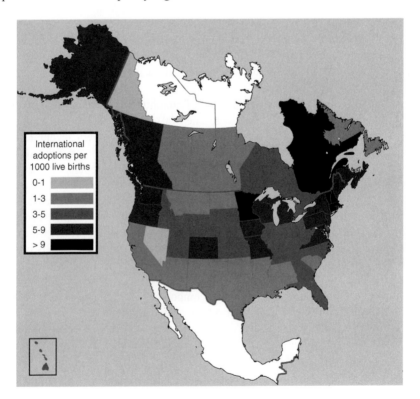

Fig. 1. International adoptions per 1000 live births.

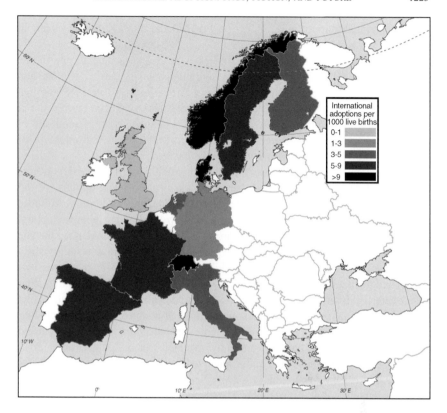

Fig. 2. International adoptions per 1000 live births.

Theresa of Calcutta vigorously promoted international adoption, consistent with her belief that "welcoming a child into one's home is like welcoming Jesus Himself" [14]. Countering this ennobled view of the practice are the statements of Lady Emma Nicholson, who, during her tenure as European Union Parliament Rapporteur for Romania, repeatedly characterized international adoption as an "international trade in children" for the purposes of "pedophilia, child prostitution or domestic servitude" [15]. A method of building families and protecting children where positions are so divided clearly deserves closer examination.

Why people adopt internationally

Although reasons vary, the fundamental motivation to adopt is the desire to parent. Irrespective of individual situations, all who venture down this path share the passion expressed by Jacob's wife Rachel in Genesis 30:1, "Give me children, or I'll die!" Why not adopt domestically, however? Most individuals who pursue international adoption want the entire spectrum of the parenting experience and therefore pursue as young a child as possible. In fiscal year 2001, only 2% of children adopted from foster care through public agencies were less than 1 year old compared with 44% of international adoptees [16]. Although independently adopting an infant or adopting through a private agency remains an option, the percentage of infants relinquished for adoption by never-married women less than 45 years old dropped from 8.7% before 1973 to 0.9% in 1989 through 1995 [17]. The shortage of adoptable children of any age is even more acute in Western Europe. In Sweden from 1995 through 1998, the number of adoptions of Swedish-born children by nonrelatives averaged 16 per year and adoption of fostered children averaged 19 per year for the entire country [18].

Adoptive parents also choose international adoption because of concerns about the child's relationship with her or his birth parents and about potential health issues in fostered children. In the 2002 National Adoption Attitudes Survey, 84% of respondents stated that if they were thinking about adopting, a major concern would be making sure that birth parents could not take the child back [7]. Other families are concerned about open adoption and wish to avoid ongoing interactions with their child's birth parent(s). Medical problems (53%) and mental health issues (63%) also are major worries when adopting from foster care [7]. International adoption does provide some degree of security that birth parents are not going to contact or reclaim their adopted child, but excluding domestic adoption in hopes of avoiding medical or behavioral problems is flawed reasoning, because the children currently available for adoption from abroad share many of the same risk factors and medical and behavioral problems as children in domestic foster care [19–23].

Other factors aside from biologic and social drives for progeny compel individuals to adopt internationally. Religious beliefs play a powerful central role in many people's decisions. Judeo-Christian tradition holds individuals who adopt in high esteem, and in Islam, taking custody of a foundling is deemed an act of piety [24]. Rescuing children from humanitarian disaster triggers resolve in many people, as was evident after the media's depiction of the plight of children in Romanian orphanages in 1990 through 1991 [25]. Family origins in the sending country or an affinity with the sending country's culture may also weigh heavily in this choice. Finally, some families seek special needs children with correctible handicaps who would otherwise not be treated, or parents may wish to share skills they acquired dealing with long-term disabilities in children with similar problems (eg, blindness, deafness).

History

International adoption is rooted in conflict and grew out of the humanitarian tragedies of World War II [26–28]. Orphaned, abandoned by their soldier-fathers, or uprooted and separated from parents, thousands of children were in need of homes. Military personnel occupying affected countries were the first to step forward to adopt these children. Between 1948 and 1962, American families adopted 1845 German, 744 Austrian, and 2987 Japanese children (Table 1)

Table 1
International adoptions to the United States (1948–2003)

Country of origin	No. children
1948–1962	
(n = 19,230)	
Korea	4162 (22%)
Greece	3116 (16%)
Japan	2987 (13%)
Germany	1845 (10%)
Austria	744 (4%)
1975	
(n = 5663)	
Korea	2913 (52%)
Vietnam	655 (12%)
Colombia	379 (7%)
The Philippines	244 (4%)
Mexico	162 (3%)
1986	
(n = 9945)	
Korea	6118 (62%)
The Philippines	634 (10%)
India	588 (9%)
Guatemala	228 (4%)
El Salvador	147 (2%)
1991	
(n = 8481)	
Romania	2594 (31%)
Korea	1818 (21%)
Peru	705 (8%)
Colombia	521 (6%)
India	445 (5%)
2003	
(n = 21,616)	
China	6859 (32%)
Russia	5209 (24%)
Guatemala	2328 (11%)
Korea	1790 (8%)
Kazakhstan	825 (4%)

[26,27]. Additional waves of adoptees arrived in the United States after the Greek Civil War (3116 children from 1948–1962), the Korean War (4162 children from 1953–1962), the Vietnam War (3267 children between 1963 and 1973), and the war in El Salvador (2083 children between 1980 and 1990) (see Table 1) [26,27].

Most of these adoptions were international and interracial. The arrival of the first wave of international adoptees during the late 1940s and early 1950s coincided with a heightened appreciation of racial issues in US society [26,28]. This era saw progress in reversing many of the more deliberate racist practices of the day, a fact that is highlighted by the Supreme Court's decision to end school segregation in Brown v. Board of Education (1954) [29]. Many families of that period saw international adoption not only as a way to build a family but to do so in a way that clearly displayed the values that directed their lives.

The "One-Family United Nations" of Helen Doss and her Methodist-minister husband Carl that graced the pages of *Reader's Digest* and the cover of *Life* in the middle of the twentieth century was the first international adoption "poster family" [30–32]. Infertile but desiring to have children, the Doss family ultimately adopted 12 children, some with special needs, who were considered unadoptable because of their mixed race parentage. The children represented Korea, Japan, the Philippines, Spain, France, Malaysia, Burma, Mexico, Hawaii, and three Native American tribes (Chippewa, Blackfoot, and Cheyenne). In "Our International Family," published in *Reader's Digest* (1949) [31] and in her best-selling book, *The Family Nobody Wanted* (1954) [32], Helen Doss articulated the interplay of religious faith and social conscience that guided their decisions:

> It is the outsiders who imagine that our family is made up of incompatible opposites. Those who have never ventured beyond the white bars of their self-imposed social cages too often take for granted that a different color skin on the outside makes for a different kind of being, not of necessity completely human, on the inside [32].
>
> If you could see our children working, playing, sharing together, dark hair against fair, black eyes laughing into blue, I'm sure you would feel as we do: when there is love and understanding and a common level of culture, artificial barriers of race or nationality disappear. Actually, we are more than an "international family." Our home, with its strong ties of mutual understanding and love, is symbolic of that most inclusive family of all, God's family [31].

Two of the most prominent figures in the early history of international adoption in the United States, Harry and Bertha Holt, shared the same evangelical roots and motivations. Already birth parents of six children, their involvement began in 1954 in response to a presentation in Eugene, Oregon, by Dr. Bob Pierce, the president of World Vision, which detailed the plight of mixed-race "GI babies" left behind after the Korean War [33]. As Bertha Holt wrote in *The Seed from the East* [34]:

> On Friday, April 15th, Harry voiced the burden on his heart.
> "I've been thinking I'd like to go to Korea."
> "I know. I've been hoping you'd go."
> "Every night when I go to bed, I see those pictures all over again. It doesn't make any difference where I am or what I'm doing. I think about those kids over there. I look out here at this beautiful playground God has so generously given us and something inside of me cries out at the thought of those poor little babies starving to death, or being thrown into dumps to be gnawed by rats. I think we ought to adopt some of the GI-children."
> "That's the way I feel, too."
> "How many do you think we could take care of?"
> I knew what I wanted to say. I had thought of it many times and I felt like bursting out with the number eight. Somehow, I lacked the courage. I knew

Harry had thought long and hard about the matter, too, and I had no idea of the number he felt would be right. Finally I answered in a far-off squeaky little voice.

"I suppose we could care for six."

"Oh my...we have plenty of room for eight...or ten...or even more."

"I felt a sudden, joyful release. Now I knew that Harry's number even surpassed mine..."

As I listened to Harry repeat almost word for word the very things I had told myself could be done, I realized that God was working in our hearts. Only God could bring about such a miracle. Simultaneously and without discussion, a highly unusual decision had been made within both our hearts.

In 1955, a special act of Congress permitted the Holts to adopt the eight children they sought [33]. This legislation permanently transformed adoption in the United States, establishing Korea as the principal source of international adoptees to the United States for the next 35 years. Embraced by people of many faiths and world views, spiritual and faith-based motivations like those of the Doss and Holt families remain solidly within the mainstream of international adoption. Health care providers must be cognizant that this decision may be as much a statement of a family's ideals as it is a desire to parent. When Holt signed copies of her book, she followed her name with a reference to Psalm 118:23, a verse that is a suitable ecumenical summary for this perspective on international adoption, "The Lord has done this, and it is marvelous in our eyes."

From 1963 through 1969 the annual number of international adoptees arriving in the United States remained stable at between 1450 and 2100 children per year [26]. However, because of a growing shortfall of adoptable infants in the United States, there was a consistent annual rise in the number of children placed, beginning in 1968 (Fig. 3). This change coincided with an era that saw increasing social tolerance and financial support for unmarried mothers and enhanced reproductive control through reliable contraceptive methods and the availability

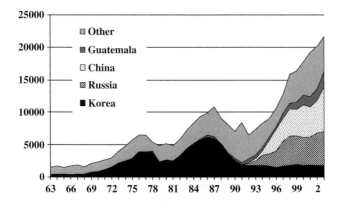

Fig. 3. Origins of international adoptees to the United States, 1963–2003.

of legal abortion services throughout the United States. The net result was that fewer infants were born to single mothers and fewer were relinquished for adoption. In 1968, an estimated 37,100 children from private agencies [35], primarily infants, and 1612 international adoptees [26] were placed in the United States. By 1975, the number of estimated placements through private agencies had decreased by 50% to 18,100 [36] and the number of international adoptees had more than tripled to 5663 (see Fig. 3; see Table 1) [26].

As the list of countries placing children in the United States grew, the number of international adoptees steadily increased over the next decade. Children from Central and South America, India, and the Philippines as well as an increasing number of children from Korea boosted the total number of international adoptees to 9945 in 1986 [26]. Faced with increasing international criticism about adoption practices, however, particularly during the 1988 Seoul Olympic Games, Korea began to limit the number of international adoptions [26]. From a high of 6188 in 1986, the number of Korean placements in the United States dropped precipitously to 1817 by 1991 and remains in that range to date (see Fig. 3; see Table 1) [26,35].

During the period from 1990 through 1995, the fall of Communism in Eastern Europe, the dissolution of the Soviet Union, and the liberalization of the Chinese adoption policy in response to population control initiatives ushered in the current era of international adoption. Although rates of adoption from Romania flared briefly in 1991 (2594 children; see Table 1), the number of children adopted from Russia and China steadily climbed during the ensuing decade [35]. By 1995, Korea had been supplanted as the top-placing country and in fiscal year 2003, China and Russia accounted for 56% of international adoption placements in the United States (see Fig. 3; see Table 1) [35].

During the past decade, the increasing number of available children coincided with a rising demand to adopt internationally. By 2000, the average American woman had her first baby at 25 years of age, 3.6 years later than in 1970 [37]. Currently, 20% of American women have their first baby after 35 years of age, and delayed childbearing brings about an increase in involuntary infertility. The probability of conceiving decreases 3% to 5% per year after the age of 30 years, and the risk of miscarriage is 50% after the age of 40 years [38]. For the first time since the end of World War II, a significant number of white children from Eastern Europe were available for adoption. Countries also were more willing to permit adoption by single parents. In fiscal year 2003, a record number of 21,616 orphan visas were issued in the United States, up 334% from the 1992 nadir (see Fig. 3; see Table 1) [35]. This phenomenon was observed in other countries as well. The number of international adoptions to Canada increased from 232 (1998) to 1874 (2001), an 8-fold increase [13], and that to Spain increased from 93 (1988) [13] to 3428, a 36-fold increase (Xavier Allué, MD, PhD, personal communication, 2001).

This increase in adoptions heralded not only a change in countries of origin but a different population of children than had been previously placed through international adoption. In the mid-1980s, most international adoptees were from

Korea. These children were relinquished by healthy women stigmatized by single parenthood, raised in foster families, provided a high level of medical care, and adopted as infants. In comparison, international adoptees today are far more likely to be abandoned by poorly nourished destitute mothers who have abused alcohol or intravenous drugs or to be cared for within institutional care settings, receive inadequate medical care, and join their adoptive families as toddlers or older children [39,40]. In large part, the increasing number of adoptees and the broad range of medical and developmental problems commonly seen in these children are responsible for the contemporary interest in international adoption medicine.

Process and participants

Why should you care about the process of international adoption? Envision your first visit with a birth family. After reviewing the chart and examining the baby, you have in-depth knowledge about the mother's medical status, prenatal course, and labor and delivery—all the factors that led up to the arrival of the child. Perhaps you also are a parent and have experienced the exhaustion and elation of a new arrival in your family through birth. Your bond with the family is strengthened by this information and your shared experiences.

Your first interaction with an adoptive parent should be just as informed. Similarities exist: parents of new international adoptees are exhausted by time zone changes and by the new responsibilities of caring for this child, who is often their first. Validating their experience by expressing understanding of the scrutiny they have endured, the lengthy waiting period, out-of-pocket expenses, distances traveled, illnesses suffered, and the inevitable frustrations of dealing with the US federal bureaucracy and a foreign government's can help to reinforce your relationship.

The process of adopting internationally is perhaps best understood by medical professionals as analogous to submitting one's first foundation or government grant, although this comparison does not fully illuminate the process that adoptive parents experience. Although the mountain of paperwork, lengthy waiting periods, anxiety, and surrender of control are similar, funding organizations are unlikely to require us to reveal intimate details of our marriage and personal life, inspect our home, request a criminal background check by the Federal Bureau of Investigation (FBI), request medical and psychiatric interviews, or examine our tax returns. One consolation is that an application to adopt internationally has a much higher likelihood of success than most funding proposals.

A recent study of 1834 families who finalized international adoptions in Minnesota during 1990 through 1998 (2291 children) found that adoptive parents were overwhelmingly white (97%), married (86% at the time of the survey), and well educated; 71% of these parents had a college degree, and 46% reported postbaccalaureate degrees [41]. Parents chose to adopt younger children. At the time the adoption was legalized in Minnesota, 64% of children were less than 12 months of age and 17% were 12 to 23 months of age. Adoptive parents were, on average, 38 years old at the time of placement and were financially advantaged. Only 15% of families had a household income less than $50,000 per year, and those of 35% exceeded $100,000 per year.

The cost of adopting internationally varies significantly but accounts for the fact that most families who adopt from abroad are economically well off. The National Adoption Information Clearinghouse lists a range of $7000 to $30,000 for international adoption. This figure includes home study expenses, dossier and immigration processing and court costs, and foreign and domestic agency fees or donations [42]. Most adoptions require one or both parents to visit the country of origin before the child's departure. Travel expenses can add significantly to these costs, depending on the number and length of visits and amount of lost wages.

Federal regulations, administered through the Department of Homeland Security and the Department of State, standardize the major steps in the process of international adoption [43,44]. Formal entry is through a state-licensed adoption agency or social worker whose principal function is to determine the prospective adoptive parent(s)' ability to care for an adopted child. The document or "home study" generated through this investigative process has set requirements under immigration law (Box 1) [45].

Before or during the home study, the parent(s) choose an agency or program to which they apply for their child. This agency may but need not be the same organization that conducts the home study. The application requirements stipulated by the foreign program are determined by considering the adoption regulations of the host country, the background and mission of the agency itself, and the agency's desire to place the child in what it believes is an optimal home environment. There is no "right to adopt." Consequently, the restrictions on marital status, length of marriage, previous divorce, income, family size, parent age, religious affiliation, fertility status, and health may limit the options of potential parents.

As soon as the home study is complete, initial application to the US Citizenship and Immigration Services (USCIS) can be made. In brief, this initial process, "Filing of the Application for Advance Processing of Orphan Petition" (I-600A), allows the federal government to determine if the parents are qualified to bring an orphan into the United States (by verifying their citizenship and reviewing their home study) and that the parent(s) and all adult members of the household are free of a criminal record (with an FBI review of fingerprints).

Once a family has accepted the referral of a specific child, the next step is to file form I-600, "Petition To Classify Orphan As An Immediate Relative," with USCIS. With this petition, the parent(s) must provide proof of the orphan's age and acceptable documentation that the child is legally available for adoption or, in other words, qualifies as an "orphan" under federal law. Assuming that all requirements are met and the petition is approved, the USCIS transmits the orphan petition and necessary supporting material to the appropriate American

Box 1. Adoption home study requirements under federal immigration law

1. At least one interview in person, and at least one home visit, with the prospective adoptive couple or the unmarried prospective adoptive parent. Each additional adult member of the prospective adoptive parents' household must also be interviewed in person at least once.
2. Assessment of the capabilities of the prospective adoptive parents to parent the orphan properly in the following areas:
   a. Assessment of the physical, mental, and emotional capabilities of the prospective adoptive parents to parent the orphan properly
   b. Assessment of the finances of the prospective adoptive parents
   c. History of abuse and/or violence
   d. Previous rejection for adoption or prior unfavorable home study
   e. Criminal history
3. Living accommodations
4. A discussion of the prospective adoptive parents' preparation, willingness, and ability to provide proper care for a special needs child if applicable
5. Summary of the counseling given and plans for postplacement counseling
6. Specific approval of the prospective adoptive parents for adoption
7. Proof the home study preparer is certified and authorized to conduct home studies
8. Documentation of review of the home study by the state of residence (if required)

consulate or to the embassy closest to the child. A consular officer then conducts an investigation to ensure that the child is indeed an orphan, arranges for the child to be examined by a physician to ensure that the child does not have significant illness or disability that is not described in the orphan petition, ensures that the prospective parent(s) have legal custody of the child, and confirms that the child has the required travel documents.

Although the administrative process of international adoption may seem beyond our purview, health care providers can actually play an important role in ensuring maximum legal protection for newly adopted children in their care. Although most US state courts do recognize the legitimacy of a foreign adoption decree, it is not a requirement, and one can only imagine the scenarios in contested divorces or in dissolutions of parental partnerships where unions lack formal recognition. Formal adoption of the child in the United States guarantees that the courts of all 50 states recognize the adoption. Once a child is adopted or readopted in state court, parents can request that a state birth certificate be issued. Having this document on file guarantees that a child can always obtain a certified copy simply by contacting the appropriate state agency. Birth certificates from abroad, once lost or destroyed, are extremely difficult to replace.

The issue of US citizenship has far more significant legal consequences. For example, nonnaturalized international adoptees whose youthful indiscretions resulted in felony convictions have found themselves before immigration judges fighting deportation, even though they have lived in this country since infancy. Currently, US citizenship is conferred immediately on entry into the United States through provisions of the Child Citizen Act of 2001 [46] as long as:

- At least one adoptive parent is a US citizen.
- The child is less than 18 years of age.
- There is a full and final adoption of the child.
- The child is admitted to the United States as an immigrant.

Children who may not qualify for immediate citizenship include those who have not been "fully and finally" adopted at the time of entry into the United States and those who may have entered the United States on medical visas rather than as immigrants. Adoptive parents, exhausted from the process and loath to incur additional expenses, may elect to postpone further paperwork and legal proceedings once the child has arrived in their home. Medical professionals should inquire about all these issues and, if appropriate, encourage consultation with knowledgeable adoption and legal professionals.

International adoption: a worldwide perspective

Although international adoption is viewed as an acceptable if not admirable method of family building in the United States and Western Europe, opinions in the international community are mixed. Whether international adoptions increase or are drastically curtailed depends on addressing the misgivings that many countries have about placing their children abroad. Concerns center in two broad areas: sensitivity toward preservation of family and culture and whether the process has sufficient integrity to act in the best interests of children and birth parents.

Preservation of family and culture

Blood relationships are the principal focal point of social legitimacy, emotional support, and cultural and religious traditions worldwide. This justifiable focus on the importance of each child's heritage is succinctly articulated in two key articles of the United Nations Convention on the Rights of the Child (UNCRC), approved by the United Nations General Assembly on November 20, 1989 [47]:

Article 7

1. The child shall be registered immediately after birth and shall have the right from birth to a name, the right to acquire a nationality and, as far as possible, the right to know and be cared for by his or her parents.

Article 8

1. States Parties undertake to respect the right of the child to preserve his or her identity, including nationality, name and family relations as recognized by law without unlawful interference.

Individuals and organizations that focus on perpetuating family and cultural identity find fault with the definition of an orphan in US immigration law, where the term is defined not only as "a child...who is an orphan because of the death or disappearance of, abandonment or desertion by, or separation or loss from both parents" but "for whom the sole or surviving parent is incapable of providing the proper care and has in writing irrevocably released the child for emigration and adoption" [48]. The Joint United Nations Program on HIV/AIDS (UNAIDS)/United Nations Children's Fund (UNICEF)/United States Agency for International Development (USAID) publication "Children on the Brink 2002" reported that almost 108 million children less than 15 years of age in 88 African, Asian, and Latin American countries had lost at least one parent. Fewer than 10% had lost both, however [49]. For children in residential care as well, the term *orphanage* is also a misnomer; most children housed in institutions are not parentless. In 252 sequential referrals from Eastern Europe orphanages evaluated for prospective adoptive families, only 9% of children were orphans as the term is commonly used (4% had lost both parents and 5% were foundlings) [39]. Most had one or two known living parents with court-terminated parental rights for neglect or abuse as the stated reason for 15% of these cases and 76% relinquished for social or economic reasons. The point made by opponents of international adoption is that making children with surviving parents eligible for international adoption diminishes emphasis and diverts resources from strengthening the family and social structure in the country of origin in favor of building families in wealthy Western countries. Irrespective of altruism, any appearance of exploiting the financial and social misfortune of others opens the door to charges of colonialism.

In recent man-made and natural disasters (eg, wars in the Balkans and West, Central, and East Africa; the sub-Saharan drought; the Indian Ocean tsunami) [50–52], there has been friction between international organizations that focus on preserving a child's identity, family, and culture and individuals who view adoption as an appropriate response to the tragedy. During humanitarian catastrophes, children may be separated from their parents but not necessarily orphaned. Under these circumstances, adoption is clearly not proper until an appropriate amount of time has passed to permit reunification with parents, extended family, or other members of the child's community. A case in point: 4 weeks after the December 2004 tsunami, UNICEF reported that of the 987 Sri Lankan children left without parents, 945 (96%) had been taken in by extended family and 1 of the remaining unidentified children was being claimed by nine couples [53]. During disasters, there also may not be a recognized or functional government to ensure that a child's legal rights are protected. Under these conditions, promulgating adoption as an appropriate first response reinforces the underlying perception of many that the motives of potential adoptive parents are more selfish than selfless.

Once placed, international adoptees lose not only their birth parents but their birth culture as well. International concern regarding this loss of identity cannot be overemphasized. Although international adoptees have many opportunities to celebrate their heritage through food, secular and religious celebrations, playmates, and language studies, for example, many continue to view international adoption as an irrevocable loss of a cultural birthright.

Adoption policy in the sending countries often centers on this issue. Some governments (eg, Greece) [54] extend preferential treatment to families who have cultural ties to their country, and some countries preclude adoption by individuals who are unlikely to raise the child in the same religious or cultural tradition. Islamic countries generally forbid adoption by non-Muslims [55] not only because Islam explicitly forbids establishing a fictive relationship of descent between the child and father, as happens under Western secular adoption law [24], but because there is absolutely no guarantee that a child's rich faith and cultural heritage are going to be respected, or even acknowledged, in Western countries, where Islam is poorly understood and underappreciated. Concerns about Western cultural sensitivity were recently reinforced when a Virginia-based Christian group, WorldHelp, attempted relocation of a group of 300 Muslim children orphaned or separated from their parents to a Christian children's home in the aftermath of the December 2004 tsunami. As reported in the *Washington Post*, the group's web site stated that WorldHelp was working to "plant Christian principles as early as possible" in the 300 Muslim children [56].

Concern and even outright anger at this loss of identity and culture emerge as international adoptees traverse the difficult years of adolescence, searching for self and their place in the world [57]. Other articles in this issue offer personal and group perspectives on this issue from Koreans adoptees—the vanguard of transracial and transcultural adoption in the United States. Even more passionate are accounts posted on the web site for transracial abductees (www.transracialabductees.org), which communicate the raw emotions at play in individual lives.

Most international adoptions are transracial, and individual families often go to great lengths to socialize their child ethnically as well as to help them develop coping skills to recognize and deal effectively with racism and discrimination. We must acknowledge, however, that national policy on this issue is of two minds. The Indian Child Welfare Act PL-95-608 was passed in 1978 expressly to prevent removal of Native American children from their tribes [58]. In the law, the congressional declaration of policy included the following statement [58]:

> The Congress hereby declares that it is the policy of this Nation to protect the best interests of Indian children and to promote the stability and security of Indian tribes and families by the establishment of minimum Federal standards for the removal of Indian children from their families and the placement of such children in foster or adoptive homes which will reflect the unique values of Indian culture...

Although we accept the importance of cultural heritage in this instance, most adoptees are placed in families with no connection to the birth culture. Preventing a white family from adopting an American Indian child while sanctioning the adoption of a Mayan Indian child from Guatemala may be legally justifiable in this country because of the special relationship between Native American tribes and the federal government, but it is difficult to explain this seeming ambivalence to the importance of culture to those living outside the United States.

Integrity of the adoption process

Safeguarding the rights of children during adoption, particularly international adoption, is specifically addressed in the UNCRC. Comparing the goals articulated in this document with the actual scope of adoption practice helps to explain why concern arises regarding the integrity of the process [47].

> Article 21
> State Parties that recognize or permit the system of adoption shall ensure that the best interests of the child shall be the paramount consideration and they shall:
> (a) Ensure that the adoption of a child is authorized only by competent authorities who determine, in accordance with applicable law and procedures and on the basis of all pertinent and reliable information, that the adoption is permissible in view of the child's status concerning parents, relatives and legal guardians and that, if required, the persons concerned have given their informed consent to the adoption on the basis of such counseling as may be necessary [47].

"Informed consent" is one of the key elements in this section of the UNCRC, and understanding the controversy surrounding this issue begins by acknowledging the asymmetries involved in the process of international adoption. In virtually all situations, birth mothers are destitute, stigmatized by their pregnancy, and rarely able to share with the birth father the burden of child bearing and rearing. They are often members of an exploited racial or ethnic minority and politically impotent. Protections afforded women and their children in these situations may be minimal. In contrast, adoptive parents are well-to-do members of a politically powerful majority in the most economically advantaged countries on earth. From this perspective, it is understandable why colonialism is again linked with international adoption.

In some countries, it is a social norm to temporarily place a child in an institution or with another family, with the expectation of future unification. The recent history of adoption in the Marshall Islands illustrates how critical the social context is to the issue of informed consent. Within the Marshallese community, all adoptions are considered "open" and the child is commonly expected to return to the birth family at a later date. As opposed to the perspective of US parents, who view adoption as a severance of ties, more than 80% of 73 Marshallese birth mothers surveyed believed at the time of placement that their child would be returned to them after the child reached adulthood [59]. These drastically different cultural perspectives on adoption led to tragic outcomes for birth and adoptive families [60].

> Article 21
> (b) Recognize that inter-country adoption may be considered as an alternative means of child's care, if the child cannot be placed in a foster or an adoptive family or cannot in any suitable manner be cared for in the child's country of origin [47].

Despite the enthusiasm of potential adoptive parents and the positive outcomes reported for children [40], international adoption has been viewed by the world community as the least desirable option, aside from institutional care, for children deprived of parental care. This statement acknowledges that a nation's children are a critical resource. It also reaffirms the importance of maintaining the cultural identity of the individual child.

> Article 21
> (c) Ensure that the child concerned by inter-country adoption enjoys safeguards and standards equivalent to those existing in the case of national adoption [47].
> (d) Take all appropriate measures to ensure that, in inter-country adoption, the placement does not result in improper financial gain for those involved in it [47].

Unfortunately, the focus on the primacy of the biologic family makes it difficult for many to understand how a child could be adequately cared for by anyone other than a birth parent or relative. This view helps to perpetuate notions that adoptive parents have ulterior motives for seeking to adopt an unrelated child. The home study process makes families adopting internationally the most scrutinized parents in the world; yet, the rare reports of abuse and even murder of international adoptees in the United States only reinforce the false concept that families who adopt are not fit parents [61]. When paired with the sums of money that change hands during the adoption process, which are easily equivalent to a decade or more of income for an average family in a sending country, it is understandable why international adoption may not be viewed as a humanitarian gesture but as child trafficking for economic gain.

Contemporary articles on international adoption inevitably highlight the large (and often inflated) dollar amounts involved and are often liberally spiced with anecdotes regarding the extravagant lifestyles of key figures in the "baby trade" [62–64]. Irrespective of this hyperbole, the actual or perceived possibility that money could corrupt every point in the process and every level of bureaucracy must be acknowledged. Although financial indiscretions most commonly are "gifts" to ensure that the adoption process goes smoothly [64], other examples include the alleged selling of children in countries without well-developed adoption safeguards (eg, Cambodia [61,64–66], Guatemala [67], India [68], Kenya [69], Romania [25,70]) and preferential placement of children for lucrative international (rather than domestic) adoption [64].

The belief that financial motives drive international adoption is so strong that outlandish rumors regarding child exploitation are easily perpetuated. At the far end of this spectrum are horrifying reports that international adoptees are being butchered to use their body parts for transplantation. These stories emerged in the mid-1980s but gained credence in the world press in January 1987 when the Secretary-General of the Honduran Committee for Social Welfare mentioned the rumor in a way that seemed to confirm its credibility. Quickly picked up by the Soviet media, the story was off and running—a full-blown urban legend. Despite the fact that it would be technically and legally impossible for clandestine organ transplantation to occur in North America or Western Europe, the rumors persisted [71–73]. In 1994, word-of-mouth allegations spread in Guatemala that eight babies had been found with their stomachs slashed open, one with a $100 bill stuck in its abdomen and a note that said in English, "Thanks for your cooperation." Frenzy over this issue led to the near-death beating of June Weinstock, a journalist from Fairbanks, Alaska, for suspected baby trafficking [74]. Two television documentaries aired in 1993, one British/Canadian and the other French, purportedly offering proof of this trafficking in baby parts. The specific cases highlighted were eventually determined to be fabrications, however [71–73]. Despite the fact that cases of this practice were never verified, in February 1993, the European Parliament's Committee on the Environment, Public Health, and Consumer Protection issued a report on trade in transplant organs that included the unsubstantiated claim that "there is evidence that fetuses, children, and adults in some developing countries have been mutilated and others murdered with the aim of obtaining transplant organs for export to rich countries" [71]. The report continued that "to deny the existence of such trafficking is comparable to denying the existence of the ovens and gas chambers during the last war" [71].

The latest iteration of the rumor came with the appointment of Lady Emma Nicholson as Rapporteur of the European Parliament to Romania from 1999 through 2004. Charged with overseeing the progress of Romania toward membership in the European Union, Nicholson devoted much of her effort to reforming the child protection system. Actions taken during her tenure not only demonstrate how rumors of financial corruption continue to plague international adoption but illustrate how the well-being of individual children can be traded for future economic benefit to a country.

Riddled with corruption, the system and the process of international adoption in Romania clearly needed transformation [75]. Nicholson spent an inordinate amount of energy promoting an outright ban on international adoption in

Romania by tarnishing the character and motives of those involved in the process, however [15,76–79]. Central to her campaign to end international placements was an effort to characterize parents seeking to adopt internationally as unfit, having been denied the option of adopting in their own countries. More outrageous were her frequently articulated, although never substantiated, charges that international adoption was an "international trade in children" controlled by criminals not only for the aforementioned "pedophilia, child prostitution or domestic servitude" but for organ transplantation as well. Appearing on Italian television on February 19, 2001, Lady Nicholson stated, "The promised dream of a perfect home in the West very often turns into sexual slavery or, even worse, mutilation and death" [76]. Nicholson refused to retract these charges, even when confronted with a statement that the United Nations Special Rapporteur on Child Prostitution believed this was an urban legend and that there were no confirmed cases anywhere in the world of children being trafficked or harvested for organs [79].

Although 37,000 Romanian children remain institutionalized and the infrastructure for foster care is inadequate [80], abandonment continues unabated at a rate of 9000 children per year [81,82], with only 1000 children per year being adopted domestically [82]. Romania was forced to placate Lady Nicholson and the European Parliament, on whose decisions its future economic well-being was dependent, by passing highly restrictive international adoption legislation in June 2004 [83,84]. Since January 1, 2005, only grandparents are eligible to adopt Romanian children internationally and, even then, only if exhaustive attempts have been made to place the child in Romania. This economic pressure is unlikely to abate in the near term. Nicholson, responding to the British Broadcasting Corporation's question on her views if Romania reasserts international adoption, said, "If Romania were to go back to the selling of children, then I believe she will be delaying her entry into the European Union for a long, long time to come." [79]

Although accorded the status of arch villain by proponents of international adoption [85,86], in Nicholson's defense, a system in which children were covertly and even openly sold for profit mandated extreme action. Yet, what is essentially a ban on international adoption, rationalized by sullying the motives and reputations of most adoptive parents, is contrary to the welfare of many children. Children with handicaps or who are members of ethnic minorities, who are difficult to place in Romanian families but readily placed abroad, currently have little hope of a permanent family [80]. In addition, slandering international adoption, particularly in a country in which adoption is not an accepted method of building a family, could have a stifling effect on domestic child placement. After all, why would families who must already overcome social obstacles to adoption willingly identify themselves with the "pedophiles and kidnappers" who adopt internationally? Disparaging some who adopt renders suspect the motives of all who adopt. Having successfully strong-armed Romania into compliance with her views, Nicholson has set her sights on new targets, such as Russia [15].

Hague convention on intercountry adoption

Two viewpoints can be distilled from this controversy: advocacy for children and advocacy for one child. Those who advocate for children, represented by such groups as UNICEF and Save the Children UK, hold many aspects of international adoption to be in direct conflict with the articles of the UNCRC [87–89]. From this perspective, sanctioning practices that downplay the value of birth family and culture and weaken legal protection for the parties involved undermines legal protection for all children. Those at the opposite pole are motivated by one of the most fundamental drives shared by human beings: protecting and nurturing the individual child. From this viewpoint, the right of a single identifiable child to grow up in a family outweighs virtually every other consideration. Reconciling these views first requires acknowledging that overly pessimistic or optimistic opinions on international adoption usually arise from limited or biased experience with the full process of identifying, placing, and raising an adoptee or from misrepresentation or ignorance of the available outcome data. Second, although these viewpoints seem to be at odds, they are both centered in the well-being of children, and within this arena, there is considerable room for thoughtful compromise.

The final portion of Article 21 of the UNCRC mandates the following [47]:

> (e) Promote, where appropriate, the objectives of the present article by concluding bilateral or multilateral arrangements or agreements, and endeavor, within this framework, to ensure that competent authorities or organs carry out the placement of the child in another country.

This challenge was taken up by the Hague Conference on Private International Law, an intergovernmental organization founded in 1893 that focuses on unifying the rule of private international law. Drafted in consultation with principal placing and accepting countries, the Hague Conference presented to its member countries a draft convention on international adoption in 1993 [90], which, as of October 18, 2004, is in force in 70 countries and is awaiting ratification by another 6 [91]. Unfortunately, 3 of the countries who have signed but not ratified or acceded to the convention are China and Russia (the 2 countries that place the largest number of children abroad) and the United States, the country that annually accepts half of worldwide intercountry placements.

Fundamental tenants of the Hague Convention on Protection of Children and Cooperation in Respect of Intercountry Adoption parallel the UNCRC in many respects, but the draft convention places international adoption in a more favorable context in other areas [90,92,93]. In brief, the major advantages of the Hague Convention are the following:

- It provides formal international and intergovernmental recognition of international adoption.
- As opposed to the UNCRC, the Hague Convention states that intercountry adoption is acceptable if a "suitable family" cannot be found in the child's

home state, thus endorsing international adoption as a viable alternative to domestic placement for many children and not as the least desirable option.

- It establishes a set of minimum requirements and procedures that apply when a child moves from one Hague Convention country to another.
- It establishes a system of cooperation among states to prevent the trafficking of children, and it requires that states amend their national adoption laws to conform to the Hague Convention's principles and guidelines, which require the sending and receiving countries to clean up corrupt adoption networks, crack down on child trafficking, and certify that children are in fact legally adoptable.
- It requires that each Hague Convention country establish a central authority to oversee the adoption process in its own territory, including the implementation of the Hague Convention's directives through new domestic legislation and coordination of adoption procedures with other states.

Future of international adoption

Interest in adopting internationally is unlikely to diminish, because the number of children available for domestic adoption in the most desirable age range is unlikely to increase in North America or Western Europe in the foreseeable future. In fact, as transracial adoption approaches the levels of acceptance observed in some areas of North America and Western Europe (see Figs. 1 and 2), international adoption is likely to become a more favorable option. Changes in sending countries, such as aggressive promotion of domestic adoption, changes in strategies for population control, better access to family planning services, and improving economic conditions, are likely to decrease the number of children available for placement abroad, however. In addition, because those adopting domestically in placing countries share a preference for younger healthy children, those available for international adoption in the future are likely to be older and to have special needs. As the risks of medical, developmental, and behavioral challenges increase, adoption must continue to be child centered but not blind to the desires, and particularly the abilities, of potential adoptive families. As medical professionals, we serve the interests of the potential adoptee best by identifying a family with resources that meet the needs of that child, helping parents to develop appropriate expectations, promptly identifying and treating postarrival problems, and supporting families through the lifelong process of raising an adopted child.

International adoption is also imperiled by the perception that the process fails to protect the rights of children. Sending countries are responsive to any reports of child trafficking, even if unsubstantiated, and often terminate international placements on any rumor of child exploitation. Because the destination of more than 50% of children adopted internationally [13] is the United States, this country has the greatest moral obligation to ensure that the adoption process meets international standards for child protection. Although the Intercountry

Adoption Act of 2000 was passed by Congress and signed into law by President Clinton on October 6, 2000, regulations to implement the Hague Convention have languished and the agreement is not currently in force. The earliest that ratification is anticipated is early 2006 [93]. In addition to implementing this agreement fully, the United States has a duty to help fund implementation of the Hague Convention in countries that are unlikely to have sufficient resources to accomplish the goals on their own. Presently, little foreign aid is earmarked for adoption and child welfare issues [92].

One program implemented by the US government in 2002 is "Adjudicate Orphan Status First," which screens potential adoptees to ascertain whether the child meets the definition of an orphan under US immigration law [94]. This screening happens before establishment of the legal relationship with adoptive parents, and the intent is to avoid situations such as the one that occurred in Cambodia in December 2001, when adoptive parents discovered at the eleventh hour that their child's status as an orphan was in question because of concerns about child trafficking [61]. Presently, the pilot program is offered only in Haiti, Honduras, the Philippines, Poland, and Sierra Leone, but it is a worthwhile if modest start to ensuring clarity in international adoption.

Additional transparency in the area of adoption practice is required, because the high cost of international adoption continues to be a touch point for criticism around the world [95]. As Kathryn Creedy discussed in her article "The Root of All Evil" [96], it is difficult to justify to an international audience why the charge for a white normal infant is significantly higher than that for a minority special needs older child. As human beings, there should be no intrinsic difference in worth, but when viewed as commodities, one is clearly more in demand by adoptive parents and thus more "marketable." Suspicion regarding the motives of adoption professionals, and even of parents, is likely to continue until fee structures are revealed and justified and profit motives are laid to rest. Quoting Creedy, "As adoption moves forward in the 21st century, this last bastion of secrecy must be breeched if we are ever going to be able to say adoption is just another way to build a family and really mean it" [96].

Receiving countries also have a responsibility to those who remain behind. Only a small number of the children who are in need of permanent families are eligible or chosen for adoption. Focusing on the development of family preservation systems, foster care, domestic adoption, and rehabilitation and reintegration of children who languish in institutional care settings is necessary to ensure a full and balanced commitment to children deprived of parental care. Criticism is justified if attention is focused only on those children eligible for international placement.

Reciprocal commitments are required from placing countries. All nations should aspire to meet the needs of their own children deprived of parental care, but this goal is not going to be reached in the near term. Allowing children to languish in institutions is unconscionable; recent work has demonstrated that significant and often permanent alternations in development occur if children are not placed within families by 6 months of age [39,40]. Foster care requires considerable social infrastructure and financial support, and adoption of unrelated children is not widely accepted in many countries. In addition, children who are older, have mental or physical handicaps, or are members of ethnic or racial minorities are likely to be difficult to place in permanent homes. Placement abroad must, and thankfully does, remain an option for these children if timely permanent placement cannot be achieved in the child's birth country [97].

Finally, developing appropriate expectations is a recurring theme for families who adopt internationally and should apply to the international community as well. A screening system has never been developed that can predict human behavior with absolute certainty. Clearly, we must focus on placing children in the best possible environment, but no amount of preadoption scrutiny or postadoption follow-up can ever prevent the isolated cases of abuse that are trumpeted in the media. Policy must be based on evidence and not on tabloids, and the data available leave no doubt regarding the positive effects of adoption. Out of calamity and loss, children recover and progress to become functionally and emotionally competent adults [40]. As stated by the distinguished adoption researcher Richard Barth [98]:

> Adoption is a time-honored and successful service for children and parents. The outcomes of adoption are more favorable for children than any social program that I know. My own research and that of my colleagues indicates that the modest difficulties experienced by children who are adopted are far outweighed by the significant benefits that they receive from having a permanent family.

References

[1] McMillan JA, DeAngelis CD, Feigin RD, et al, editors. Oski's pediatrics. 3rd edition. Philadelphia: Lippincott, Williams & Wilkins; 1999.

[2] Hoekelman RA. Primary pediatric care. 4th edition. St. Louis: Mosby; 2001.

[3] Rudolph CD, Rudolph AM, Hostetter MK, et al, editors. Rudolph's pediatrics. 21st edition. New York: McGraw-Hill; 2003.

[4] Behrman RE, Kliegman RM, Jenson HB, editors. Nelson textbook of pediatrics. 17th edition. Philadelphia: WB Saunders; 2004.

[5] Wiener JM, Dulcan MK. Textbook of child and adolescent psychiatry. 3rd edition. Arlington, VA: American Psychiatric Publishing; 2004.

[6] Kreider R. Adopted children and stepchildren: 2000. US Department of Commerce, US Census Bureau. October 2003. Available at: http://www.census.gov/prod/2003pubs/censr-6.pdf. Accessed February 18, 2005.

[7] National adoption attitudes survey. Dave Thomas Foundation for Adoption, Evan B. Donaldson Adoption Institute. June 2002. Available at: http://www.adoptioninstitute.org/survey/survey_intro.html. Accessed March 4, 2005.

[8] Congressional Coalition on Adoption Institute. Members of Congress page. Available at: http://www.ccainstitute.org/. Accessed March 4, 2005.

[9] How many children were adopted in 2000 and 2001? US Department of Health and Human Services, Administration for Children and Families National Adoption Information Clearinghouse page. August 2004. Available at: http://naic.acf.hhs.gov/pubs/s_adoptedhighlights.cfm. Accessed March 4, 2005.

[10] Martin JA, Hamilton BE, Ventura SJ, et al. Births: final data for 2001. Natl Vital Stat Rep 2002;51(2):1–103. Available at: www.cdc.gov/nchs/data/nvsr/nvsr51/nvsr51_02.pdf. Accessed March 4, 2005.

[11] International adoptions. Citizenship and immigration Canada. The Monitor 2003;Fall:5. Available at: http://www.cic.gc.ca/english/monitor/issue03/06-feature.html. Accessed March 4, 2005.

[12] Births 2001. Statistics Canada. The Daily. August 11, 2003. Available at: http://www.statcan.ca/Daily/English/030811/d030811a.htm. Accessed March 4, 2005.

[13] Selman P. The demographic history of intercountry adoption. In: Selman P, editor. Developments, trends and perspectives. London: British Agency for Adoption and Fostering; 2000. p. 15–37.

[14] Mother Theresa. Spiritual poverty and the breakdown of peace. Origins 1994;23:616.

[15] Nicholson N. Red light on human traffic. Guardian Unlimited. July 1, 2004. Available at: http://society.guardian.co.uk/adoption/comment/0,8146,1250913,00.html. Accessed March 4, 2005.

[16] Kinder N. International adoption: trends and issues. Child Welfare League of America. November 2003. Available at: http://ndas.cwla.org/research_info/publications/. Accessed March 4, 2005.

[17] Miller BC, Coyl DD. Adolescent pregnancy and childbearing in relation to infant adoption in the United States. Adoption Quarterly 2000;4:3–25.

[18] Anderson G. Intercountry adoption in Sweden: the perspective of the Adoption Center in its 30th year. In: Selman P, editor. Intercountry adoption: developments, trends and perspectives. London: British Agency for Adoption and Fostering; 2000. p. 346–67.

[19] Chernoff R, Combs-Orme T, Risley-Curtiss C, et al. Assessing the health status of children entering foster care. Pediatrics 1994;93(4):594–601.

[20] Halfon N, Mendonca A, Berkowitz G. Health status of children in foster care: the experience of the Center for the Vulnerable Child. Arch Pediatr Adolesc Med 1995;149:386–92.

[21] Takayama JI, Wolfe E, Coulter KP. Relationship between reason for placement and medical findings among children in foster care. Pediatrics 1998;101:201–7.

[22] Simms MD, Dubowitz H, Szilagyi MA. Health care needs of children in the foster care system. Pediatrics 2000;106:909–18.

[23] Murphy Garwood M, Close W. Identifying the psychological needs of foster children. Child Psychiatry Hum Dev 2001;32(2):125–35.

[24] Pollack D, Bleich M, Reid Jr CJ, et al. Classical religious perspectives of adoption law. Notre Dame Law Rev 2004;79(2):693–753.

[25] Hunt K. The Romanian baby bazaar. New York Times Magazine March 24, 1991;140:24–53.

[26] Altstein H, Simon RJ. Introduction. In: Alstein H, Simon RJ, editors. Intercountry adoption: a multinational perspective. New York: Praeger; 1991. p. 1–13.

[27] International adoption facts. Evan B. Donaldson Adoption Institute. January 2002. Available at: http://www.adoptioninstitute.org/FactOverview/international.html. Accessed March 4, 2005.

[28] Herman E. International adoptions. University of Oregon, The Adoption History Project. 2005. Available at: http://darkwing.uoregon.edu/~adoption/topics/internationaladoption.htm. Accessed March 4, 2005.

[29] US Supreme Court. Brown v Board of Education. 347 US 483 (1954). Available at: http://www.nationalcenter.org/brown.html. Accessed March 4, 2005.

[30] Herman E. The family nobody wanted. University of Oregon, Adoption History Project. 2005. Available at: http://darkwing.uoregon.edu/~adoption/topics/familynobodywanted.htm. Accessed February 18, 2005.

[31] Doss H. Our international family. Readers Digest 1949;55:58–9. Available at: http://darkwing.uoregon.edu/~adoption/archive/DossOIF.htm. Accessed February 18, 2005.

[32] Doss H. The family nobody wanted. Boston: Little, Brown and Company; 1954. p. 165. Available at: http://darkwing.uoregon.edu/~adoption/archive/DossTFNW.htm. Accessed March 1, 2005.

[33] Herman E. Bertha and Harry Holt. University of Oregon, Adoption History Project. 2005. Available at: http://darkwing.uoregon.edu/~adoption/people/holt.htm. Accessed March 1, 2005.

[34] Holt B, Wisner D. The seed from the east. Los Angeles: Oxford Press; 1956. p. 44–5. Available at: http://darkwing.uoregon.edu/~adoption/archive/HoltSFE.htm. Accessed March 1, 2005.

[35] Immigrant visas issued to orphans coming to the US, 2004. US Department of State, Bureau of Consular Affairs. Overseas Citizens Services, Office of Children's Issues. Available at: http://travel.state.gov/family/adoption/stats/stats_451.html. Accessed March 1, 2005.

[36] Placek PJ. National adoption data. In: Marshner C, Pierce WL, editors. Adoption factbook III. Alexandria, VA: National Council for Adoption; 1999. p. 24–68.

[37] American women are waiting to begin families. US Department of Health and Human Services, Centers for Disease Control and Prevention, National Center for Health Care Statistics. December 11, 2002. Available at: http://www.cdc.gov/nchs/pressroom/02news/ameriwomen.htm. Accessed March 1, 2005.

[38] Barad D. Age and female fertility. American Fertility Association. Available at: http://www.theafa.org/faqs/afa_ageandfemaleinfertility.html. Accessed March 1, 2005.

[39] Johnson DE. Medical and developmental sequelae of early childhood institutionalization in international adoptees from Romania and the Russian Federation. In: Nelson C, editor. The effects of early adversity on neurobehavioral development. Mahwah, NJ: Lawrence Erlbaum Associates; 2000. p. 113–62.

[40] Johnson DE. Adoption and the effect on children's development. Early Hum Dev 2002;68: 39–44.

[41] Gunnar M. First findings from International Adoption Project, February, 2002. Available at: http://education.umn.edu/icd/iap/Results4.25.htm. Accessed July 25, 2005.

[42] Costs of Adopting. A fact sheet for families, 2004. US Department of Health and Human Services, Administration for Children and Families National Adoption Information Clearinghouse. Available at: http://naic.acf.hhs.gov/pubs/s_cost/index.cfm. Accessed March 1, 2005.

[43] Intercountry adoptions. US Department of Homeland Security, US Citizenship and Immigration Services. Available at: http://uscis.gov/graphics/services/index2.htm. Accessed March 1, 2005.

[44] International adoption. US State Department, Bureau of Consular Affairs. Overseas Citizens Services, Office of Children's Issues. Available at: http://travel.state.gov/family/adoption/notices/notices_473.html. Accessed March 1, 2005.

[45] Orphans. US Department of Homeland Security, US Citizenship and Immigration Services, Sec. 204.3. August 1, 1994. Available at: http://uscis.gov/lpBin/lpext.dll/inserts/slb/slb-1/slb-9985/slb-12552/slb-13006?f=templates&fn=document-frame.htm#slb-8cfrsec2043. Accessed March 1, 2005.

[46] Information for adoptive parents. US Department of Homeland Security, US Citizenship and Immigration Services, Child Citizenship Act. February 27, 2001. Available at: http://uscis.gov/graphics/publicaffairs/backgrounds/cbground.htm. Accessed March 1, 2005.

[47] Convention on the rights of the child. UNICEF. Available at: http://www.unicef.org/crc/crc.htm. Accessed March 1, 2005.

[48] Immigration services and benefits, appendix B, glossary/definitions. US Department of Homeland Security, US Citizenship and Immigration Services. Available at: http://uscis.gov/graphics/services/appen.htm#b. Accessed March 1, 2005.

[49] Children on the brink 2002: a joint report on orphan estimates and program strategies. UNAIDS/UNICEF/USAID. July 2002. Available at: http://www.unicef.org/publications/index_4378.html. Accessed March 1, 2005.

[50] BAAF advice about the adoption of tsunami victims. British Association for Adoption and Fostering. January 6, 2005. Available at: http://www.adoption-net.co.uk/news/2005/January/060105tsunami.htm. Accessed March 1, 2005.

[51] Friess S. Adoption not best way to help victims now, experts say. USA Today. January 10, 2005. Available at: http://www.usatoday.com/news/world/2005-01-09-tsunami-adoption_x.htm. Accessed March 1, 2005.

[52] Update on adoption of December 26 tsunami victims. US Department of State, Bureau of Consular Affairs. Overseas Citizens Services, Office of Children's Issues. Available at: http://travel.state.gov/family/adoption/notices/notices_2017.html. Accessed March 1, 2005.

[53] Sengupta S. For tsunami orphan, no name but many parents. New York Times. January 26, 2005. Available at: http://www.nytimes.com/2005/01/26/international/worldspecial4/26orphan.html?oref=regi. Accessed March 1, 2005.

[54] International adoption. Greece. US Department of State, Bureau of Consular Affairs. Overseas Citizens Services, Office of Children's Issues. Available at: http://travel.state.gov/family/adoption/country/country_387.html. Accessed March 1, 2005.

[55] Other Near East/Asia international adoption. US Department of State, Bureau of Consular Affairs. Overseas Citizens Services, Office of Children's Issues. Available at: http://travel.state.gov/family/adoption/country/country_431.html. Accessed March 1, 2005.

[56] Cooperman A. Tsunami orphans won't be sent to Christian home. Washington Post. January 14, 2005. Available at http://www.washingtonpost.com/wp-dyn/articles/A7535-2005Jan13.html. Accessed March 1, 2005.

[57] Freundlich M, Lieberthal JK. The gathering of the first generation of adult Korean adoptees: adoptees' perceptions of international adoption. Evan B. Donaldson Adoption Institute. June 2000. Available at: http://www.adoptioninstitute.org/proed/korfindings.html. Accessed March 1, 2005.

[58] Indian Child Welfare Act of 1978, PL 95–608, Title 25 USC. Chapter 21 1901, 1902. Available at: http://www.law.cornell.edu/uscode/html/uscode25/usc_sup_01_25_10_21.html. Accessed March 1, 2005.

[59] Roby J, Matsumura S. If I give you my child, aren't we family? A study of birthmothers participating in Marshall Islands-US Adoptions. Adoption Quarterly 2002;5(4):7–31.

[60] Roche Jr WF. A duel for a daughter agonizes two families. Baltimore Sun. November 3, 2003. Available at: http://www.baltimoresun.com/news/nationworld/bal-te.adopt03nov03,0,4753333.story. Accessed March 1, 2005.

[61] Working R, Rodriguez A. Rescue of boy ends in tragedy. Chicago Tribune May 21, 2004:6.

[62] Mainville M. Prospective parents flock to Russia to adopt, but some balk at westerners 'buying' children. New York Sun November 16, 2004;120(149):9.

[63] Adoption of Russian children is profitable business. Russian Journal. November 16, 2004. Available at: http://www.russiajournal.com/news/cnews-article.shtml%3Fnd=46358. Accessed March 1, 2005.

[64] Wheeler C. Babies-for-sale trade faces a global crackdown. Guardian Unlimited. November 21, 2004. Available at: http://observer.guardian.co.uk/international/story/0,1356054,00.html. Accessed March 1, 2005.

[65] Important update regarding Cambodian adoptions. US Department of State, Bureau of Consular Affairs. Overseas Citizens Services, Office of Children's Issues. Available at: http://travel.state.gov/family/adoption/country/country_361.html. Accessed February 12, 2002.

[66] Cambodia babies sold for $20. Associated Press. March 5, 2004. Available at: http://abclocal.go.com/wpvi/news/3504-cambodia.html. Accessed February 18, 2005.

[67] Adoption and the rights of the child in Guatemala. Latin American Institute for Education and Communication/UNICEF. 2000. Available at: http://www.iss-ssi.org/Resource_Centre/Tronc_DI/ilpec-unicef_english_report_2000.PDF. Accessed March 8, 2005.

[68] Katz G. No place to call home. Dallas Morning News. March 22, 2004. Available at: www.dallasnews.com/sharedcontent/dws/spe/2004/adoption/stories/032104dnadopt4.7d48f011.html. Accessed March 4, 2005.

[69] Bogan S. Miracle worker or baby thief? Times Online. September 3, 2004. Available at: http://www.timesonline.co.uk/printFriendly/0,1-7-1243799,00.html. Accessed March 4, 2005.

[70] Loyd Roberts S. Shopping for Romanian babies. BBC News. March 3, 2000. Available at: http://news.bbc.co.uk/2/hi/programmes/from_our_own_correspondent/664916.stm. Accessed March 4, 2005.

[71] Leventhal T. The "baby parts" myth: the anatomy of a rumor. Washington, DC: United States Information Agency; 1984. p. 1–12.

[72] Frankel M, Barry J, Schrieberg D. Too good to be true. Newsweek June 26, 1995:20–2.

[73] Barry J, Schrieberg D. Too good to check. Newsweek June 26, 1995:33.

[74] Lopez L. Dangerous rumors. Time April 18, 1994:48.

[75] Ambrose MW, Coburn AM. Report on intercountry adoption in Romania. US Department of Health and Human Services, Administration for Children and Families, The Children's Bureau. January 22, 2001. Available at: http://www.acf.hhs.gov/programs/cb/publications/romanadopt.htm. Accessed March 4, 2005.

[76] Mitu F. Interview granted by Baroness Emma Nicholson. TELE7ABC Italy. February 19, 2001. Available at: http://www.peds.umn.edu/iac/pdf/ABCtranscript.pdf. Accessed March 3, 2005.

[77] Nicholson has proof on children abused by adopting foreigners. ZIUA. March 13, 2004. Available at: http://www.ziua.net/display.php?id=7019&data=2004-03-13. Accessed March 4, 2005.

[78] Damian G. Romania has been destroyed by internal corruption. ZIUA. March 29, 2004. Available at: http://www.ziua.net/display.php?id=8733&data=2004-03-29. Accessed March 4, 2005.

[79] Interview with Baroness Emma Nicholson MEP. BBC News. September 18, 2004. Available at: http://www.adoptachild.org/Messageboard/forum_posts.asp?TID=93&TPN=2&dlimit=1. Accessed March 4, 2005.

[80] Richards SE. Dispatches from Romania: the babies left behind. December 1, 2004. Available at: http://slate.msn.com/id/2109971/entry/2109977//. Accessed March 4, 2005.

[81] UNICEF. Babies still abandoned in Romanian hospitals: pattern unchanged for 30 years, says UNICEF. January 20, 2005. Available at: http://www.unicef.org/media/media_24892.html. Accessed March 4, 2005.

[82] Partlow J. Lives caught in limbo on two sides of the globe. Washington Post. March 9, 2005. Available at: http://www.washingtonpost.com/wp-dyn/articles/A18704-2005Mar8.html. Accessed March 15, 2005.

[83] Traynor I. Romania bans adoptions in other countries. Guardian Unlimited. June 16, 2004. Available at: http://www.guardian.co.uk/eu/story/0,7369,1239785,00.html. Accessed March 4, 2005.

[84] Romania bans foreign adoptions. Deutsche Welle. June 22, 2004. Available at: http://www.dw-world.de/dw/article/0,1564,1243642,00.html. Accessed March 4, 2005.

[85] Romania's new adoption laws. Deutsche Welle. June 27, 2004. Available at: http://www.dw-world.de/dw/article/0,1248088,00.html. Accessed March 4, 2005.

[86] Kunz D, Reese D. A one-woman war against intercountry adoption. Wall Street Journal Europe February 4–6, 2005;XXIII(5).

[87] Intercountry adoption. UNICEF International Child Development Center. December 1998. Available at: www.unicef-icdc.org/publications/pdf/digest4e.pdf. Accessed March 4, 2005.

[88] Position on international adoption of children from Bulgaria. Save the Children UK. October 2003. Available at: http://www.europarl.eu.int/meetdocs/delegations/bulg/20040316/08en.pdf. Accessed March 4, 2005.

[89] Dillon S. Making legal regimes for intercountry adoption reflect human rights principles: transforming the United Nations Convention on the Rights of the Child with the Hague Convention on Intercountry Adoption. Boston University International Law Journal 2003;21(2): 179–257.

[90] Convention of 29 May 1993 on Protection of Children and Co-operation in Respect of Intercountry Adoption. Hague Conference on Private International Law. Available at: http://hcch.e-vision.nl/index_en.php?act=conventions.text&cid=69. Accessed March 4, 2005.

[91] Status table. Hague Conference on Private International Law. October 18, 2004. Available at: http://hcch.e-vision.nl/index_en.php?act=conventions.status&cid=69. Accessed March 4, 2005.

[92] Kapstein EB. The baby trade. Foreign Affairs 2003;82(6):115–25. Available at: http://www.foreignaffairs.org/20031101faessay82611/ethan-b-kapstein/the-baby-trade.html. Accessed March 4, 2005.

[93] Hague Convention on Intercountry Adoption. US Department of State, Bureau of Consular Affairs. Overseas Citizens Services, Office of Children's Issues. Available at: http://travel.state.gov/family/adoption/convention/convention_459.html. Accessed March 4, 2005.

[94] Adjudicate orphan status first pilot program. US Department of Homeland Security, US Citizenship and Immigration Services. Available at: http://uscis.gov/graphics/services/orphan_pilot.htm. Accessed March 4, 2005.

[95] Freundlich M. Adoption and ethics: the market forces in adoption. Washington, DC: Child Welfare League of America; 2000.

[96] Creedy K. The root of all evil. Adoption Quarterly 2002;5(4):77–87.

[97] Mitchell A. Too many kids, not enough parents. Associated Press. January 2, 2005. Available at: http://www.twincities.com/mld/twincities/news/nation/10534780.htm?1c. Accessed March 4, 2005.

[98] Duke ML. Groups seeking to eliminate adoption. In: Marshner C, Pierce WL, editors. Adoption factbook III. Washington, DC: National Council for Adoption; 1999. p. 222.

ELSEVIER
SAUNDERS

PEDIATRIC CLINICS
OF NORTH AMERICA

Pediatr Clin N Am 52 (2005) 1247–1269

Preadoption Opportunities for Pediatric Providers

Jennifer Chambers, MD, MPH & TM

*Department of Pediatrics, University of Alabama, International Adoption Clinic, MCT 201,
1600 7th Avenue South, Birmingham, AL 35233, USA*

As the number of couples choosing to adopt internationally increases, almost every pediatric practice cares for an internationally adopted (IA) child. Pediatricians are often asked for advice by parents who are thinking about adopting internationally, or are asked to review medical records for a potential adoptee and offer guidance to parents in making this monumental decision. What is the pediatrician's role before adoption? Typical questions posed to pediatricians include the following:

How do we start the international adoption process?
From which country should we adopt?
What are the problems commonly seen in IA children?
Can you review the child's medical information before we make a
    final decision?

These basic questions are enough to leave a pediatrician reeling, even guessing, and surely looking for answers. This article addresses how to interpret the limited information provided about children available for international adoption based on experience gained from reviewing hundreds of medical reports and from the research of experts practicing in international adoption clinics. What can and cannot be determined about a particular child before adoption is discussed, and information that is important for medical professionals to convey to parents before they adopt is reviewed.

E-mail addresses: adoption@peds.uab.edu, jnobles@peds.uab.edu

Parent expectations

Parents often want a pediatrician to review the adoptive child's medical report for potential medical problems before they make the decision to adopt. Others have already decided to adopt the child but seek advice on what to expect once they bring him or her home. In either case, the medical reviewer's job is to provide a risk assessment for long-term prognosis and to explain what the postadoption needs of the child may be. After reviewing the child's medical information, the pediatrician may categorize the child as average, above average, or high risk compared with information available on similarly aged children from the same background. The reasons for the assigned risk category should be explained to the parents, along with intervention options, so that the family can decide whether they are going to be able to provide this care. Parents are then in a better position to make informed decisions and to prepare for the child's arrival.

IA children should never be considered low risk. These children have suffered abandonment and long periods of deprivation, leading to significant emotional turmoil, developmental delays, and health concerns. Although many adoptive families perceive that IA children have fewer risk factors than children in foster care here in the United States, this simply is not true. IA children often come from chaotic and stressful home situations and are then placed in institutions that are typically underfunded and understaffed. Their past medical and social history is difficult to obtain. These children also are uniquely vulnerable to the emotional void, medical hazards, and developmentally stifling environments that are found in orphanages [1].

Although services for families adopting internationally are improving, parents may still receive little or no preadoption education regarding what to expect and how to care for their child after adoption. It is best not to assume that because parents know about the adoption process in general, they know about the needs of postinstitutionalized children. The goal of preadoption education should be to help parents set realistic expectations so as to decrease postadoption disappointment and stress.

Parent self-evaluation

An important early step for parents in the adoption process is to evaluate their resources honestly. Is this a one- or two-parent household? Are one or both parents returning to work immediately after the adoption is completed? Are they financially strained after having paid the typical $10,000 to $30,000 in adoption fees? What health care resources are available in their area? For example, it may be too stressful for a single parent who must return to work immediately to adopt a sibling group or for a couple in a remote area without easy access to health care to adopt a child with fetal alcohol syndrome (FAS). Although not much is known about any particular child before adoption, we do know enough about the general needs of these children to aid families during this part of the decision process. It is helpful to the pediatrician to know where parents are in this self-evaluation process and what conclusions they have reached before discussing with them the referral information regarding a specific child.

Adoption process

For preadoption counseling, pediatricians should be familiar with the components of the adoption process:

1. Adoption agencies: agencies process the paperwork necessary to facilitate the adoption. Key factors in choosing an agency are dependability and ethical practices. A family is best served by a well-established agency that has a good reputation with past clients, works in several countries (in case one country closes its doors to international adoption), and provides thorough parent education and follow-up.
2. The home country: the adoption agency educates the family about adoption policies, which differ among countries that offer children for adoption. Some countries have exclusion criteria that may narrow the family's choices (eg, practices of accepting few single parents, parental age, length-of-marriage requirements).
3. International adoption clinics: these interdisciplinary clinics are often composed of one or more of the following: a pediatrician with expertise in international pediatrics or child development; an occupational, physical, or speech therapist; and a psychologist or social worker. Many offer comprehensive pre- and postadoption services and serve as excellent resources for adoptive parents and pediatricians. Most clinics review medical information and counsel adoptive parents during the preadoption phase and then provide medical and developmental evaluations after the family returns from abroad.
4. Resources: the international adoption community is a close-knit group with many resources in print and on the Internet. A list of resources that are useful to parents during the preadoption stage is provided in Appendix 1.

Reviewing the medical information

Medical reports on adoptees are often difficult to interpret unless the physician is accustomed to evaluating such information. A physician must review at least 100 medical reports from orphanages in multiple countries before he or she can begin to feel comfortable with the nuances of these reports. The thoroughness of the report, the accuracy and the terminology, and the source of the information all must be taken into consideration. Reviewing preadoption medical reports is like putting together a puzzle with many missing pieces—each small addition clarifies the picture a little bit more. Pieces of that puzzle may include any of the following:

1. Written information about the child's medical history
2. Photograph(s)
3. Videotaped footage of the child
4. Verbal reports from the orphanage
5. Reviewer's own cultural and medical knowledge of the area

Most commonly, agency intermediaries, orphanage workers, and doctors collect the information and send it for review while the family is still in the United States. In some countries (eg, Ukraine and parts of Russia), parents travel to see the child and are given information only on arrival. These trips are referred to as "blind trips." Once in-country, families can take pictures and collect information for medical professionals in the United States to review via the Internet. In these cases, families usually have only approximately 24 hours to decide whether to adopt that particular child; thus, it is a good idea for them to contact or meet with the medical professional who is going to be reviewing the information before they leave the United States.

During the pretravel visit, the medical professional should review with the family what questions should be asked about the child once they arrive at the orphanage (Fig. 1), give instructions on how to use a growth chart and review normal and abnormal facial features, and show them how to photograph or videotape the child. The family should be given written instructions on how to contact and send information to the medical reviewer while in-country. Parents also should be advised to arrange backup plans for communication and review in case the electronic mail or telephone connection is down or if the primary reviewer is unavailable or unreachable. The importance of this pretravel visit in decreasing the stress and increasing the knowledge of the adoptive family cannot be overemphasized. The author's clinic refers to this type of evaluation as a "parent-directed medical evaluation," because it is our goal for parents to have an educated rather than blind trip.

What should the medical information include?

The child information questionnaire included in Fig. 1 lists information that is often included in a written medical report. Some diagnoses may be accurate, whereas others may be unsupported by clinical, radiologic, or laboratory evidence or not congruent with the rest of the information in the medical report or in the photographs or videotape. It is important to remind the family that the child may have diagnoses that are not included in the medical information.

CHILD INFORMATION QUESTIONNAIRE

Child Name:
Date of Birth:
Current Age:
Region:
Orphanage:

CHILD SOCIAL HISTORY
Date to orphanage:
Age upon arrival:
Reason for placement in orphanage (voluntary
  release or termination of parental rights?):
Pre-orphanage history (time in birth home?
  Foster care? Hospital?):

MATERNAL INFORMATION
Age of mother at birth of child:
Number of pregnancies:
Number of deliveries:
Other children:
Maternal use of alcohol or drugs?
Prenatal care?
Other health information:

PATERNAL INFORMATION

BIRTH INFORMATION
Gestation (prematurity?):
APGAR (1-10):
Place of birth (home or hospital):
Other significant birth information or diagnoses:

GROWTH INFORMATION	Weight	Height	Head circumference
Birth			
Current			

MEDICAL HISTORY
Hospitalizations:
Illnesses:
Vaccines given:

BLOOD OR IMAGING TESTS

HIV	Date _____	Result _____
Hepatitis B	Date _____	Result _____
Hepatitis C	Date _____	Result _____
Syphilis	Date _____	Result _____

If syphilis positive, was it treated with penicillin?
  For how many days?
Other blood or imaging tests:

SOCIAL
Is there a particular person that the child is attached to
  in the orphanage?

LANGUAGE/COGNITION
Can the child say any words or phrases? How many?
If so, what is the longest sentence that the child can
  say (how many words)?
What type of questions or commands does the child
  understand?
Is the child's pronunciation of words age-appropriate?
How does child compare with same age children in
  orphanage?

MOTOR
Is the child sitting? Crawling? Standing? Walking?

Fig. 1. Child information questionnaire. (© 2004 University of Alabama at Birmingham International Adoption Clinic.)

Interpreting the written information

Growth

The most consistently available and objective data available about a child before adoption are growth parameters. US growth charts (http://www.cdc.gov/growthcharts) are sufficient for nearly all IA children because they are standardized tools for assessment of growth patterns and velocity. Even Asian children typically have growth parameters between the 3% and 50% on the US growth chart. Usually, current measurements and growth parameters obtained when the child entered the institution are available. Institutionalization can have a dramatic and predictable effect on a child's growth, leading to abnormal growth curves [2–4]. In many orphanages, there is obvious malnutrition attributable to lack of food, poor feeding techniques, or loss of appetite because of neglect. If this is the case, like any other child with nonorganic growth failure, the growth curve should first reflect deficiencies in weight percentiles; next, those in height; and, finally, a slowing of head circumference growth. If all growth parameters are equally delayed from birth, it is more likely that the child's growth failure is attributable to some type of syndrome (in this population, FAS is most common), poor prenatal conditions, or extreme neglect.

There is a degree of neglect in all orphanages, because it is impossible to provide one-on-one care for each child. Neglect alone, even in the presence of adequate calories, can cause global growth failure, but it affects height most drastically [5–7]. In general, for every 3 months a child spends in a neglectful situation, he or she loses 1 month of linear growth [8], a phenomenon referred to as psychosocial short stature [9]. Parents often ask whether their child's height is going to catch up after adoption. A study of Romanian adoptees whose arrival height was more than 2 SDs below the mean demonstrated that postarrival height velocity z scores were markedly (+5.5) elevated after adoption [9]. The longer a child remains in a state of emotional and nutritional deprivation, however, the less likely it is for catch-up growth to occur to within the normal range [5,6].

Mild to moderate growth delays can be overcome with good caloric intake and attention from a loving parent; these delays usually do not affect the child's cognition. Severe malnutrition is defined by weight that is less than 2 SDs for a child half that child's chronologic age. If severe malnutrition is not corrected before the age of 2 to 3 years, we can see long-term cognitive deficits [10]. Also, other causes of persistent growth failure (eg, chronic infectious diseases, genetic and metabolic conditions) must be considered.

Microcephaly is seen in 30% of IA children [4]. In general, parents should be reminded that if the head is not growing normally, neither is the brain [11]. Microcephaly places a child at high risk for long-term cognitive difficulties, even if the cause is malnutrition. Neglect alone can also cause microcephaly. Long-term observation of Romanian adoptees in the United Kingdom confirmed that cognitive outcome was clearly related to head size at the time of adoption [12].

The prevalence of low birth weight (LBW) in IA countries is 10% to 40%, compared with 2% to 3% in developed countries [13]. The cause is usually unknown, but, as in the United States, it is believed to be multifactorial— attributable to congenital infections and malformations; genetic causes; behaviors like maternal smoking, alcohol, and drug abuse; poor nutrition; and placental insufficiency leading to poor growth in utero.

Birth information and maternal history

Prematurity is reported in 25% of preadoption medical reports [14]. Generally, the exact gestation is unknown, because most birth mothers who place their children for adoption receive no prenatal care. It is common to see multiple pregnancies with relatively few deliveries, because elective abortion is the primary method of birth control in many countries. Maternal alcohol use may also be mentioned in the report. As discussed later in this article, these perinatal risk factors significantly increase the risk to the child. In a study of 2814 preadoption medical reviews, Jenista [15] found a high incidence of these risk factors in birth and maternal histories (Table 1).

Child social history

Knowing the child's preorphanage history and length of time spent in the orphanage is helpful in predicting developmental outcomes. In general, a child in foster care or in his or her birth home receives more environmental stimulation, and thus has fewer developmental delays, whereas a child in an orphanage is much more likely to have developmental delays. Extensive hospitalizations (eg, tuberculosis treatment can take 9–12 months in a hospital setting) contribute to further decreased stimulation, and thus more delays. Although rarely mentioned in

Table 1
Parental- and pregnancy-related risk factors found in preadoption medical reports

Risk factor	Percentage
No prenatal care	15%
More than five pregnancies	20%
Syphilis	14%
Premature delivery	25%
Small for gestational age	40%
Poverty	28%
Single parent	25%
Involuntary termination of parental rights for abuse or neglect	25%
Parental alcoholism	12%
Drug use	2%
Incarceration	2%
Schizophrenia	2%

medical reports, physical and sexual abuse occur in this population, particularly as children age out of baby homes at 3 to 4 years of age and enter orphanages for older children. Parental rights may have been terminated for abuse or neglect. In these cases, the child certainly has experienced emotional or physical trauma.

Medical history

Major hospitalizations and illnesses are likely to be listed in the medical reports. A list of common diagnoses and their frequency is provided in Table 2 [15].

Preadoption laboratory tests

Preadoption medical reports usually contain at least some laboratory test results for infectious diseases. Most reports provide HIV and hepatitis B results. Many also include test results for syphilis (often referred to as TRUST in China or Reaction Wasserman [RW] in Eastern Europe) and hepatitis C. A few, such as those from China, also include a complete blood cell count (CBC), urinalysis, and liver function test results. It is reassuring when these test results are normal, but we must convey to parents that we do not know much about the quality control standards in many of these laboratories. The timing of the laboratory tests must also be considered. For example, the hepatitis B virus can have an incubation period of 12 weeks. If laboratory samples are drawn before 3 months of age, as they often are, an infected child may still have a negative hepatitis B surface antigen test result. Parents must be informed that until the laboratory tests are repeated in the United States, we cannot be certain of their accuracy. Most parents want to know whether the test results are normal and what the long-term prognosis is if they are not. For example, this may involve a discussion of the possibility of liver disease if the child tests positive for hepatitis B surface antigen or the short-term nature and treatment of anemia.

Table 2
Medical diagnoses found in preadoption medical reports

Medical diagnosis	Percentage
Severe growth retardation	13%
Severe microcephaly	23%
Mild to moderate growth delay	50%
Mild to moderate developmental delay	86%
Rickets	41%
Anemia	68%
Hip dysplasia	11%
Cardiopathy	12%
Open foramen ovale	27%
Hypermetropia	17%
Alcoholic fetopathy	2%

Reviewing a picture of a child

Another objective piece of information is a photograph of the child. The most helpful photograph is one in which the child has a neutral facial expression and is taken at his or her eye level. These views allow the examiner to see the form of the lips, philtrum, eyes, nose, and mouth. The most common syndrome seen in children adopted from orphanages is FAS. Maternal alcohol use has been cited in 12% to 41% of preadoption medical reports from Eastern Europe and the former Soviet Union [15–17]. Other studies by Aronson [18] and Abel and Sokol [19] examined the records of IA children and found that the rate of fetal alcohol spectrum disorder (FASD) was, respectively, 8 and 47 times the worldwide rate. In another study, maternal alcoholism was mentioned in 17% of adoption referral documents [9]. It is imperative that the pediatric provider who reviews pre-adoption medical reports be well versed on the characteristics of FASD and have a high index of suspicion for this disorder. It is also important to inform the family that maternal prenatal alcohol use is associated with a wide range of outcomes [20,21] and that affected children may not have the classic facial features associated with FASD. Normal facial features do not rule out significant prenatal alcohol exposure. Conversely, an isolated facial anomaly may not be indicative of FASD or another syndrome, because 14% of the population has one minor anomaly that is not associated with any syndrome [22]. Epicanthal folds and a flattened nasal bridge, which are commonly found in infants (particularly in Asian faces), are not necessarily indicative of a syndrome.

Reviewing a videotape of a child

Often, a videotape accompanies the preadoption medical report, or parents are allowed to take their own videotape footage and send it for review from abroad. A videotape is an excellent way to gather developmental, neurologic, and behavioral information, but it has significant limitations as well. Common problems include poor videotape resolution and inadequate length for collecting interpretable information. The videotape may also only show the child in one position or be out of focus in the close-up shots of the face. Videographers sometimes forget to report the age of the child at the time of filming, thus limiting our assessment of age-appropriate skills. Videotaping is not a common occurrence in orphanages, so children are often afraid of the camera and the videographer. In addition, the viewer cannot know the circumstances under which the videotape was taken (eg, what the child's mood was during the taping, whether he or she had just been awakened from a nap). These circumstances must be taken into consideration if the videotape seems to portray a child's lack of skills.

Despite these limitations, the skills observed in videotapes can be helpful. The reviewer must consider whether the videotape provides sufficient developmental information and adequate images to assess facial features. If parents are going to be filming the videotape, it is important to instruct them on what to tape. Facial views from the front, 45° turn, and 90° turn are essential. It is also helpful to give the parents a copy of a developmental milestones checklist, such as the Denver Developmental Screening Test [23]. Using this checklist, they can videotape the child performing developmental tasks for the reviewer to assess.

From a video assessment, the reviewer can evaluate the developmental stage of the child. The author's clinic uses the Hawaii Early Learning Program (HELP) to assess development from videotape footage. In infants and toddlers, a videotape can give the reviewer some sense of the child's fine and gross motor skills. It is important to remember, however, that good fine and gross motor development may not indicate normal cognitive function. Expressive and receptive speech development is more predictive of cognitive skills [4], but these developments are rarely captured adequately in the footage. Speech is the most common delay in postinstitutionalized children, largely because of the paucity of reciprocal communication and the lack of speech models in an orphanage. Unidentified and untreated ear infections often lead to impaired or transient hearing. In addition, the lack of opportunity to suck from a normal nipple impairs the oral motor development needed to create speech sounds. A group of Russian psychologists found that 60% of 2-year-old children from orphanages lacked any expressive language [24]. In contrast, older children often do speak on these videotapes, but unless they are reciting a poem or are speaking in long sentences, it is difficult to assess their language development.

Neurologic maturity can sometimes be assessed from videotape footage. For instance, the neurologic immaturity of an infant with FAS may be exhibited as tremulousness. Asymmetry and quality of movement in the extremities may indicate cerebral palsy. It is not uncommon for children to present with hypotonicity, especially of the trunk, secondary to excessive time spent on their backs in cribs and in walkers.

Videotapes may provide clues about social development, especially if the child is videotaped alongside another child or a familiar caregiver. It is helpful to see the child interacting with toys as well. Many children exhibit what is referred to as "orphanage passivity," a lack of reaction to their surroundings that develops over time from lack of an adult figure to teach and stimulate them to interact with their environment. Conversely, children may appear to be quite alert and active. Unfortunately, the level of alertness and activity on a videotape has not consistently proven to be predictive of future cognitive skills.

Parents should be counseled to expect developmental delays in institutionalized children [25]. As a rule of thumb, for every 3 months a child spends in an institution during the first year of life, he or she loses 1 month of motor and language development; thus, the reviewer must adjust his or her developmental expectations. The child's age at placement in an institution and the preplacement environment also have a significant impact on development. As mentioned earlier, the child most likely receives more developmental stimulation in a birth or foster home than in an orphanage, but it seems that the worst place for a child, developmentally speaking, is in a hospital, where caregiver attention is minimal. Thus, the social information provided in the medical report can have a significant impact on the reviewer's expectations for developmental performance.

This is an opportune time to remind parents that although many of their child's delays are going to fade once a nurturing home is provided, some require short-term specialized interventions and some result in lifelong learning differences. When they arrive in the United States, it is important for these children to receive a developmental evaluation from someone experienced with postinstitutionalized children. Too often, children do not receive needed therapy because well-meaning professionals are not cognizant of the typical expected catch-up rate in international adoptees.

Country-specific medical reports

Currently, China and Russia place the largest numbers of children in the United States. Specific considerations for reviewing medical reports from these and other commonly represented countries are discussed at length in this section.

China

Because of China's widely publicized one-child policy and its traditional preference for boys, healthy children adopted from China are almost always girls. Although most come from orphanages, a small but growing percentage come from foster homes that are overseen by orphanage staff. On average, these little girls are 8 to 24 months of age. China currently has the most standardized medical reports, which typically include one or two photographs, results of at least one physical examination, laboratory studies, limited social information, and the child's daily schedule. The results of the physical examination are usually normal unless the child is listed as a special needs child. China is careful not to label the child healthy unless her or his physical examination is normal, so unexpected diagnoses are uncommon. The adoption agency gives the family the Chinese medical report and its English translation. It is helpful to have both when reviewing information, even if you are not fluent in Chinese, because translation errors are common. Arabic numerals, laboratory studies, and the Chinese characters for negative and positive are generally easy to read and interpret.

The social information provided for a typical Chinese adoptee states when and where the child was found. In China, an unwanted child is first abandoned in a public area and found by strangers before being placed in the orphanage. If the child was placed in foster care, this is conveyed in the medical report as well. Most of the time, no information is left with the child when he or she is found, so the actual date of birth and the child's medical and family history are un-known. Chinese orphanage workers usually estimate the child's age and assign a birth date based on the state of the umbilical cord development and on growth information. The first physical examination is typically a few months after the child's entrance into the orphanage and generally contains updated measurements. The developmental part of the report is a checklist that sometimes correlates with true development but does not always. Laboratory studies include hepatitis B and C, syphilis (TRUST), CBC, HIV, and, often, a liver panel and urinalysis. There is often a description of the temperament of the child and his or her interaction with the other children. Children from China who are listed as having special needs have similar medical reports, but these also include limited information about the child's diagnosis. Special needs can range from the benign (eg, a simple hemangioma) to major defects, such as a congenital heart defect.

Russia and other Eastern European countries

In Russia, children available for adoption are usually abandoned or voluntarily relinquished in the immediate postpartum period. Children also enter orphanages because of profound poverty or, less commonly, because of the death or incarceration of parents [9]. Court-ordered termination of parental rights may be attributable to neglect or abuse. This process is also required when mothers abandon their children without relinquishing their rights in writing. Prenatal information is often scarce; however, the birth mother typically receives no prenatal care. More boys than girls are available for adoption from these countries.

The medical record is fairly standardized but can be frustrating to the Western physician because of the paucity of useful information and the use of diagnoses that a Western doctor would consider catastrophic or require immediate medical attention. An ominous medical report may be accompanied by a videotape of a healthy-appearing child with no obvious medical illness, leaving the reviewer to question the discrepancy. Eric Downing, a Western-trained physician working in Russia, explains that the major difficulty with interpreting reports from Russia and other Eastern European countries stems from the nature of the medical systems in these countries. For example, diagnostic categories, concepts of pathophysiology, methods of assessment, and the psychology of physicians are different from Western traditions. The average North American doctor assumes that the child is healthy unless there are obvious physical signs; in most cases, diagnoses are only made after confirming testing has been conducted. Conversely, Russian doctors diagnose the child before the testing. In the first years of their lives, Russian children are examined on a regular basis and given a list of diagnoses during this time. Diagnostic terms and therapy are often different from those used in Western medicine (www.russianadoptions.org).

It is not uncommon in Russia for a healthy child to see multiple subspecialists during infancy and childhood. Thus, Russian medical reports tend to contain a variety of opinions. All children are seen by a neurologist who may only have limited post–medical school training. Neurologic diagnoses, such as perinatal encephalopathy (PE) and pyramidal insufficiency, are common. These diagnoses do not have the same meaning and prognosis as they would if used by a Western doctor. They are usually not supported by the physical examination findings or by laboratory or radiologic verification. Appendix 2 contains common diagnoses and definitions seen in Eastern European reports. Although overdiagnosis is common, underdiagnosis can be a more serious problem [3]. Parents must be made aware of this reality.

Korea

Most children adopted from Korea are cared for in foster homes. Medical care in Korea is comparable to that in Western countries, and the social and medical records are typically thorough and fairly accurate. The medical report includes the child's medical history, laboratory test results, and any medical complications or medications administered. The social history provides information about the birth parents, including age, religion, education, occupation, and marital status. There is also some detail on the child's birth and background about the circumstances under which the child was placed for adoption.

Guatemala

Foster care is also common in Guatemala. Many families adopting from Guatemala are matched within the first month of the child's life; at this time, they receive the medical report and photographs. The adoption is finalized 5 to 6 months later. In many cases, families have the option during this period to receive updates or to visit their child in Guatemala. Medical records are fairly accurate, although limited, because of the young age of the child. Additional information is not difficult to obtain if needed.

When more information is required

Often, there is not enough information about the child to make even an educated guess about his or her health and developmental status. A common scenario is a child who appears healthy, with the exception of one alarming detail listed in the medical report. In many cases, the reviewer can make a list of questions about the child for the family to ask the agency. These questions must be focused, straightforward, and worded simply because they are going to be translated, e-mailed, or faxed to the country of origin and go through two to three people before the questions are actually posed to the person who can answer them. Questions should also be limited to issues that can help the family to make the decision to adopt. For example, if the child is growing well but the last head circumference measurement has not increased appropriately, it would be appropriate to ask for a recent measurement.

Adopting an older child

Families adopting older children need individualized preadoption education, because there are many facets to the transition of the older child into the family that are best thought through and prepared for in advance. These children deserve well-educated and prepared parents. Many parents think that older child adoption is the "easier route" because they will have bypassed the diapers and irregular infant sleep patterns. On the contrary, older adoptees are a much higher risk population. A survey of families who had adopted in Minnesota over a 9-year period looked at child outcomes versus the number of preadoption risk factors and age at adoption [26]. Within this group of children, the longer a child is in an orphanage setting, the more risk factors he is likely to have. Nearly 50% of the children placed at 24 months of age or older had four or more of the following risk factors: prebirth exposure to alcohol or drugs, maternal malnutrition during pregnancy, prematurity, institutionalization for longer than 6 months, neglect of social needs, neglect of physical needs, and physical abuse. Also, as age and the number of risk factors increased, school difficulties increased, the number of behavioral problems increased, and participation in talented and gifted programs decreased. Of all IA children in this survey, 17% fell behind in some or all subjects. This number jumped to 44% in children who were poorly cared for before adoption and to 42% in children who spent at least 2 years in an institution.

Families adopting older children also need more preadoption education to make sure they collect valuable information while visiting the orphanage during the adoption process. Once adopted, these children lose their native language abilities quickly (6–8 weeks) yet are not fluent enough for testing in English for 6 to 12 months [27], making it difficult to assess school readiness and cognitive skills during the initial period after their adoption. Although it is best to get this information once the child arrives in the United States from a speech pathologist fluent in the child's birth language or from a bilingual translator, not all medical providers are able to provide a skilled translator. At adoption, parents often have the opportunity to ask orphanage workers about the child's language and educational skills. In these cases, parents may use the questionnaire developed by Sharon Glennen, PhD, to ask language and cognitive questions of the child's orphanage workers (http://pages.towson.edu/sglennen/index.htm).

Finally, special consideration is necessary for parents to determine appropriate school placement in the first year of an older child's life with his new family. Older IA children are at risk for such extensive cultural deprivation and may not be ready for school in the traditional sense for months or years. In addition, it is helpful to remember that school makes cognitive and social demands and that children may have different abilities in these two separate areas. Finding and implementing an education plan is also difficult, because most schools are unfamiliar with the needs of IA children. Generally unaware of the recommendations made by experts in this field, schools may instead rely on educational guidelines for immigrant children, which recommend that children be placed in the grade appropriate for their age. In contrast, school placement for the IA child varies depending on the history of the child, and placement behind age level is often recommended. In some cases, home schooling is the best option for at least the first year after adoption. Families need time to investigate school options before adoption. This subject is addressed in detail in a separate article in this issue.

Adopting multiple children or children with special needs

In some cases, multiple children may be adopted at one time. This is often done to keep biologic siblings together and, under these circumstances, is usually in the best interest of the children. Adopting two unrelated children at the same time, however, is not in either child's best interest. As mentioned previously, any child being adopted from an orphanage has unique needs that need time and resources to overcome. In the case of unrelated children, it is in the best interest of each child that adoptions be spaced apart by at least 1 year so as to give each child the needed attention and opportunity to integrate well into the family.

In the case of a child who has been identified as having special needs, prospective parents want to know what the postadoption needs of the child may be. For example, a child with a cleft palate may require multiple operations, is at risk for eustachian tube dysfunction, and has speech delays that require therapy. The child also needs to be followed by an interdisciplinary cleft palate clinic. Information like this can help families to schedule the amount of time off from work they need to take and the emotional and financial preparations they need to make to care for this child.

Parent education issues that need to occur before adoption

Postadoption parent education should begin during the preadoption phase, counseling parents about the interventions that are available to their post-institutionalized child. There is an ample amount of "waiting time" before an adoption takes place, and pediatricians should view this as an opportunity to provide most of the education the family needs regarding postadoption issues. Once the child is with the family, stress and emotion levels rise, diluting educational efforts. Further, high stress levels in the family can negatively affect the attachment process, and thus the development of the child. It is therefore imperative to prepare parents before adoption and to help them know what to expect so that the transition can go smoothly. The following is an abbreviated list of necessary topics to be covered before adoption. The substance of each topic is included in other articles in this issue.

Topics of focus for preadoption education

1. Timing of the first postadoption visits, which should be 1 to 2 weeks after arriving in the United States and again the following month, to address new questions

2. Common transition illnesses, such as upper respiratory tract or ear infections, diarrhea, vomiting, impetigo, scabies or lice, and feeding or sleeping issues
3. Laboratory screening needed at the first visit [28]
4. Normal growth and development as a basis of comparison
5. Normal postinstitutional development, including rapid catch-up and leveling off by around 6 to 12 months after adoption
6. Importance of 6-month postadoption developmental assessment by a clinician experienced in international adoption to assess the rate of catch-up and attachment
7. Frequency of speech delays
8. Ways to facilitate attachment, especially during the first few months

Initial attachment

Attachment of the child to the family and vice versa is an important issue to discuss before adoption. It is an area in which the parents play the role of sole facilitators; thus, their preadoption research and attention should be focused in this area. Attachment is the tie of affection and emotion between people that continues indefinitely over time and lasts even when people are geographically separated. Attachment issues in IA children range from mild to severe, but few children are truly "unattached" once integrated into the family. Initial post-adoption visits help to provide a baseline to assess future progress. Infants and young children usually demonstrate attachment progress within the first weeks and months. Older children often progress more slowly, and it can take several months or more to form enduring attachments. Bringing an IA child home can be challenging, because many children grieve or exhibit orphanage behaviors. The following is a list of ways in which children may respond during this transition from the orphanage to first postadoption visit:

- May appear extremely passive (often termed *orphanage passivity*)
- May be overly active like a wind-up toy (overstimulated)
- May cry desperately; if he or she had little or no attachment previously, may have little outward expression of loss
- May not sleep, eat, or toilet normally (grief can affect all these)
- May reach for other people and search for previous caregivers
- May not make eye contact or may arch his or her back when held or bat at the parent's face when they are close

Many parents do not know how to handle these behaviors or feel unable to facilitate a sound integration of the child into their family. Box 1 lists parenting techniques that parents can use to facilitate attachment during the transition period. Helping parents initiate attachment style parenting from the beginning

Box 1. Parenting techniques that parents can use to facilitate attachment during the transition period

- Do not allow your child to be passed around to multiple caregivers until attachment to you has become more secure so as not to promote indiscriminate attachment.
- Hold and carry your child as much as possible. Keep stroller time to a minimum.
- Maintain close proximity to your child.
- Keep your life low key for 4 to 6 months after you get home.
- Only parents should hold, feed, and nurture. Friends and extended family need to wait.
- Provide high levels of nurture and structure.
- Reparent your child as if he or she is younger.
- Maintain eye contact during bottle feedings with infants and toddlers.
- Cradle your child in your arms and sing or use loving words, as you would an infant.
- Help with sleep issues, and do not let your child ''cry it out.'' Go to the child or sleep near the child until he or she feels more secure.
- Baby games like peek-a-boo and patty cake work well to facilitate the initial interactions.
- Skin-to-skin contact is helpful; use swimming and bathing as opportunities to increase attachment.
- Be your child's primary caregiver for as long as you can. Six months to a year is helpful.
- Have realistic expectations, and ask for help if things do not seem right or if you do not feel warmth between you and your child.

and helping them to prepare in advance for this integration lower stress for the parent and child and begin the life of the family in a positive way. These lists are hardly comprehensive; before receiving their child, the parents and their pediatrician should read at least one book on attachment from an adoption perspective (see Appendix 1).

Summary

International adoption pairs the most vulnerable and high-risk pediatric population with the lowest risk parent group. IA parents typically are financially established, well educated, and have only a 3% divorce rate [26]. Thus, these adoptions offer a wonderful combination with excellent potential for a lifetime family bond.

International adoption also presents unique and rewarding challenges for primary care pediatricians. After receiving information from the medical reviewer, a parent must determine whether or not this child is "their child." The decision to adopt a particular child is ultimately that of the parent. The position of the medical reviewer is to provide the family with as much information as possible about the health status of the child by explaining the terminology in the report and assessing the photograph or videotape. It is also the reviewer's job to guide the parent's expectations of the adoption by explaining the inherent differences in the development of children in institutions. In the preadoption phase, we must remember that our ultimate goal is to aid in the permanent placement of a child with a family that has realistic expectations and is well prepared to aid that child to reach his or her fullest potential. The irony is that we must accomplish this task while at the same time knowing:

> Although very many important things about human beings may be approached by scientific quantification, the most important things about human beings are neither measurable nor predictable.—Unknown

Although this dichotomy is not comfortable, it is inevitable and worthwhile to face for the cause of placing children into their forever families.

Appendix 1. Resources

International adoption web sites

American Academy of Pediatrics: www.aap.org/sections/adoption/adopt-states/adoption-map.html. Map of pediatricians who specialize in international adoption

Families with Children from China: www.fwcc.org. Resources for families adopting from China

Families for Russian and Ukrainian Adoption: www.frua.org. Resources for families adopting from Russia and Ukraine

Eastern European Adoption Coalition: www.eeadopt.org. Resources for families adopting from Romania and other Eastern European countries

Fetal Alcohol Syndrome (support, training, advocacy, and resources): www.fasstar.com. Resources for families regarding FASP disorder

International Adoption Clinic at the University of Minnesota: www.umniac.org. Web site of Dr. Jane Aronson: www.orphandoctor.com. Web sites created by international adoption clinics that contain articles on medical and developmental issues in postinstitutionalized children

International Adoption Clinic at the University of Alabama at Birmingham: http://adoption.chsys.org

Joint Council on International Children's Services: www.jcics.org. Legal and government information about adoption issues

Korean Focus: www.koreanfocus.org. Adopting from Korea: www.adopt korea.com. Resources for families adopting from Korea

Latin American Parents Association: www.lapa.com. Resources for families adopting from Central and South America

National Council on Adoptable Children: www.nacac.org. General resources for adoptive families

National Adoption Information Clearinghouse: http://naic.acf.hhs.gov/. General resources for adoptive families

Parents Network for the Post Institutionalized Child: www.pnpic.org. Articles on the medical and developmental issues of postinstitutionalized children

General adoption issues

Miller M, Ward N. Eyes wide open. (Workbook for parents adopting international children older than 1 year of age). St. Paul (MN): Children's Home Society of Minnesota; 2001.

Hopkins-Best M. Toddler adoption: the weaver's craft. (Specific information about a toddler's adjustment from an orphanage or foster home into a family). Indianapolis (IN): Perspectives Press; 1998.

Mascew T. Our own. (Specific information about adopting older children). Morton Grove (IL): Snowcap Press; 2003.

Attachment

Keck G. Adopting the hurt child. (Realistic look at how trauma and disruptions affect the postinstitutionalized child's development and integration into the family). Colorado Springs (CO): NAV Press Publishing; 1998.

Eshleman L. Becoming a family. (Easy-to-read book on how to promote healthy attachments between a family and their adopted child). Lanham (MD): Taylor Trade Publishing; 2003.

Gray D. Attaching in adoption. (Comprehensive guidebook for easing the adopted child's transition and attachment into a family). Indianapolis (IN): Perspectives Press; 2002.

Normal development

Brazelton TB. Touchpoints: your child's emotional and psychological development. (Normal child development that is especially helpful for first-time parents). Cambridge (MA): Da Capo Lifelong Books; 1992.

Losquadro Liddle T, Yorke L. Why motor skills matter. (Explains the impact that motor skills have on the child's neurodevelopment). New York: McGraw Hill; 2003.

Appendix 2. Common diagnoses in Eastern European medical evaluations

Additional (abnormal) heart chordae (or trabeculae) refers to "extra" muscle tissue in the wall of the heart, usually the left ventricle. This is an "incidental finding" that does not cause symptoms or disease and is found by doing an echocardiogram of the heart.

Australian antigen is the classic name in Russian for the hepatitis B surface antigen test.

Bacillus Calmette-Guérin (BCG) vaccination is the vaccination against tuberculosis, which is mandatory in most countries outside the United States. The BCG vaccination is usually given at birth.

Dysbacteriosis is loose or diarrhea-like stool after lack of breastfeeding, illness, or use of antibiotics, presumably attributable changes in the normal bacterial flora of the intestine. This condition is treated first with antibiotics to decontaminate the gastrointestinal tract and then with enzymes and probiotics, similar to treatment with lactase and/or lactobacillus.

Hip dysplasia is an unsatisfactory term that usually indicates little more than a "suspected" problem with a hip joint. Usually, there is little information indicating the basis of the diagnosis or whether ultrasound or radiologic tests have been performed. It refers to perceived instability of the hip joint; however, without elaboration, it is difficult to determine whether the physician meant instability or frank dislocation. Observation is usually the only treatment, and the diagnosis is often removed at some point in the first year of life. Hips that are truly unstable are usually splinted.

Hyperexcitability syndrome, or syndrome of increased reflexes, is occasionally mentioned in the medical reports and does not correlate with true pathologic findings. An exception is seen in the child with drug withdrawal because of maternal drug use, which often additionally notes abstinence syndrome.

Hypertensive-hydrocephalic syndrome, hypertensive syndrome, and hydrocephalic syndrome all refer to the same frequently diagnosed condition. Often, this diagnosis is made after a cranial ultrasound scan looking for dilation of the ventricles or ischemia. In most children, it is considered to be a transient condition secondary to the birth process. Treatment consists of certain vitamins, diuretics, and/or other drugs to improve blood flow to the brain. The diagnosis and treatment are theoretic only. Surgical shunting is rare. This is almost never true hydrocephalus.

Hypostature means short stature. Past the first year of life, it may be termed *alimentary nanism*.

Hypotrophy means the child is small for his or her age. If used for a neonate, it means small for gestational age. If applied to a child who is older, it is less specific and may refer to a child who is failing to thrive.

Hypoxia (hypoxy) of the newborn is lack of oxygen at or before delivery and is usually diagnosed if there was a difficult pregnancy, labor, or delivery and refers to hypoxia in utero. It rarely means that there was true hypoxia. If the infant needed resuscitation at birth because of an obstetric complication, the diagnosis of asphyxia is used and APGAR scores are low as well.

"Mother had syphilis" is rather common in Russian medical reports. Syphilis has been on the rise in Russia for several years, and Russian pediatricians are alert to the possibility of maternal infection. Mothers are routinely screened in the third trimester of pregnancy, and proper treatment is given. If the maternal history is unknown, the possibility of congenital syphilis is considered and the infant is tested. Subsequent treatment and follow-up are generally adequate. The most common difficulty encountered in interpreting the Russian medical reports is a lack of detail concerning the precise treatment received or the diagnostic evaluation undertaken. On adoption, these children should be screened for syphilis to confirm that the infection has cleared, even though the possibility of continued infection is low. The RW test is equivalent to the Western VDRL test for syphilis.

"No comment" regarding maternal use of alcohol and drugs. Concerning the possibility of FASD, it is interesting how seldom information concerning maternal alcohol use is provided. Prenatal records and hospital records often are not transmitted to the orphanage in detail at the time the child is transferred to the orphanage. A similar problem exists when trying to obtain family history.

Patent oval window refers to an open foramen ovale, the normal embryologic connection between the two upper chambers (atria) of the heart. It is generally not considered a heart defect (ie, not the same as atrial septal defect).

PE is the single most common medical diagnosis and is noted in the medical reports of more than 95% of children in some regions of Eastern Europe. It is considered to be attributable to "chronic intrauterine hypoxia," which is not to be confused with asphyxia. Typically, PE is described as ischemic, chemical, traumatic, or of mixed origin. Usually, the diagnosis is stated without corroborating medical evidence—physical findings are not noted, and laboratory or diagnostic studies are not mentioned. The medical theory behind this diagnosis is based on Russian concepts of pathophysiology in the newborn period. Most consultants questioned have not been able to give a clear explanation of the term. It can be applied solely on the basis of history (known or suspected during pregnancy). Physicians often mention tremor of the fingers or chin when the child is crying, which is considered a sign of PE (although in the West, this might be termed a *fussy baby*). PE does not correspond to the Western diagnosis of cerebral palsy, nor is it used as a Western-trained physician would use the term *hypoxic-ischemic encephalopathy*.

Rickets (rachit or rachitis) and iron-deficient anemia are extremely common diagnoses in Russian orphanages because of vitamin D and iron deficiencies. These diagnoses can be accurate and usually can be treated by a balanced diet, iron supplementation, and, sometimes, supplemental vitamin D and calcium. With most diseases, Russian medical practice considers the mildest form of a disease to be stage 1 and the most severe to be stage 4, although classification into one or another stage is at the individual physician's discretion.

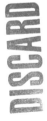

Spastic tetraparesis or paraparesis, muscular hypertonus, pyramidal syndrome, pyramidal insufficiency syndrome, prenatal insult of the central nervous system, and natal trauma of the cervical spine are frequently used expressions that also arise from Russian pathophysiologic concepts. These terms all basically refer to the same "disorder," which is associated with the belief that there is cranial and spinal cord trauma at the time of birth and that trauma manifests itself through changes in muscle tone. It is generally treated conservatively and is considered to have a good prognosis. This disorder does not correspond to the Western diagnosis of cerebral palsy. It is frequently used as a contradiction to giving immunizations with the thought that vaccinations may exhaust the immune system and prevent complete resolution of the condition. This diagnosis does not correlate with true pathologic findings and is not actually a contraindication to immunizations.

References

[1] Frank DA, Klass PE, Earls F, et al. Infants and young children in orphanages: one view from pediatrics and child psychiatry. Pediatrics 1996;97:569–78.

[2] Johnson DE, Miller LC, Iverson S, et al. The health of children adopted from Romania. JAMA 1992;268:3446–51.

[3] Albers L, Johnson DE, Hostetter M, et al. Health of children adopted from the former Soviet Union and Eastern Europe: comparison with pre-adoptive medical records. JAMA 1997;278: 922–4.

[4] Miller LC. Initial assessment of growth, development, and the effects of institutionalization in internationally adopted children. Pediatr Ann 2000;29(4):224–32.

[5] Rutter M for the English and Romanian Adoptees (ERA) Study Team. Developmental catch-up, and deficit, following adoption after severe global early deprivation. J Child Psychol Psychiatry 1998;39:465–76.

[6] Ames EW, et al. The development of Romanian orphanage children adopted to Canada: Final report, Romanian adoption project. Burnaby, British Columbia: Simon Fraser University; 1997. p. 1–138.

[7] Widdowson EM. Mental contentment and physical growth. Lancet 1951;1:1316–8.

[8] Johnson D, Miller L, Iverson S, et al. The health of children adopted from Romania. JAMA 1992;268:3446–51.

[9] Johnson DE. Medical and developmental sequelae of early childhood institutionalization in international adoptees from Romania and the Russian Federation. In: Nelson C, editor. The effects of early adversity on neurobehavioral development. Mahwah, NJ: Lawrence Erlbaum Associated; 2000. p. 113–62.

[10] Loyd-Still J. Clinical studies on the effects of malnutrition during infancy and subsequent physical and intellectual development. In: Malnutrition and intellectual development. Littleton, MA: Publishing Sciences Group; 1976.

[11] Winick M, Rosso P. Head circumference and cellular growth of the brain in normal and marasmic children. J Pediatr 1969;74:774–8.

[12] Rutter M, O'Connor TG. Are there biological programming effects for psychological development? Findings from a study of Romanian adoptees. Dev Psychol 2004;40:81–94.

[13] Villar J, Belizan JM. The relative contribution of prematurity and fetal growth retardation to low birth weight in developing and developed societies. Am J Obstet Gynecol 1982;143:793–8.

[14] Jenista J. Pre-adoption review of medical records. Pediatr Ann 2000;29(4):212–5.

[15] Jenista JA. Findings from foreign medical records. Adoption/Medical News 1999;10:1–6.

[16] Johnson D, Albers L, Iverson S, et al. Health status of US-adopted Eastern European (EE) orphans. Pediatr Res 1996;39:134A.

[17] McGuinness T, McGuiness J, Dyer G. Risk and protective factors in children adopted from the former Soviet Union. J Pediatr Health Care 2000;14(3):109–17.

[18] Aronson JE. Prevalence of fetal alcohol syndrome and fetal alcohol effect in pre-adoptive evaluations of children in Russian orphanages. Presented at the Evan B. Donald Institute Conference: Adoption and Prenatal Alcohol and Drug Exposure: The Research, Policy and Practice Challenges. Alexandria, VA, October, 1997.

[19] Abel EL, Sokol RJ. Incidence of fetal alcohol syndrome and economic impact of FAS-related anomalies. Drug Alcohol Depend 1987;19:51–70.

[20] Streissguth AP, Barr HM, Sampson PD. Moderate prenatal alcohol exposure: effects on child IQ and learning problems at age 7.5 years. Alcohol Clin Exp Res 1990;14:662–9.

[21] Streissguth AP, Barr HM, Sampson PD, et al. Maternal drinking during pregnancy: attention and short-term memory in 14 year old offspring—a longitudinal prospective study. Alcohol Clin Exp Res 1994;18:202–18.

[22] Marden PM, Smith DW, McDonald MJ. Congenital anomalies in the newborn infant, including minor variations. J Pediatr 1964;64:357–71.

[23] Frankenburg WK. Denver II developmental screening manual. Denver, CO: Developmental Materials; 1990.

[24] Dubrovina I. Psichologicheckoe razvitie vospitanikov v detskom dome [Psychological development of children in orphanages]. Moscow: Porveschenie Press; 1991.

[25] Miller L, Keirnan M, Mathers M, et al. Developmental and nutritional status of internationally adopted children. Arch Pediatr Adolesc Med 1995;149:40–4.

[26] 2002 IAP Newsletter. Available at: http://education.umn.edu/ICD/IAP. Accessed March 14, 2005.

[27] Gindis B. Language-related issues for international adoptees and adoptive families. In: Tepper T, Hannon L, Sandstrom D, editors. International adoption: challenges and opportunities. Meadowlands, PA: Parent Network for the Post Institutionalized Child; 1999. p. 98–108.

[28] Pickering LK. Medical evaluation of internationally adopted children for infectious diseases. In: Pickering LK, editor. Red book. Report of the Committee on Infectious Diseases. 26th edition. Elk Grove Village, IL: American Academy of Pediatrics; 2003. p. 173–80.

ELSEVIER
SAUNDERS

PEDIATRIC CLINICS
OF NORTH AMERICA

Pediatr Clin N Am 52 (2005) 1271–1286

Prevention of Travel-Related Infectious Diseases in Families of Internationally Adopted Children

Elizabeth D. Barnett, MD[a,b],*, Lin H. Chen, MD[c,d]

[a]Maxwell Finland Laboratory for Infectious Diseases, Room 503, Boston Medical Center, 774 Albany Street, Boston, MA 02118, USA
[b]Department of Pediatrics, Boston University School of Medicine, Boston, MA 02118, USA
[c]Travel Medicine Center, Division of Infectious Diseases, Mount Auburn Hospital, 330 Mount Auburn Street, Cambridge, MA 02238, USA
[d]Department of Medicine, Harvard Medical School, Boston, MA 02115, USA

Prevention of travel-related infectious diseases for adoptive families starts before and extends beyond the travel period. Many families adopting internationally travel to their child's birth country at least once before bringing their new family member home. Most commonly, families are traveling to the republics of the former Soviet Union, China, Guatemala, or other developing countries in Asia, Central or South America, or Africa. Family members who travel and family and close contacts of the child who remain at home all need information about protecting themselves during travel and preventing acquisition of diseases that could be transmitted by the internationally adopted child after arrival in the United States.

Travel for adoption presents risks that are different from those encountered by the tourist or business traveler or those travelers who travel to visit friends and relatives (VFR travelers). Although the application to adopt internationally usually requires at least 1 or 2 years of preparation, families may be notified about travel within 2 to 3 weeks of departure. Adoptive families may not have a choice in their travel destination or itinerary, the time of travel, or accommodations during the trip. They may not speak the local language or have regular

* Corresponding author. Maxwell Finland Laboratory for Infectious Diseases, Room 503, Boston Medical Center, 774 Albany Street, Boston, MA 02118.
E-mail address: ebarnett@bu.edu (E.D. Barnett).

0031-3955/05/$ – see front matter © 2005 Elsevier Inc. All rights reserved.
doi:10.1016/j.pcl.2005.06.002   pediatric.theclinics.com

access to interpreters and may be apprehensive about accommodations, visa requirements, and overseas procedures. They may be inexperienced first-time parents or may be traveling with other children who require attention to their own needs.

Travel for adoption may lead to prolonged and unexpected stays in the country, possibly with accommodation in nontourist facilities, such as local apartments, hostels, or their child's orphanage. Because of a desire to please the many individuals with power over the adoption process (eg, facilitators, interpreters, court and government officials, agency and orphanage personnel), families may accept risks they would ordinarily avoid, such as eating local foods or drinking potentially unsafe water, drinking more or different types of alcohol, seeking medical care in rural health facilities, or using local means of transport without seat belts or car seats. Families may be exposed to extreme air pollution, farm animals, second-hand cigarette smoke, or infectious agents, such as tuberculosis, that they might otherwise avoid were it not for the adoption process.

As the field of travel medicine evolves, distinct groups of travelers with specific risks have been identified, such as VFR travelers. It is possible that the families and close contacts of internationally adopted children comprise such a group. Better description of these risks through systematic study may lead to improved interventions in this population in the future. This article addresses the current body of knowledge and recommendations for preventing travel-related illness in this group (see Appendix).

Preparation for international travel

Individuals traveling to arrange adoptions or pick up their child should receive standard travel advice appropriate for their destination (including stops along the way), length of travel, immunization history, medical history, and types of exposures that might occur. It is helpful to elicit as much information as possible about type of accommodation expected, mode of travel between destinations, and anticipated activities. Many sources of pretravel advice are available (Table 1) [1–3]. The US Centers for Disease Control and Prevention (CDC) make their recommendations available in print or on line (www.cdc.gov/travel) [4]. Adoptive families may also receive information from agencies, travel agents, airlines, and embassies; it is prudent for families to verify any information about possible outbreaks or other local situations with reliable and authoritative sources such as the CDC or World Health Organization (WHO). For example, a measles outbreak in a Chinese orphanage led the CDC to suspend adoptions from the affected orphanage temporarily [5]. During the severe acute respiratory syndrome (SARS) outbreak in 2003, the CDC provided up-to-date information and released travel advisories that were instrumental in informing families and adoption agencies about the status of the epidemic. Although the SARS outbreak resulted in suspension of adoptions from several countries, disruption of plans

Table 1
On-line resources to guide families planning international adoption

Web site	Highlight
http://travel.state.gov/family/adoption/ adoption_485.html	International adoption booklet; information on US visa requirements; travel warnings
http://www.cdc.gov/nie/menus/groups.htm#intl	General health information regarding international adoption
http://www.immunize.org/adoption/index.htm	Link to journal articles and recommendations on international adoption; link to numerous resources for parents and providers
http://www.istm.org	Travel clinic directory
http://www.cdc.gov/travel	Travel health warning and precautions; outbreaks; travel health recommendations

of many adoptive families, and household isolation of some newly adopted children, no cases were reported in internationally adopted children.

Immunizations for international travel

The two steps involved in providing immunizations for international travel are updating routine immunizations and providing immunizations specific for the travel destination (Table 2). Immunization records of each traveler should be reviewed to assess if the individual is up to date with routinely recommended vaccines. For adopting parents, attention should be paid to updating the 10-yearly tetanus-diphtheria (Td) booster, verifying immunity to measles and varicella, and providing vaccine to those who are susceptible [6]. For children who may travel, routine and catch-up recommendations are also available [7,8]. Missing doses or booster doses that are due can be administered at this time.

Additional doses of some routine vaccines may be needed for international travel depending on presence of diseases or outbreaks in the destination country. For example, travelers to Asia have required preparation for exposure to measles; adult travelers to West Africa, India, and other countries where polio still occurs should receive a booster dose of polio vaccine [4]; and individuals susceptible to complications of influenza should receive this vaccine per current recommendations [9]. Today's travelers to Asia may need information about avoiding exposure to avian influenza. In the past, diphtheria outbreaks in the newly independent republics of the former Soviet Union, the SARS epidemic, and outbreaks of meningococcal meningitis have led to a need for specific travel advice for families traveling to affected countries.

Recommendations for travel vaccines are based on the destination countries, length of travel, medical history, and types of exposures that might occur. Hepatitis A vaccine is recommended for almost all individuals traveling to arrange adoptions or pick up children outside the United States, because the risk of hepatitis A is intermediate to high in most countries from which children are adopted [4]. Hepatitis A vaccine is highly effective, and a two-dose schedule

Table 2
Vaccines for families adopting internationally

Vaccines for those who travel	Standard dose/route	Comment
Update all childhood vaccines for any children in household		
Routine vaccines for adults (administer as needed according to standard schedules and recommendations)		
Hepatitis B	1.0 mL IM, 3 doses at 0, 1, 6 months	
Influenza	0.5 mL IM, according to season	
Measles, mumps, rubella	0.5 mL SC, documented 2 doses separated by ≥1 month	
Pneumococcal polysaccharide	0.5 mL SC or IM	
Polio	0.5 mL SC	For travel to areas with transmission of polioviruses
Td or TdaP	0.5 mL IM	
Varicella	0.5 mL SC, 2 doses separated by 4–8 weeks	
Special vaccines for travel to high- or intermediate-risk areas		
Hepatitis A	1.0 mL adult/0.5 mL pediatric IM, 2 doses at 0, 6 months	
Typhoid	0.5 mL IM or 4 capsules PO	
Travel to high-risk areas or required by destination		
Japanese encephalitis	0.5 mL ages 1–2, 1.0 mL ages ≥3 SC, 3 doses on days 0, 7, 30	For travel to parts of Asia
Meningococcus	0.5 mL SC	For travel to endemic and outbreak areas
Rabies	1.0 mL IM, 3 doses on days 0, 7, 21 or 28	For longer term travel, remote destinations
Yellow fever	0.5 mL SC	For travel to parts of South America and Africa

Abbreviations: IM, intramuscular; PO, by mouth; SC, subcutaneous; Td, tetanus diphtheria; TdaP, tetanus-diphtheria-acellular pertussis.

offers long-term protection [10]. Adults who need protection against hepatitis A and B may receive the combination vaccine Twinrix (Hepatitis A Inactivated and Hepatitis B [Recombinant] vaccine; Glaxo SmithKline, Research Triangle Park, North Carolina) [11,12]. Typhoid vaccine should be considered for travel to many of these countries, because this disease is also contracted by exposure to contaminated food and water [4]. Protection afforded by typhoid vaccines is incomplete, however, and all travelers to countries where a risk of contracting diseases associated with contaminated food and water is present should be counseled about appropriate dietary precautions. These include drinking only boiled or safe drinking water (chlorinated water, bottled water from a reliable source, or carbonated water), eating only cooked or freshly peeled fruits and vegetables, and avoiding raw or undercooked meat and seafood [13].

Other travel vaccines are destination specific. Individuals traveling to parts of South America or Africa where yellow fever is present are candidates for yellow fever vaccine. A single dose of vaccine administered at least 10 days before travel and documented on the WHO International Certificate of Immunization is valid for 10 years [14]. Yellow fever vaccine must be administered at a Yellow Fever Vaccine Center. Consultation with a travel medicine provider can be helpful in determining which travelers are candidates for this vaccine.

Japanese encephalitis vaccine may be indicated for travel to some destinations in Asia. The risk to short-term (< 4 weeks) travelers and those who remain in urban centers is low, and the disease is seasonal in occurrence. Adoptive parents who may spend extended periods of time in rural areas, make repeated trips to endemic areas in transmission season, or plan extended travel in the region, especially to rural areas, may be candidates for this vaccine. The three-dose series is given on days 0, 7, and 30, and the series should be completed at least 10 days before travel because of the rare occurrence of delayed allergic reactions to vaccine requiring medical attention. An accelerated schedule is available for those with imminent departures [15].

Meningococcal vaccine may be indicated for some travelers, especially in areas where outbreaks are occurring. Yearly outbreaks take place in sub-Saharan Africa, and sporadic outbreaks may occur in other areas. Consultation with a travel medical provider may be helpful in providing the most recent information. Information about disease outbreaks is available (http://www.cdc.gov/travel/outbreaks.htm).

Malaria prevention

Travelers to destinations where malaria is present should receive detailed information about malaria, including methods of prevention, signs and symptoms of disease, and when to seek medical attention. Malaria chemoprophylaxis should be offered, with a detailed description of the options of medications available for the destination, how to take the drug, and adverse events potentially associated with the medication. Many excellent sources of information about malaria prevention are available [16–18]. Brochures are available from the CDC suitable for patient handouts, giving detailed information about malaria and options for prevention and treatment [19]. Adherence to an appropriate regimen of chemoprophylaxis is the most important determinant of successful malaria prevention.

The drug of choice for prevention of malaria for travelers to regions of the world where chloroquine resistance is absent is chloroquine. The dose for adults is base, 300 mg (salt, 500 mg) once weekly beginning 1 to 2 weeks before travel, continuing during travel, and for 4 weeks after return. Chloroquine is usually tolerated well, but minor gastrointestinal disturbance, headache, and other symptoms may occur; these usually do not require stopping the medication. Chloroquine may exacerbate psoriasis.

Options for prevention of malaria for those traveling to chloroquine-resistant areas include atovaquone-proguanil, mefloquine, and doxycycline. Mefloquine is taken weekly, whereas the others require daily dosing. Decisions about appropriate antimalarials involve attention to the medical history of the traveler, destination, and length of travel. A fourth option, primaquine, is available to travelers who do not have G6PD deficiency and are unable to tolerate other alternatives; consultation with travel medicine experts is recommended if this alternative is considered [16].

Children traveling to meet new siblings require pretravel preparation as well. Similar attention should be paid to updating routine immunizations according to current schedules and risk of diseases at their destination, and travel vaccines should be administered according to current recommendations [20,21]. For some children, this may mean administering some primary or booster doses at shortened intervals or according to accelerated vaccine schedules [7,8]. For example, a sibling traveling to meet the adopted child should receive two doses of measles-containing vaccines administered at least 4 weeks apart; a sibling who is less than 12 months of age and has not received the first dose of measles, mumps, and rubella (MMR) vaccine should receive a dose of measles vaccine if traveling to an area where exposure to measles may occur [4].

General advice

Although the focus of much of a pretravel consultation is on administration of vaccines and prevention of malaria, accidents and other infectious diseases, such as diarrhea and upper respiratory infections, are more common causes of morbidity during travel. All travelers can benefit from information about dietary precautions, oral rehydration, general safety precautions, sun protection, jet lag, motion sickness, animal hazards, swimming hazards, road safety, seat belt and car seat use, and what medical supplies to bring with them. Traveling to receive a child puts additional burdens on travelers, especially those becoming parents for the first time, who may never have traveled long distances with a small child. When siblings travel, attention must be paid to their needs as well as to those of the new adoptee. Bringing along another adult to care for siblings is often helpful, especially if only one parent is traveling [22]. Many sources of detailed travel advice for children are available [20–28].

Traveler's diarrhea affects approximately 50% of travelers to less developed parts of the world [29]. Prevention of diarrhea depends on careful attention to food and water precautions. Travelers can be advised to drink boiled water or carbonated beverages and to avoid tap water, ice, and bottled water from questionable sources. Piping hot food and thick-skinned fruits that are peeled by the traveler are safest; raw seafood, vegetables and fruits like lettuce and berries with surfaces that can contain infectious organisms, and unpasteurized dairy products are least safe. Food that has been sitting at room temperature for prolonged periods or that could be set on by flies or other insects should also be avoided.

Treatment of traveler's diarrhea in adults can be accomplished with oral rehydration, antimotility agents, and judicious use of self-treatment with antibiotics [2,29,30]. For mild diarrhea that does not affect usual activities, maintaining hydration status is the most important step. When there are mild or moderate symptoms and one to two loose stools per day without blood in the stool, an antimotility agent can be added. When distressing symptoms or more frequent stools are present, an antibacterial agent can be added to the regimen. Antibacterial agents shown to be effective in traveler's diarrhea include the fluoroquinolones, although resistance rates are increasing in some areas and antibiotic-associated diarrhea is a potential side effect of concern. Azithromycin and rifaximin are also effective treatments for traveler's diarrhea [31–33]. If self-treatment does not result in improvement or if there is continued high fever, blood in the stool, dehydration, persistent vomiting, copious diarrhea, or abdominal pain, travelers must seek medical attention.

Those traveling to adopt a child may be faced with managing diarrhea in their new child or in siblings who have traveled with them. Antimotility agents are not recommended for infants or children less than 6 years of age and should be used judiciously in older children [23]. Instead, oral rehydration is the mainstay of therapy for mild to moderate symptoms. Antibacterial agents that can be used for children are limited by resistance rates to common antibacterial agents and lack of approval of fluoroquinolones in children. At this time, azithromycin is the drug of choice for treatment of most traveler's diarrhea in children, and a dose of 10/mg/kg/d for up to 3–5 days is a reasonable option, although no studies have been done to ascertain the optimal dose or length of therapy. Parents should monitor the child's condition carefully. If high fever, blood in the stool, persistent symptoms, or worsening dehydration occurs, families should seek immediate medical attention. Parents should also be aware that diarrhea in the adopted child may represent infections or conditions other than acute traveler's diarrhea, such as chronic diarrhea related to parasitic infections or malabsorption syndromes. Medical care should be sought for acutely ill children in the country where the adoption is occurring. Additional evaluation for causes of chronic diarrhea can be undertaken during the child's initial medical assessment in the United States.

Jet lag occurs almost universally in travelers who cross two or more time zones, and symptoms can last a week or more. Families may find it helpful to know that it may take approximately 1 day for each hour of time change for full acclimatization to the new time zone. Although there are no documented curative remedies, many approaches have been reported as helpful for some travelers, including light exposure, adjusting the sleep-wake cycle, and melatonin [2,34]. If possible, adding a few days to their travel itinerary for adjustment to the new time zone may be helpful for families when traveling for the purpose of adoption so as to maximize alertness for negotiating legal and bureaucratic tasks and caring for the child.

Parents traveling to meet and bring home their child should receive some preparation about what to do if their child is ill or becomes ill. Meeting with a pediatrician before the trip can be helpful in preparing a family for such an event. New parents want to know tasks, such as how to take a child's temperature, count the child's respiratory rate, and monitor a child's hydration status. Information can be given to parents about health care providers in the area of travel, available through the directory of the American Academy of Pediatrics or from the US consulate in major cities. A means of communication with a physician in the United States, available at all hours, is reassuring for parents. Families may also find it helpful to arrange with a relative or friend to be available at all times in the United States throughout their trip. This person can then track down medical contacts, legal advice, or travel help or can take care of other time-consuming tasks that are difficult to manage from outside the United States. Although the availability of electronic mail and international telephone service has improved dramatically as a result of enterprises like Internet cafes, families traveling to remote regions may find it helpful to rent a satellite telephone for the duration of their trip.

Additional travel advice about sun protection, swimming hazards, and insect precautions should be provided pertinent to the destination country [1]. All travelers should be provided information about general safety, including animal bites, use of car seats and seat belts, and personal safety. Parents may be able to find out from other recently traveling families or the adoption agency whether car seats are available or can be used. In many countries, their use may be limited by lack of seat belts in available vehicles. Emergency evacuation insurance is recommended for families, especially for prolonged trips, although whether or at what point the policy would cover the adopted child should be clarified with the insurance company. Similarly, parents should inquire from their health insurance

---

Box 1. Medical supplies for adoptive family members traveling to meet child

Oral antibiotic for traveler's diarrhea
Antimotility drug
Anti-inflammatory/antipyretic
Antihistamine
Decongestant
Topical antibiotic, steroid, antifungal
Scabicide
Adhesive bandages
Thermometer
Insect repellant
Sunscreen (if indicated)
Hand sanitizer
Oral rehydration packets
Needles/syringes/oral syringes
Bulb syringe, nasal saline spray
Pediatric formulations of medications
First time parents: consider medical kit for adopted child

plan (and get in writing) assurances of the exact date or point in the adoption process that the child becomes eligible for emergency medical coverage.

Most families, especially those who are becoming first-time parents, request guidance about what medical supplies to bring for themselves and for their child. Parents and accompanying travelers should bring all the medications and equipment they would normally use for their own medical needs, such as medications, syringes for insulin, contact lens cleaning solution, and other personal items. Although the availability of these supplies worldwide has improved in the last decade, it is usually far more convenient and reassuring for the traveler to use familiar items.

Suggested supply lists for the needs of the newly adopted child are available from many sources and depend to some extent on the destination and length of the trip [23]. General items include waterless hand sanitizer, a thermometer, diapers, oral rehydration packets, sunscreen (if indicated), insect repellant, diaper rash cream, antibacterial ointment, amoxicillin or azithromycin, oral syringes for measurement of doses and administration of medications, band-aids, antihistamines, and antipyretics (acetaminophen or ibuprofen) (Box 1).

Travel with a child with special needs

Adoptive parents of a child with special needs can benefit from having a carefully constructed plan (designed with the primary pediatrician or specialist) about expected needs and possible complications. Parents need to obtain from the orphanage a full supply of any chronic medication, such as antiseizure medications, heart medications, or other drugs taken regularly by the child. Continuing these medications until the child is in the United States is usually more advisable than changing medications because of the risk of allergic reactions, adverse events to new medications, or changes in drug levels attributable to different formulations of the same drug. If there is a need for oxygen on the trip, this must be arranged in advance with the airlines, and parents must provide their own tubing and appropriately sized face masks. A child who needs oxygen for a long flight or at relatively high flow rates needs special tanks, because those routinely available on aircraft are not adequate to meet these needs. Written documentation and advance preparation are almost always required for these arrangements.

Potential for transmission of infectious diseases by internationally adopted children

Internationally adopted children typically are exempted from preimmigration blood tests, radiographic examinations, and immunizations during their overseas visa medical examination. If immunizations are not up to date according to US recommendations, parents must sign a waiver stating that they are going to begin updating immunization within 30 days of arrival in the United States. Newly adopted children should, however, have a medical evaluation within 2 weeks after arrival and begin immunizations as soon as possible.

Data collected from institutions where significant numbers of internationally adopted children are seen have identified infectious diseases with potential for transmission to the family and community [35–39]. Some of the diseases identified during the health assessment may be reportable to US public health authorities (eg, tuberculosis, *Giardia*, measles) and require investigation of the household. Rarely, such as during the SARS outbreak in 2003, household isolation has been required for internationally adopted children. Preparation for these situations and explanation of the role of the public health system in identifying contacts of the child so as to prevent additional infections are helpful for parents and may reduce anxiety. Health care professionals seeing internationally adopted children should also involve public health authorities in the event of severe or unusual diseases in these children, because the public health authorities may be able to provide additional diagnostic or epidemiologic information in the event of a unique outbreak or new agent, such as SARS or avian influenza.

Hepatitis B, hepatitis A, tuberculosis, measles, and *Salmonella* have been transmitted to family members or close contacts of children adopted internationally [5,40–46]. Those involved in the care of internationally adopted children also describe transmission of *Giardia*, lice, scabies, *Shigella*, pertussis, and cytomegalovirus (CMV) as well as other respiratory, gastrointestinal, and dermatologic conditions (Jerri Jenista, MD, personal communication, 2005). CMV transmission has not been reported formally in families of internationally adopted children, but the high rates of CMV shedding in adoptees and the documentation of child-to-parent transmission suggests that the potential exists for this to occur [35,47,48]. Families may also be at increased risk of pertussis, influenza, and pneumococcal disease, especially if no other young children are living in the household [49–51].

Prevention of disease that may be transmitted by adoptees

Hepatitis A and hepatitis B vaccines should be offered to family members and close contacts (eg, live-in child care providers) before the adopted child arrives in the household (Table 3) [52]. Review of the potential contacts' status of immunity to measles, mumps, rubella, and varicella can provide an opportunity to offer MMR and varicella vaccines to nonimmune individuals. Those who are candidates for pneumococcal and influenza vaccines should receive these vaccines per current recommendations [6].

Avoiding transmission of diseases not prevented by vaccines requires providing information about how these diseases are transmitted and what can be done to prevent them. Prevention of tuberculosis depends on testing, assessment, and treatment of infected individuals. Parents must be informed of the importance of completing recommended treatment for tuberculosis if their child has a positive tuberculin skin test result or has tuberculosis. Currently, the vaccine

Table 3
Vaccines for nontraveling family members and close contacts

Vaccine	Standard dose/route
Update all childhood vaccines for any children in household	
Vaccines for adults (administer as needed according to standard schedules)	
Hepatitis A	1.0 mL adult/0.5 mL pediatric IM, 2 doses at 0, 6 months
Hepatitis B	2.0 mL IM, 3 doses at 0, 1, 6 months
Influenza	0.5 mL IM, according to season
Measles, mumps, rubella	0.5 mL SC, documented 2 doses separated by ≥1 month
Pneumococcal polysaccharide	0.5 mL SC or IM
Td or TdaP	0.5 mL IM
Varicella	0.5 mL SC, 2 doses separated by 4–8 weeks

Abbreviations: IM, intramuscular; SC, subcutaneous; Td, tetanus diphtheria; TdaP, tetanus-diphtheria-acellular pertussis.

against tuberculosis, Bacille Calmette-Guérin (BCG), is not used routinely in the United States and is not recommended for adoptive families.

An acellular pertussis vaccine, in combination with tetanus and diphtheria toxoids, was licensed recently in the US and is available in Canada and some European countries. Prevention of pertussis also involves early recognition of disease and timely provision of antibiotic prophylaxis to exposed family members [53]. CMV is usually transmitted by contact with body fluids, especially urine, of children who are carriers. Prevention of transmission involves careful hand washing, especially when changing diapers. Because routine screening for CMV is not recommended for internationally adopted children and a substantial proportion of asymptomatic children may be carriers, such advice should be given to all families. Some experts recommend testing adoptive mothers and providing targeted advice to those who are antibody-negative and who could potentially become pregnant [54].

A number of gastrointestinal pathogens have been identified on screening of internationally adopted children, including *Giardia*, *Salmonella*, *Campylobacter*, *Shigella*, and *Clostridium difficile* [35,38,39]. Transmission to family members is possible for these gastrointestinal pathogens [47]. Prevention of transmission of gastrointestinal pathogens as well as skin infections involves identification of these conditions in the adoptee and treating them appropriately as well as emphasizing hand washing and careful attention to hygiene during this process.

Summary

Pretravel consultation before international adoption must encompass standard advice for those who travel, advice for those who are exposed to the newly adopted child, and information about caring for a new child during travel.

. who travel to meet siblings may need special accommodations before
during travel. Data on the health of internationally adopted children illustrate
risk of exposing family members and close contacts to some infectious
diseases during or after international adoption. Parents, family members, and
close contacts of the newly adopted child should be given advice to reduce their
own and their child's risk. Targeted preadoption counseling, close attention to
hygiene and safety advice, and prompt identification and treatment of infections
lead to the safest and most trouble-free adoption travel experience.

Appendix: Checklist for families planning international adoption

Before travel

Consult international adoption clinic to consider review of child's medi-
cal history.
Consult travel medicine center several months before anticipated travel.
Choose pediatrician.
Prepare travel medical supplies.
Prepare travel supplies for child, including car seat, child carrier, stroller,
clothing, diapers, formula and bottles, baby food or snacks, and toys.

During travel

Consult a medical professional if you suspect a serious illness or a contagious disease. Fever, lethargy, the appearance of difficulty in breathing, and
severe diarrhea or vomiting with possible dehydration would require immediate
medical evaluation.

Basic management if your child is ill
Nasal congestion (commonly caused by viruses)
- Encourage oral fluids.
- For babies, you may use saline nasal spray and bulb syringe.
- For older children, you may use an oral decongestant.
- Seek medical evaluation if your child has a fever or if the symptoms
  are prolonged (>2 weeks), especially if accompanied by yellow or
  green discharge.
Cough (commonly caused by viruses)
- Encourage oral fluids.
- For older children, you may administer a cough suppressant.
- Seek medical evaluation if your child has a fever or respiratory difficulty,
  symptoms seem severe (associated with vomiting), or the cough is pro-
  longed (>2 weeks).

Diarrhea
- Encourage oral fluids.
- Check and change diapers frequently.
- Apply diaper rash ointment to prevent breakdown of skin.
- Seek medical evaluation if your child has a fever, appears lethargic or dehydrated, has abdominal pain, or if the diarrhea is prolonged (>3 days).

Vomiting
- Encourage oral fluids.
- You may use oral rehydration solutions.
- Seek medical evaluation if your child has a fever, appears lethargic or dehydrated, has abdominal pain, or if vomiting lasts longer than 1 day.

Rash
- You may treat localized superficial skin infection with a topical antibiotic.
- You may treat suspected ringworm with a topical antifungal.
- You may treat localized itchy rash that may be allergic in nature with a topical steroid.
- Seek medical evaluation if your child has a fever, the rash is diffuse, or you suspect a highly contagious cause, such as scabies.

Fever
- Seek medical evaluation.
- Encourage oral fluids.
- You may administer pediatric acetaminophen to control the temperature.

After child arrives in the United States

Medical evaluation of child within 2 weeks of arrival
Update immunizations for child within 30 days of arrival

Important telephone numbers

US Consulate _____
International Adoption Clinic _____
Pediatrician _____
Travel Medicine Center _____
Adoption Agency Contact _____

References

[1] Jong EC, McMullen R. The travel and tropical medicine manual. Philadelphia: Elsevier Science; 2003.
[2] Ryan ET, Kain KC. Health advice and immunizations for travelers. N Engl J Med 2000; 342:1716–25.
[3] Spira AM. Preparing the traveler. Lancet 2003;361:1368–81.
[4] Centers for Disease Control and Prevention. Health information for international travel

2006. Atlanta: US Department of Health and Human Services, Public Health Ser-
; 2005.
enters for Disease Control and Prevention. Multistate investigation of measles among adoptees
from China—April 2004. MMWR Morb Mortal Wkly Rep 2004;53:309–10. Available at: http://
www.cdc.gov/mmwr/preview/mmwrhtml/mm53d409a1.htm. Accessed July 12, 2005.

[6] Centers for Disease Control and Prevention. Recommended adult immunization schedule—United States, October 2004–September 2005. MMWR Morb Mortal Wkly Rep 2004;53(45):Q1–4.

[7] Centers for Disease Control and Prevention. Recommended childhood and adolescent immunization schedule. MMWR Morb Mortal Wkly Rep 2005;53(51/52):Q1–3. Available at: http://www.cdc.gov/mmwr/preview/mmwrhtml/mm5351-Immunizational.htm. Accessed July 12, 2005.

[8] Centers for Disease Control and Prevention. Recommended childhood and adolescent immunization schedule for children and adolescents who start late or who are >1 month behind, United States 2005. Available at: http://www.cdc.gov/nip/recs/child-schedule.htm#catchup. Accessed July 12, 2005.

[9] Centers for Disease Control and Prevention. Prevention and control of influenza: recommendations of the Advisory Committee on Immunization Practices (ACIP). MMWR Morb Mortal Wkly Rep 2003;52(RR08):1–36.

[10] Werzberger A, Mensch B, Kuter B, et al. A controlled trial of a formalin-inactivated hepatitis A vaccine in healthy children. N Engl J Med 1992;327:453–7.

[11] Anonymous. Twinrix: a combination hepatitis A and B vaccine. Med Lett Drugs Ther 2001; 43:67–8.

[12] Thoelen S, Van Damme P, Leentvaar-Kuypers A, et al. The first combined vaccine against hepatitis A and B: an overview. Vaccine 1999;17(13–14):1657–62.

[13] Quick R, Beach M. Centers for Disease Control and Prevention. Risks from food and drink. In: Arguin PM, Kozarsky PE, Navin AW, editors. Health information for international travel 2005–2006. Atlanta: US Department of Health and Human Services, Public Health Service; 2005. p. 29–35.

[14] Centers for Disease Control and Prevention. Yellow fever vaccine; recommendations of the Advisory Committee on Immunization Practices (ACIP). MMWR Morb Mortal Wkly Rep 2002; 51(RR-17):1–11.

[15] Centers for Disease Control and Prevention. Inactivated Japanese encephalitis virus vaccine. Recommendations of the Advisory Committee on Immunization Practices (ACIP). MMWR Morb Mortal Wkly Rep 1993;42(RR-1):1–15.

[16] Parise M, Barber A, Mali S. Centers for Disease Control and Prevention. Malaria. In: Arguin PM, Kozarsky PE, Navin AW, editors. Health information for international travel 2005–2006. Atlanta: US Department of Health and Human Services, Public Health Service; 2005. p. 189–212.

[17] Kain KC, Shanks GD, Keystone JS. Malaria chemoprophylaxis in the age of drug resistance part I. Clin Infect Dis 2001;33:226–34.

[18] Kain KC, Shanks GD, Keystone JS. Malaria chemoprophylaxis in the age of drug resistance part II. Clin Infect Dis 2001;33:381–5.

[19] Centers for Disease Control and Prevention. Prevention of malaria in travelers. A guide for travelers to malaria-risk areas. Available at: http://www.cdc.gov/malaria/pdf/travelers.pdf. Accessed July 12, 2005.

[20] Weinberg N, Weinberg M, Maloney S. Centers for Disease Control and Prevention. Traveling safely with infants and children. In: Arguin PM, Kozarsky PE, Navin AW, editors. Health information for international travel 2005–2006. Atlanta: US Department of Health and Human Services, Public Health Service; 2005. p. 434–46.

[21] Mackell SM. Vaccinations for the pediatric traveler. Clin Infect Dis 2003;37:1508–16.

[22] Miller LC. Travel and transition to the adoptive family. In: The handbook of international adoption medicine. New York: Oxford University Press; 2005. p. 135–51.

[23] Mackell SM. Travel advice for pediatric travelers: infants, children, and adolescents. In: Jong EC, McMullen R, editors. The travel and tropical medicine manual. Philadelphia: Elsevier Science; 2003. p. 167–85.

[24] Fisher PR. Travel with infants and children. Infect Dis Clin North Am 1998;12(2):355–68.

[25] Stauffer WM, Konop RJ, Kamat D. Traveling with infants and young children. Part I: anticipa tory guidance: travel preparation and preventive health advice. J Travel Med 2001;8(5):254–9.

[26] Stauffer WM, Kamat D. Traveling with infants and children. Part II: immunizations. J Travel Med 2002;9(2):82–90.

[27] Stauffer WM, Konop RJ, Kamat D. Traveling with infants and young children. Part III: travelers' diarrhea. J Travel Med 2002;9(3):141–50.

[28] Stauffer WM, Konop RJ, Kamat D. Traveling with infants and children. Part IV: insect avoidance and malaria prevention. J Travel Med 2003;10(4):225–40.

[29] Ericsson CD. Traveler's diarrhea: epidemiology, prevention, and self-treatment. Infect Dis Clin North Am 1998;83:285–303.

[30] Connor BA. Centers for Disease Control and Prevention. Travelers' diarrhea. In: Arguin PM, Kozarsky PE, Navin AW, editors. Health information for international travel 2005–2006. Atlanta: US Department of Health and Human Services, Public Health Service; 2005. p. 278–87.

[31] Shanks GD, Smoak BL, Aleman GM. Single dose of azithromycin or three-day course of ciprofloxacin as therapy for epidemic dysentery in Kenya. Clin Infect Dis 1999;29:942–3.

[32] Adachi JA, Ericsson CD, Jiang Z-D, et al. Azithromycin found to be comparable to levofloxacin for the treatment of US travelers with acute diarrhea acquired in Mexico. Clin Infect Dis 2003;37:1165–71.

[33] DuPont HL, Jiang Z-D, Ericsson CD, et al. Rifaximin versus ciprofloxacin for the treatment of traveler's diarrhea: a randomized, double-blind clinical trial. Clin Infect Dis 2001;33:1807–15.

[34] Bezruchka SA. Disequilibrium: jet lag, motion sickness, and heat illness. In: Jong EC, McMullen R, editors. The travel and tropical medicine manual. Philadelphia: Elsevier Science; 2003. p. 112–25.

[35] Hostetter MK, Iverson S, Thomas W, et al. Medical evaluation of internationally adopted children. N Engl J Med 1991;325:479–85.

[36] Johnson DE, Miller LC, Iverson S, et al. The health of children adopted from Romania. JAMA 1992;268:3446–51.

[37] Albers LH, Johnson DE, Hostetter MK, et al. Health of children adopted from the former Soviet Union and Eastern Europe: comparison with pre-adoptive medical records. JAMA 1997;278(11): 922–4.

[38] Miller LC, Hendrie NW. Health of children adopted from China. Pediatrics 2000;105(6):e76. Available at: http://www.pediatrics.org/cgi/content/full/105/6/e76. Accessed July 12, 2005.

[39] Saiman L, Aronson J, Zhou J, et al. Prevalence of infectious diseases among internationally adopted children. Pediatrics 2001;108(3):608–12.

[40] Friede A, Harris JR, Kobayashi JM, et al. Transmission of hepatitis B virus from adopted Asian children to their American families. Am J Public Health 1988;78:26–9.

[41] Sokal EM, Van Collie O, Buts JP. Horizontal transmission of hepatitis B from children to adoptive parents [letter]. Arch Dis Child 1995;72:191.

[42] Wilson ME, Kimble J. Posttravel hepatitis A: probable acquisition from an asymptomatic adopted child. Clin Infect Dis 2001;33:1083–5.

[43] Hershow RC, Hadler SC, Kane MA. Adoption of children from countries with endemic hepatitis B: transmission risks and medical issues. Pediatr Infect Dis J 1987;6:431–7.

[44] Centers for Disease Control and Prevention. Measles outbreak among internationally adopted children arriving in the United States, February–March 2001. MMWR Morb Mortal Wkly Rep 2002;51:1115–6.

[45] Curtis AB, Ridzon R, Bogel R, et al. Extensive transmission of Mycobacterium tuberculosis from a child. N Engl J Med 1999;341:1491–5.

[46] Centers for Disease Control and Prevention. Multiresistant Salmonella and other infections in adopted infants from India. MMWR Morb Mortal Wkly Rep 1982;31:285–7.

[47] Adler SP. Molecular epidemiology of cytomegalovirus: viral transmission among children attending a day care center, their parents, and caretakers. J Pediatr 1988;112:366–72.

[48] Pass RF, Little EA, Stagno S, et al. Young children as a probable source of maternal and congenital cytomegalovirus infection. N Engl J Med 1987;316:1366–70.

[49] Centers for Disease Control and Prevention. Pertussis in an infant adopted from Russia—May 2002. MMWR Morb Mortal Wkly Rep 2002;51:394–5.

[50] Whitney CG, Farley MM, Hadler J, et al. Decline in invasive pneumococcal disease after the introduction of protein-polysaccharide conjugate vaccine. N Engl J Med 2003;348:1737–46.

[51] Hendley JO, Sande MA, Stewart PM, et al. Spread of *Streptococcus pneumoniae* in families. I. Carriage rates and distribution of types. J Infect Dis 1975;132:55–61.

[52] Chen LH, Barnett ED, Wilson ME. Preventing infectious diseases during and after international adoption. Ann Intern Med 2003;139:371–8.

[53] American Academy of Pediatrics. Pertussis. In: Pickering LK, editor. Red book: 2003 report of the Committee on Infectious Diseases. 26th edition. Elk Grove Village, IL: American Academy of Pediatrics; 2003. p. 472–86.

[54] Hostetter MK. Internationally adopted children and cytomegalovirus. Pediatrics 1989;84: 937–8.

ELSEVIER
SAUNDERS

Pediatr Clin N Am 52 (2005) 1287–1309

PEDIATRIC CLINICS
OF NORTH AMERICA

Immunizations and Infectious Disease Screening for Internationally Adopted Children

Elizabeth D. Barnett, MD

*Maxwell Finland Laboratory for Infectious Diseases, Room 503, Boston Medical Center,
774 Albany Street, Boston, MA 02118, USA*

Internationally adopted children are at increased risk of lacking some routine childhood immunizations and having certain infectious diseases compared with American-born children. US immigration law requires that internationally adopted children begin immunizations within 30 days of arrival in the United States, and the American Academy of Pediatrics (AAP) recommends a comprehensive health assessment within the first 2 weeks of arrival. Several centers specializing in the care of internationally adopted children have gathered data that can be used to inform health care professionals about immunizing and screening such children for infectious diseases. This article discusses approaches to providing immunizations and evaluating internationally adopted children for symptomatic and asymptomatic infectious diseases.

Immunization issues for internationally adopted children

Immunizations are a major concern for families with newly adopted children. US visa regulations require that internationally adopted children begin receiving immunizations within 30 days of arrival in the United States. Families are highly motivated to begin this process but also anxious about exposing their new child to this stressful and potentially painful process so soon after arrival. Families may have heard conflicting information about the status of immunizations in their child's birth country, may have concerns about adverse events after immunization, or may have views about approaches to immunization that are not in agreement with current recommendations. The US health system regards immu-

---

E-mail address: elbarnett@bu.edu

nizations as a high priority for all children, especially immigrant and internationally adopted children, who may be lacking vaccines given routinely in the United States. Health care professionals must be prepared to provide families of internationally adopted children with information about the status of vaccines and immunization documents from overseas; US immunization recommendations, including requirements for child care and school entry; vaccine adverse events; and how immunizations can be provided in a way that protects the child from vaccine-preventable diseases and additional trauma from the immunization process itself.

This section examines the interpretation and validity of immunization records for internationally adopted children, correlation of measured antibody with documentation of vaccination, relation of vaccine response to stress and nutritional status, current recommendations for immunization of internationally adopted children, and rational and cost-effective approaches to immunization of adoptees. Future directions for research are also addressed.

Risk of vaccine-preventable diseases in internationally adopted children

Internationally adopted children rarely contract vaccine-preventable diseases in the United States after adoption. One of the earliest reports describing medical problems in this population described two cases of varicella and one case each of mumps and rubella occurring at or within the first month of arrival, but it is not clear where disease exposure occurred [1]. Several recent outbreaks of measles related to exposures outside the United States have been described in adopted children from China during or on arrival, which were associated with documented transmission within the United States [2,3]. A case of pertussis in a child adopted from Russia was diagnosed on arrival in the United States [4].

To date, there are no reports of vaccine-preventable diseases contracted by adoptees in the United States attributed to inadequate immunization. The fact that internationally adopted children do not seem to be at increased risk of vaccine-preventable diseases after arrival in the United States compared with a US-born cohort is likely attributable to successful timely immunization of adoptees on arrival as well as to the relatively low risk of exposure to vaccine-preventable diseases in the United States compared with their countries of origin.

Risk of vaccine-preventable diseases in families of internationally adopted children

Family members of internationally adopted children are at risk of contracting vaccine-preventable diseases from adopted children. Measles, hepatitis A, and hepatitis B have been transmitted to caretakers of internationally adopted children [2,3,5–8]. Tuberculosis has been transmitted from an internationally adopted child to a family member and to numerous community contacts [9]. In most cases, transmission occurred because of failure to provide appropriate immunizations to family members before travel or failure of health care providers to screen or to treat adoptees with infectious diseases on arrival in the United States. Before the adoption, health care providers need to provide family members and other close contacts with information about preventing transmission of infectious diseases and obtaining appropriate pretravel immunizations. Screening and treating internationally adopted children for transmissible infectious diseases at their initial health assessment decrease the risk of disease transmission after arrival.

Assessment of vaccine records of internationally adopted children

Two issues need to be addressed when assessing records of internationally adopted children. The first is the validity of the record itself: does the record document accurately the type and dose of vaccine given and the date it was administered? Questions about validity of immunization records might arise when vaccine doses are recorded before a child's birth, vaccines are documented on the same date in consecutive months, all vaccines are recorded in the same handwriting and color of ink, the vaccine administered was not available in the country at that time, or there is concern that vaccine doses are being diluted to allow immunization of greater numbers of children.

Some of these concerns have been validated, but for others, alternative explanations have been identified. Dates may have been transposed during copying (eg, 12/3 becomes 3/12), records may look "too good to be true" if copied neatly in preparation for adoption, and, in some situations, scheduled immunizations do occur on specific days of the month as routine practice. The extent of falsification of immunization records for internationally adopted children, alteration of dates on these records, and administration of inadequate doses of vaccine is probably never going to be known. Schulte and colleagues [10] evaluated the acceptability and completeness of overseas records for 504 internationally adopted children, of whom 35% had written immunization records. Ninety-four percent of the records were valid (eg, had dates of administration and no doses recorded before the child's date of birth) and had some vaccine doses that were acceptable and up to date by current immunization schedules. Three records (<1%) had one or more doses given before the child's date of birth. In most cases, it is possible to accept as valid immunization doses given at appropriate ages and intervals and documented in an apparently valid written record [11]. Health care professionals may need to allow extra time to explain immunization records to parents, especially when doses documented on a valid record are not accepted in the United States (eg, measles, mumps, and rubella [MMR] vaccine before the age of 1 year), when a child has received excess doses of some vaccines (eg, oral polio vaccine in countries in the former Soviet Union), or when the child has received vaccines not administered routinely in the United States (eg, Japanese encephalitis vaccine).

Relation of written vaccine records and protection against disease for internationally adopted children

The second issue is the relation of the documented immunization to the development of adequate protection against the disease for which the child has been immunized. Concern about protection of adoptees against diseases for which they had documentation of immunization was raised in 1998, with the presentation of data on 26 adoptees from China, Russia, and Eastern Europe. Investigators compared results from children adopted from orphanages with those of children adopted from noninstitutional settings, primarily family-based foster care. Protective titers to diphtheria and tetanus were found in only 12% of children living in orphanages who had received three or more doses of diphtheria-pertussis-tetanus (DPT) vaccine; 78% of the nine children living in foster homes had protection against the two diseases. The authors speculated on a number of reasons for their results: falsification of records, decreased potency of vaccine distributed to orphanages, and poor immune response because of prolonged institutionalization [12]. Based on these findings, the AAP supported repeating previously documented immunizations if there were questions about validity of the vaccine record [13].

Several additional reports have addressed the issue of protection against disease in relation to receipt of vaccine in internationally adopted children. A 1999 report documented suboptimal protection against polio vaccine in 4 children adopted from Lithuania, Russia, and China who had documentation of 3–6 doses of polio vaccine [14]. Subsequent work by the same investigator explored the possible relation between nutritional status and vaccine response as well as the potential for differences in response to vaccines administered in orphanages compared with those given to children living in the community. Although lack of antibody ranged from 3% for tetanus and diphtheria to 50% for pertussis, no relation was found between the presence of antibody and nutritional status (as measured by z scores for height, weight, and head circumference); residence in an orphanage; or medical problems of the child, including the presence of parasitic infections, anemia, rickets, or a positive tuberculin skin test result. The authors proposed measuring antibody to vaccine-preventable diseases as a method of guiding decisions about immunization of international adoptees [15]. Subsequent studies of the correlation between vaccine records and presence of protective antibody in internationally adopted children have yielded conflicting results. Different cutoff values and methods used to detect antibody add to the challenge of comparing results from different studies. A study from the Netherlands documented antibody levels to tetanus and diphtheria similar to those from Dutch children in adoptees from all countries except China and suboptimal levels of antibody to diphtheria, tetanus, and polio in 98 children adopted from China. The authors recommended testing for antibody in children adopted from China but could not recommend repeating vaccines without testing because of unknown long-term consequences of repeated immunizations [16]. Most internationally adopted children from 11 countries evaluated in Cincinnati who had documentation of two or more doses of DTP and hepatitis B vaccines were found to be protected adequately against diphtheria, tetanus, and hepatitis B. The authors identified measurement of antibody as a useful method of ensuring proper immunization and avoiding excess doses of vaccine [17].

Risks attributable to excess immunization of internationally adopted children

Repeating immunizations is generally safe, although it is recommended that children receive no more than six doses each of tetanus and diphtheria toxoids before the age of 7 years because of the potential for local and systemic adverse events [18]. The primary deterrents to repeating immunizations may be the extra costs and health care visits required as well as the pain associated with injections [19]. In an era of unpredictable vaccine supply, it is also important to use vaccine resources judiciously.

Cost-effectiveness of screening versus immunization for internationally adopted children

Cost-effectiveness studies are lacking and could be helpful in informing providers whether testing or repeating immunizations is the most appropriate strategy for specific vaccines. One study examining screening refugees for varicella antibody demonstrated the cost-effectiveness of screening children 5 years of age and older before immunization [20]. Studies are unavailable for internationally adopted children and for other vaccines.

Recommendations for immunization of internationally adopted children

Current standards for immunization of internationally adopted children include the following options: (1) repeating all doses of vaccines when available immunization records cannot be relied on, (2) accepting as valid those immunizations for which there is documentation of doses of vaccines administered according to current US vaccine schedules, and (3) judicious use of serotesting to assess a child's immunity to vaccine-preventable diseases and making decisions about what vaccines to administer based on these results [21]. Primary care providers determining the best approach to completing a child's immunizations need to consider the number of doses of vaccines needed if the child repeats all doses, number of visits required to repeat doses, availability of serologic tests, costs of testing, and barriers to school or child care entry for the child while awaiting test results. The risk of contracting a vaccine-preventable disease while completing immunizations may also be a factor. For example, children are at less risk of contracting polio, which has been eradicated in North America, than

Table 1
Recommended and alternative approaches to immunizations for internationally adopted children by vaccine

Vaccine	Recommended (R) and alternative (A) approaches		Supporting information	Challenges
Hepatitis B	R	Test for HBSAg, HBSAb, and HBcoreAb before immunizing. If HBSAg positive, no vaccine needed. If HBSAb positive, complete series; no additional vaccine if three doses. If HBcoreAb positive, may have acute, resolved, or chronic infection; can give one dose vaccine and retest in 1 month (see text)	Consensus regarding screening for hepatitis B [21]	Children with HBSAg require additional evaluation to assess status of infection [60]. Children with less than three documented doses who are screened and have positive results for HBSAb still must complete the series for long-term protection
	A	Begin vaccine series at the same time as sending above tests; continue or stop vaccine accordingly		
DTaP	R	Continue age-appropriate immunizations; test for antibody to tetanus and diphtheria toxoids if severe local reactions	Severe local reactions may be related to high antibody concentrations at the time of immunization [18]	Serologic tests may not be available in all areas
	A_1	Test for antibody to tetanus and diphtheria toxoids before immunizing for children with three or more documented doses (especially those adopted from China)	Most children with three or more doses documented have protection against diphtheria and tetanus [15–17]	Assessment of pertussis immunity not available [72]
	A_2	Administer single DTaP dose, then test in one month and continue immunization appropriately for children with three or more doses	Children adopted from China may be at increased risk for lack of protective antibody against tetanus and diphtheria [16]	Single antigen pertussis vaccine not available; must give DTaP to protect against pertussis in children less than 7 years old
	A_3	Repeat all doses without screening when serologic testing is not available and receipt of immunologic vaccine cannot be assured		
Polio	R	Accept documented does of vaccine and complete immunization with IPV per recommended schedule		Serologic tests may not be available in all areas

		Recommendation		Comments
	A	For children with three or more doses, measure antibody to polioviruses types 1, 2, and 3. Give single dose IPV and then measure antibody to poliovirus types 1, 2, and 3. If antibody present to all three serotypes, complete immunization with IPV per recommended schedule; if antibody absent, consider repeating the series		Cost of testing may be prohibitive. No consensus about number of additional doses needed if antibody lacking for three or fewer serotypes
MMR	R	Age-appropriate immunization with MMR		If immunity is not documented well, children may face barriers to child care and school entry if fewer than the required number of MMR doses are documented
	A₁	Test for measles antibody; if present, give a single dose MMR (children ≥1 year of age)	A₁	Although school systems may accept a single dose of mumps and rubella vaccines, two doses are recommended by the AAP [73,74]
	A₂	Test for all three antibodies and immunize accordingly (children ≥1 year of age)		
Varicella	R	Serologic testing, followed by age-appropriate immunization if antibody negative (children ≥1 year of age)	R	Cost-effectiveness of screening for refugees 5 years of age and older [20]
	R	Age-appropriate immunization	R	History of varicella may be less reliable in immigrants [75]
	R	If scarring because previous varicella infection present, no vaccine needed		If documentation of presence of antibody or presence of scarring caused by varicella is not done adequately, children may face barriers to child care or school entry
Haemophilus influenzae type B	R	Age-appropriate immunization		
Pneumococcus		Age-appropriate immunization		

Abbreviations: DTaP, diphtheria and tetanus toxoids and acellular pertussis vaccine; HBcoreAb, hepatitis B core antibody; HBSAb, hepatitis B surface antibody; HBSAg, hepatitis B surface antigen; IPV, inactivated polio vaccine; MMR, measles, mumps, and rubella vaccine.

pertussis, varicella, or pneumococcal disease, and providers may want to plan the schedule accordingly. Table 1 lists options for immunization and serologic testing for specific antibodies by vaccine. These options can be discussed with adoptive parents, and the best option can be chosen for the individual child.

Relation between response to vaccine and stress and nutritional status of adoptees

The relation between stress, nutritional status, and response to immunization is receiving international attention. Psychologic status and recent stress were found to be related to immune response to vaccination in a study of healthy young women [22]. In malnourished children, secretory IgA antibody was delayed in appearance and did not achieve levels comparable to those observed in healthy controls after immunization with oral polio and live-attenuated measles vaccines [23]. Coadministration of vitamin A to Indian infants at the time of immunization with oral polio vaccine enhanced the response to poliovirus type 1 [24]. In contrast, response to hepatitis B vaccine was not impaired in 31 infants with protein calorie malnutrition [25]. Detailed investigation of specific markers of immune response and the relation to specific and nonspecific nutritional deficiencies are lacking, but data demonstrating improved response to vaccines after vitamin administration in HIV-infected patients suggest that this is an area of potential investigation [26].

Future directions for research

Future directions for research could include continued development of combination vaccines to permit a reduction in the number of immunizations, standardized and more widely available testing for antibody to vaccine-preventable diseases, and cost-effectiveness studies to inform decisions about screening versus immediate immunization. A recent abstract highlighted a rapid diagnostic test for identification of antibody to vaccine-preventable diseases that has the potential to be used in a clinical setting for on-site decisions about immunizations [27]. Although it is imperative to immunize children rapidly on arrival to the United States, the interaction between repletion of nutritional status and response to vaccine is not well understood; it is likely that antibody response would be enhanced by providing nutritional supplementation before providing vaccines.

Primary care providers for internationally adopted children are still left with the challenge of determining an appropriate immunization strategy for each new adoptee. Repeating every vaccine dose is the most conservative approach to ensure immunity but may have unintended consequences or additional costs. Accepting valid records may be appropriate for most adoptees, but it is important to identify the situations when it is not. Building a body of knowledge about the quality of immunization records, cost-effectiveness of various immunization and serotesting strategies, vaccine response and nutritional status, and acceptability of various strategies by parents and adoptees can inform future vaccine recommendations for internationally adopted children.

Screening for infectious diseases

Children adopted from countries outside the United States may present with symptomatic or asymptomatic infectious diseases on arrival home with their new families. Children who are ill on arrival to the United States require thorough and immediate assessment for diseases present in their country of origin as well as for those they may have contracted during their journey or soon after arrival. Additional screening tests to identify certain asymptomatic diseases contracted overseas are recommended within 2 weeks of arrival. Although testing may have been done overseas to identify these conditions, most experts recommend repeating these tests in the United States for many reasons, including lack of standardization of overseas tests, testing while the child may be experiencing ongoing exposure to the condition being tested for, and concern about reliability of test results. Screening to identify infectious diseases is important to promote the long-term health of a child and to prevent transmission to family members and other close contacts in the periadoptive period. In addition to reports of transmission of vaccine-preventable diseases, such as hepatitis A, hepatitis B, and measles from international adoptees to their US caretakers, documentation of transmission of tuberculosis by an internationally adopted child to many community contacts emphasizes the importance of screening and appropriate follow-up of test results after adoption [9].

The AAP provides recommendations for screening internationally adopted children for infectious diseases [21]. These recommendations are based on epidemiologic studies of infectious diseases identified by systematic screening of internationally adopted children and on clinical experience of experts in the field [1,28–33]. Recommended screening tests are listed in Table 2. Detailed information about these tests, prevalence of infection in international adoptees, interpretation of tests, and treatment considerations are reviewed in the disease-specific sections that follow.

Tuberculosis

The prevalence of tuberculosis reached an all-time low in the United States in 2002. Currently, more than half the tuberculosis cases identified in this country are in foreign-born individuals [34]. Continued reduction in the incidence of tuberculosis in the United States depends on identification and treatment of cases in immigrants, including internationally adopted children [35]. Tuberculosis is prevalent in many of the countries from which children are adopted, and rates of positive tuberculin skin tests range from 3% to 19% [28–32].

Table 2
Screening tests for infectious diseases recommended for internationally adopted children

Test	Population to be screened	Additional testing or considerations
Tuberculin skin test	All adoptees	Consider repeating in 2–3 months or when nutritional status is improved if negative on initial screen
Hepatitis serology Hepatitis B surface antigen (HBSAg) Hepatitis B surface antibody (HBSAb) Hepatitis B core antibody (HBcoreAb)	All adoptees	Consider repeating in 6 months
Complete blood cell count with differential, red blood cell indices, and platelet count	All adoptees	Some findings may suggest, in combination with clinical signs and symptoms, that additional evaluation is necessary as follows: Eosinophilia: parasitic infections Anemia/thrombocytopenia: malaria Thrombocytopenia: CMV Leukopenia: HIV
Syphilis serology Nontreponemal test (RPR, VDRL, ART) Treponemal test (MHA-TP, FTA-ABS)	Nontreponemal tests for all adoptees Treponemal tests if non-treponemal tests are reactive; if clinical signs and/or symptoms of syphilis are present	Children with positive test results and those diagnosed and/or treated in their birth country need additional testing (see text)
Stool examination for ova and parasites (three specimens) Stool specimen for antigen for *Giardia lamblia* and *Cryptosporidium parvum* (one specimen)	All adoptees	Repeat in those with persistent symptoms Repeat to confirm elimination of parasites after treatment
HIV 1 and 2 ELISA (consider DNA PCR in infants)	All adoptees	Consider repeating in 6 months if negative on initial screen
Hepatitis C	Adoptees from China, Russia, Eastern Europe, and Southeast Asia Adoptees with risk factors for infection	Consider repeating in 6 months if negative on initial screen

Abbreviations: ART, automated reagin test; CMV, cytomegalovirus; ELISA, enzyme-linked immunosorbent assay; FTA-ABS, fluorescent treponemal antibody absorption; MHA-TP, microhemagglutination test for *Treponema pallidum*; PCR, polymerase chain reaction; RPR, rapid plasma reagin; VDRL, Venereal Disease Research Laboratory (test).

Most cases of tuberculosis in children adopted internationally are asymptomatic and can be classified as latent tuberculosis infection (LTBI). One highly publicized case of infectious tuberculosis in an adoptee from the Republic of the Marshall Islands, resulting in infection of as many as 56 contacts, highlights the imperative of appropriate diagnosis and treatment of internationally adopted children with positive tuberculin skin test results [9]. All children should be tested with a properly applied tuberculin skin test soon after arrival in the United States. The size of the reaction should be measured and interpreted according to standard methods [36]. Skin test reactions measuring less than 5 mm are negative; reactions larger than 5 mm are interpreted based on risk factors for disease. For internationally adopted children, a reaction 10 mm or larger is always positive; a reaction from 5 to 9 mm is positive if a child is immune compromised; has been exposed to tuberculosis; or has signs or symptoms of tuberculosis disease, including an abnormal chest radiograph [37]. Although specific exposures to tuberculosis may be unknown for these children, orphanage caretakers have been found to be infected with active tuberculosis. Careful evaluation of children with tuberculin skin test results in the 5- to 9-mm range is necessary, with treatment given if there is concern about a possible exposure to tuberculosis at any time before the adoption.

Many children have received the bacillus Calmette-Guérin (BCG) vaccine in their country of origin. The BCG vaccine is not a contraindication to tuberculin skin testing. Skin test reactions should be interpreted regardless of receipt of the BCG vaccine, because a positive skin test reaction from the BCG vaccine cannot be distinguished from a positive reaction attributable to exposure to *Mycobacterium tuberculosis*. In fact, positive skin test reactions attributable to the BCG vaccine are rare after 6 months of age in children given the BCG vaccine at birth [38].

When a positive purified protein derivative (PPD) is identified, the child should be evaluated with a chest radiograph and a physical examination focusing particularly on potential sites of extrapulmonary tuberculosis, including the lymph nodes, bones, central nervous system (CNS), genitourinary tract, and abdomen. Children are at higher risk of developing extrapulmonary disease than adults, and clinically apparent disease may not manifest until a year or more after infection. In addition, children with clinically apparent disease, especially if malnourished or immune compromised, may have negative tuberculin skin test results.

Combination therapy for treatment of tuberculosis should be initiated while awaiting culture results in cases in which there is a high clinical suspicion of active disease [39]. Because of the prevalence of multidrug-resistant tuberculosis in many of the countries from which children are adopted, consultation with experts in the diagnosis and management of tuberculosis is advised when active tuberculosis is diagnosed. Notification of public health authorities and the adoption agency facilitates notification of other families of the potential for tuberculosis in children adopted from the same orphanage.

If no active disease is found on thorough evaluation of adoptees with positive tuberculin skin test results, a 9-month course of isoniazid (INH) is indicated for treatment of LTBI. The effectiveness of INH compared with placebo in reducing the incidence of active tuberculosis ranged from 25% to 92% (averaging 60%), with greater effectiveness associated with better adherence to treatment, in a compilation of studies involving large numbers of patients from a variety of populations [40]. The single study evaluating different lengths of treatment with INH found that 6 months of treatment was 65% effective and 12 months of therapy was 75% effective, but these rates did not differ statistically. The optimal duration of INH therapy has been determined to be 9 months, based on review and assessment of data from multiple studies [41,42]. Treatment for LTBI is recommended for all children and adolescents because of the risk of progression to disease and safety of the drugs and because infection is likely to have been recent [43].

A high index of suspicion is necessary when considering the diagnosis of tuberculosis in internationally adopted children. Expert consultation is helpful when the diagnosis is in question or when the diagnosis has been made, because adherence to treatment regimens is challenging and is critical for the success of treatment. An excellent discussion of aspects of management of tuberculosis in internationally adopted children is available [44].

Hepatitis B virus

Hepatitis B infection occurs overall in approximately 5% to 7% of internationally adopted children, although higher rates have been reported, especially in adoptees from Romania [29]. The risk also may be greater in older children and those adopted from countries in Asia and sub-Saharan Africa, especially in countries in which hepatitis B vaccine is not administered routinely. Not identifying children who are carriers of hepatitis B can result in transmission to family members and other close contacts and loss of the opportunity to monitor the child for potential complications of chronic hepatitis B infection, such as chronic liver disease or hepatocellular carcinoma [6–8,45,46]. Children identified as having hepatitis B infection have often had negative test results for this infection in their birth country [47].

Diagnostic tests for hepatitis B recommended for all internationally adopted children include hepatitis B surface antigen (HBSAg), hepatitis B surface antibody (HBSAb), and hepatitis B core antibody (HBcoreAb), which can help to distinguish between infection (presence of HBSAg) and immunity to hepatitis B (presence of HBSAb alone). The presence of HBcoreAb can indicate acute, resolved, or chronic infection. Interpretation of the results of hepatitis B testing is described in Table 3. Children who have antibody to HBSAg without other markers of infection and have received no vaccine or three doses of vaccine are immune and need no additional doses of vaccine. One exception is infants who may have the presence of maternal antibody; these children should be retested to determine the need for vaccine. Children who have antibody to HBSAg (and are HBSAg-negative and HBcoreAb-negative) and have received fewer than three

Table 3
Screening for hepatitis B, interpretation of results, and suggested immunization action

Hepatitis B test	Result	Interpretation	Action
Surface antibody Core antibody Surface antigen	Negative Negative Negative	Susceptible	Offer vaccine
Surface antibody Core antibody Surface antigen	Positive Negative Negative	1. Immune (from vaccine or disease) 2. Maternal antibody	1. No vaccine needed 2. Retest to assess loss of maternal antibody; if lost, immunize
Surface antibody Core antibody Surface antigen	Positive Positive Negative	1. Immune (from disease) 2. Maternal antibody	1. No vaccine needed 2. Retest to assess loss of maternal antibody; if lost, immunize
Surface antibody Core antibody Surface antigen	Negative Negative Positive	Chronic infection or carrier	No vaccine needed Immunize household and other contacts
Surface antibody Core antibody Surface antigen	Negative Positive Positive	Acute or chronic infection	No vaccine needed Immunize household and other contacts
Surface antibody Core antibody Surface antigen	Negative Positive Negative	1. Recovering from acute infection[a] 2. Immune; surface antibody BDL[a] 3. False-positive core antibody: susceptible[a] 4. Chronic infection; Undetectable HBSAg[a] 5. Maternal antibody	1. No vaccine needed 2. No vaccine needed 3. Vaccine needed 4. No vaccine needed 5. Retest to assess loss of maternal antibody; if lost, immunize

Abbreviations: BDL, below detectable limits; HBSAg, hepatitis B surface antigen.
  [a] Five possible interpretations for these findings; repeat testing may help to clarify the situation.

doses of vaccine need to complete the vaccine series to develop long-term immunity. Children who have received three or more doses of hepatitis B vaccine but have no detectable antibody (and are HBSAg-negative and HBcoreAb-negative) can be managed by giving a single dose of vaccine and measuring antibody in 1 month. If antibody is detectable, no additional doses are needed. If no antibody is detected, the three-dose series can be completed and antibody measured 1 month after the third dose. If no antibody is detected at that time, the child is unlikely to respond to additional doses. At that time, appropriate counseling about decreasing the risk of contracting hepatitis B can be given.

Children who have only core antibody to hepatitis B may be recovering from acute infection, may develop chronic infection, or may have persistent maternal antibody. This result may represent undetectable levels of surface antigen or antibody. Several approaches are possible. First, the test may be repeated in 1 to 2 months. Alternatively, a dose of hepatitis B vaccine could be given, with testing again in 1 month; if undetectable levels of HBSAb were present initially, the dose of vaccine should boost them to the detectable range. Finally, and especially if repeat testing yields the same result, testing for hepatitis B viral DNA load by polymerase chain reaction (PCR) could be helpful in identifying the status of infection.

Children infected with hepatitis B require further testing to clarify the status of their infection. Additional tests may include hepatitis B e antigen and e antibody (markers of infectivity), liver function tests (to identify the presence of liver disease), hepatitis B viral load, and serum α-fetoprotein level. Some experts recommend testing for hepatitis D virus if the assay is available. Ultrasound of the abdomen is also appropriate for children with liver disease. Referral to specialists in the treatment of hepatitis B is warranted for children with liver disease attributable to hepatitis B because of the rapid evolution in treatment protocols and options for these children.

Children with hepatitis B infection should receive immunization against hepatitis A, and families should be counseled about reducing their child's risk of further damage to the liver. Family members and other close contacts (eg, baby-sitters, day care providers) should be immunized against hepatitis B before the child enters the United States. If this has not been completed before adoption, immunization is crucial for families of children infected with hepatitis B to prevent additional cases of infection.

Diagnosis of chronic hepatitis B in an internationally adopted child may be devastating for some families. All families can benefit from support to address concerns about social stigma or issues that might arise concerning transmission in the child care or school setting or, for the older child, as a result of sexual activity. Web sites (eg, www.pkids.org) or organizations like the Hepatitis B Coalition may also be helpful to these families.

Parasitic diseases

Screening with a stool examination for ova and parasites is warranted in almost every child adopted internationally, with the possible exception of children adopted from foster care settings in Korea [48]. Most children with parasites are asymptomatic. Intestinal parasites have been reported in approximately 25% of adoptees, with *Giardia lamblia* the most common pathogen. A single stool sample for *Giardia* and *Cryptosporidium* antigen detection and three stool samples (collected over several days) for microscopic examination are optimal for identification of most intestinal parasites. Children who remain symptomatic after identification and treatment for pathogens found on initial evaluation require additional testing, because pathogens not identified on first testing may be revealed [49].

Children with unexplained eosinophilia require additional testing to identify parasitic infection. Serology for *Strongyloides stercoralis* is warranted in all adoptees with eosinophilia and for those without eosinophilia who are immune compromised or who require steroids or other medical therapy that may render the child immune compromised. Treatment of *Strongyloides* infection should be completed before initiating any immunosuppressive therapy. Some experts recommend serologic testing for antibody to *Toxocara* in children with eosinophilia. Other tests that may be helpful in identifying parasites associated with eosinophilia include serology for schistosomiasis and filariasis, depending on the epidemiology of these diseases in the child's country of origin.

Sources of information about diagnosis and treatment of intestinal parasites are available widely [50,51]. Eradication of *G lamblia* may be especially challenging in internationally adopted children and may require multiple courses of medication. Treatment of asymptomatic internationally adopted children is warranted, because infection may be chronic or may be associated with subtle nutritional deficiencies. Families appreciate being informed that public health personnel may be notified about *Giardia* infection and may contact the family. Additional testing for gastrointestinal parasites is warranted for children who continue to have diarrhea, poor growth, poor appetite, chronic abdominal pain, flatulence, or other nonspecific symptoms despite initial treatment [52].

Other gastrointestinal infections

Diarrhea may be caused by bacterial or viral pathogens, although the more chronic the diarrhea, the less likely this is to be the case. Culture of the stool for bacteria is warranted for children with diarrhea occurring at the time of arrival in the United States or soon thereafter, especially if systemic signs of illness are present. Because of increasing antimicrobial resistance in *Salmonella*, *Campylobacter*, and other bacteria, susceptibility testing should be used to guide therapy when these pathogens are found [53,54]. Testing of the stool for rotavirus may also yield a cause for acute diarrhea.

Internationally adopted children are at high risk of infection with *Helicobacter pylori* for many reasons, including lack of breastfeeding, crowded living conditions, residence in orphanages, presence of nutritional deficiencies and gastrointestinal pathogens, and high prevalence of infection in countries from which many children are adopted. Children infected with *H pylori* may be asymptomatic or may have abdominal pain, recurrent vomiting, hematemesis, or growth failure. Infection with *H pylori* has been associated with malnutrition, increased susceptibility to enteric infections, and iron-deficiency anemia unresponsive to treatment. Long-term sequelae include chronic gastritis, duodenal ulcers, and gastric cancers.

Diagnosis of *H pylori* infection is challenging in young children. A definitive diagnosis can be made by endoscopy and biopsy, and the [13]-C-urea breath test is sensitive and specific in children older than 6 years of age [55]. Use of serologic tests is problematic in young children, because antibodies may not be present until many months after infection and sensitivity and specificity are suboptimal in young children [56]. Stool antigen tests and PCR diagnostic methods are under investigation and are becoming more widely available. For these reasons, routine screening of internationally adopted children for infection with *H pylori* is not recommended at this time. Selected children with symptoms suggestive of *H pylori* infection for which no other cause has been identified may be candidates for testing. A serologic test plus another method of diagnosis is appropriate, such as the [13]-C-urea breath test for children old enough to cooperate with the procedure. Some children may require endoscopy to confirm the diagnosis.

Treatment of children with *H pylori* is controversial. Some experts reserve treatment for those with documented sequelae of infection, whereas others believe that the risk of infection and long-term sequelae in internationally adopted children is high enough to warrant treatment for all infected children and consideration of empiric treatment in those with positive serology and symptoms compatible with *H pylori* infection [57,58]. Typically, treatment consists of two antibacterial agents (eg, amoxicillin, clarithromycin, or metronidazole) and a proton-pump inhibitor for 14 days [57]. Lack of response to treatment may indicate resistance to the antibacterial agents or inability to complete the drug regimen because of medication adverse events. In this event, management of the infection in collaboration with gastrointestinal or infectious disease specialists may be warranted.

Syphilis

Although syphilis is diagnosed rarely in internationally adopted children (<2% of adoptees), the consequences of undiagnosed syphilis are significant enough to warrant testing of all children on arrival. Enormous increases in rates of syphilis have been reported from republics of the former Soviet Union and from China in the past couple of decades [59,60]. Children who have been diagnosed with and treated for syphilis in their countries of origin based on maternal studies or assessment of the child require close follow-up to identify cases in which diagnostic assessment may have been incomplete (eg, no cerebrospinal fluid [CSF] examination in children with positive treponemal studies) or treatment may have been inadequate. In some cases, treatment may not have been initiated early enough to prevent late complications, such as hearing loss, dental abnormalities, or interstitial keratitis.

Testing of internationally adopted children for syphilis is complicated by the inability to compare test results with those of the mother to distinguish maternal antibody from that of the child. All children should be tested initially with a nonspecific treponemal test. If the result of this test is negative in an asymptomatic child, no additional testing is needed.

Children who have been treated adequately for congenital syphilis before adoption require close clinical evaluation and testing with a nonspecific treponemal test at 1, 2, 3 or 4, 6, and 12 months of age, in addition to hearing and vision evaluations and assessment for dental, neurologic, and development abnormalities. Specific treponemal test results remain positive for life, whereas nonspecific test results become nonreactive over time.

Symptomatic children and those with positive test results should have specific treponemal tests (fluorescent treponemal antibody absorption [FTA-ABS] or microhemagglutination test for *Treponema pallidum* [MHA-TP]) performed as well as lumbar puncture if there is suspicion of neurosyphilis, if there are physical examination findings consistent with syphilis, if there is a positive darkfield or fluorescent antibody test result on body fluids (eg, nasal discharge), or if there is untreated syphilis of more than 1 year's duration [61]. Additional testing may include long bone films, a complete blood cell count, and other testing as indicated by clinical status.

Treatment of children with syphilis depends on the child's age and presence of neurosyphilis. Standard protocols are available [61]. It is often helpful to manage these children in consultation with infectious disease specialists.

HIV 1 and HIV 2

HIV infection is diagnosed in less than 1% of internationally adopted children; however, it is an almost universal concern of adoptive parents [62]. For this reason, and because many adopted children have multiple risk factors for HIV, including maternal HIV infection, testing for HIV 1 and HIV 2 is recommended for all internationally adopted children on arrival. Most experts recommend repeat testing 6 months after arrival, although no cases of infection identified by this second test have been reported. Infants require specialized testing to distinguish infection from passively acquired maternal antibody. When collected from infants from 1 to 36 months of age, a single blood specimen tested with a DNA PCR assay has a sensitivity of 95% and specificity of 97%. HIV infection can be excluded in infants when the results of two DNA PCR assays performed at or beyond 1 month of age and a third performed at 4 months of age or older are negative. When HIV antibody testing is used in children older than 6 months of age, the results of two negative antibody tests performed at an interval of at least 1 month may be used to exclude infection [63]. Management and treatment of HIV in the rare adoptee found to be infected are best undertaken in consultation with experts in the care of HIV-infected children.

Hepatitis C virus

Hepatitis C is reported rarely in internationally adopted children (0%–2.5%) in published studies. Recommendations for screening continue to evolve as more data become available about the prevalence of disease in countries from which children are adopted and treatment options become available for children. Children with standard risk factors for hepatitis C, such as blood transfusions, and those children born to hepatitis C–infected mothers or mothers with risk factors, such as intravenous drug use, should be tested [64]. Screening is also recommended for children adopted from China, Russia, Eastern Europe, and Southeast Asia because of the increased prevalence of disease in these regions of the world [21]. Because maternal risk factors are not always known and most children are adopted from countries with a higher prevalence of hepatitis C, most international adoption experts recommend screening all adoptees at the time of arrival and 6 months later. No data have been published to identify whether infections have been diagnosed by testing at 6 months in children with negative test results on arrival.

The initial screening test for hepatitis C is an antibody test. Because antibody tests do not distinguish between active and past infection and false-positive tests are not uncommon, especially in populations with low seroprevalence, all positive test results require confirmation with recombinant immunoblot assays. Testing is complicated further by the persistence of maternal antibody for as long as 12 to 15 months [65]. Qualitative PCR assays can be useful in confirming infection in these cases, and testing of liver function may provide additional information about the presence of liver disease [66]. Management of children with hepatitis C infection or children in whom the diagnosis is uncertain is best performed with the consultation of experts in the field of hepatitis C. Treatment options change frequently, and those active in the field are most likely to have access to and be most knowledgeable about current treatment protocols. Immunization with hepatitis A and hepatitis B vaccines is recommended for children infected with hepatitis C and those for whom the diagnosis is uncertain.

Cytomegalovirus

Routine screening for cytomegalovirus (CMV) is not recommended. Although children adopted from orphanages have a high prevalence of CMV infection, this rate of infection is comparable to that of US-born children attending group day care [28,67]. Clinical examination and audiologic screening may identify conditions potentially associated with congenital CMV infection (hearing loss, neurologic abnormality, or developmental delay). CMV may be found in the urine of these children, but differentiation between unrelated asymptomatic shedding of CMV and congenital CMV infection is still problematic.

Families may be informed about the potential for CMV infection and asymptomatic virus shedding and the means to prevent transmission, primarily good hand washing. Alternatively, some experts recommend testing for CMV immunity in adoptive mothers with any potential to become pregnant [68].

Other infectious diseases

Routine screening for other infectious diseases is not recommended routinely. Although transmission of hepatitis A from an internationally adopted child has been reported, routine screening for hepatitis A is not usually helpful [5]. Instead, emphasis has been placed on preventing disease transmission by immunizing family members and close contacts with hepatitis A vaccine.

Other diagnostic tests may be appropriate when clinical signs or symptoms suggest diagnoses compatible with a child's country of origin. For example, testing for malaria is indicated in a child with fever adopted from a malaria-endemic country, and evaluation for neurocysticercosis would be appropriate in a child with a seizure accompanied by a cystic brain lesion. Rashes and skin infestations are common in new adoptees; scabies should be considered in any new arrival with a pruritic rash. Many infections that are unusual in the United States, such as tungiasis or *Pneumocystis carinii* pneumonia, have been described in internationally adopted children, requiring a high index of suspicion and careful clinical evaluation for such conditions [69–71]. Evaluations appropriate to the specific symptoms, country of origin, and history of the child may be facilitated by consultation with specialists in infectious diseases or tropical medicine.

Summary

Health care professionals play a critical role in providing age-appropriate immunizations and assessing newly arrived internationally adopted children for infectious diseases. A systematic approach to screening for infectious diseases combined with assessment of signs and symptoms that could be related to diseases prevalent in the child's country of origin supports children's long-term health and that of their new families.

Acknowledgments

The author thanks Susan Maloney, Lisa Albers, and Jerri Jenista for their helpful comments on this manuscript.

References

[1] Jenista JA, Chapman D. Medical problems of foreign-born adopted children. Am J Dis Child 1987;141:298–302.
[2] Centers for Disease Control and Prevention. Measles outbreak among internationally adopted children arriving in the United States, February–March 2001. MMWR Morb Mortal Wkly Rep 2002;51:1115–6.
[3] Centers for Disease Control and Prevention. Multistate investigation of measles among adoptees

from China—April 2004. MMWR Morb Mortal Wkly Rep 2004;53:309–10. Available at: http://www.cdc.gov/mmwr/preview/mmwrhtml/mm53d409a1.htm. Accessed July 10, 2005.

[4] Centers for Disease Control and Prevention. Pertussis in an infant adopted from Russia—May 2002. MMWR Morb Mortal Wkly Rep 2002;51:394–5.

[5] Wilson ME, Kimble J. Posttravel hepatitis A: probable acquisition from an asymptomatic adopted child. Clin Infect Dis 2001;33:1083–5.

[6] Friede A, Harris JR, Kobayashi JM, et al. Transmission of hepatitis B virus from adopted Asian children to their American families. Am J Public Health 1988;78:26–9.

[7] Hershow RC, Hadler SC, Kane MA. Adoption of children from countries with endemic hepatitis B: transmission risks and medical issues. Pediatr Infect Dis J 1987;6:431–7.

[8] Sokal EM, Van Collie O, Buts JP. Horizontal transmission of hepatitis B from children to adoptive parents [letter]. Arch Dis Child 1995;72:191.

[9] Curtis AB, Ridzon R, Bogel R, et al. Extensive transmission of *Mycobacterium tuberculosis* from a child. N Engl J Med 1999;341:1491–5.

[10] Schulte JM, Maloney S, Aronson J, et al. Evaluating acceptability and completeness of overseas immunization records of internationally adopted children. Pediatrics 2002;109:e22. Available at: http://pediatrics.aappublications.org/cgi/content/full/109/2/e22. Accessed July 10, 2005.

[11] Centers for Disease Control and Prevention. General recommendations on immunization. MMWR Morb Mortal Wkly Rep 2002;51(RR-2):1–35. Available at: http://www.cdc.gov/mmwr/preview/mmwrhtml/rr5102a1.htm. Accessed May 20, 2005.

[12] Hostetter MK, Johnson DJ. Immunization status of adoptees from China, Russia, and Eastern Europe [abstract]. Pediatr Res 1998;43:147A.

[13] American Academy of Pediatrics. Medical evaluation of internationally adopted children for infectious diseases. In: Pickering LK, editor. 2000 Red book: report of the Committee on Infectious Diseases. 25th edition. Elk Grove Village, IL: American Academy of Pediatrics; 2000. p. 148–52.

[14] Miller LC. Internationally adopted children—immunization status [letter]. Peditarics 1999; 103:1078.

[15] Miller LC, Comfort K, Kelly N. Immunization status of internationally adopted children. Pediatrics 2001;108:1050–1.

[16] Schulpen TWJ, van Seventer AHJ, Rumke HC, et al. Immunisation status of children adopted from China. Lancet 2001;358:2131–2.

[17] Staat MA, Daniels D. Immunization verification in internationally adopted children [abstract]. Pediatr Res 2001;49:468A.

[18] Rennels MB, Deloria MA, Pichichero ME, et al. Extensive swelling after booster doses of acellular pertussis-tetanus-diphtheria vaccines. Pediatrics 2000;105:e12.

[19] Feikema SM, Klevens RM, Washington ML, et al. Extraimmunization among US children. JAMA 2000;283:1311–7.

[20] Figueira M, Christiansen D, Barnett ED. Cost-effectiveness of serotesting compared with universal immunization for varicella in refugee children from 6 geographic regions. J Travel Med 2003;10:203–7.

[21] American Academy of Pediatrics. Medical evaluation of internationally adopted children for infectious diseases. In: Pickering LK, editor. Red book: 2003 report of the Committee on Infectious Diseases. 25th edition. Elk Grove Village, IL: American Academy of Pediatrics; 2003. p. 173–80.

[22] Snyder BK, Roghmann KJ, Sigal LH. Effect of stress and other biopsychosocial factors on primary antibody response. J Adolesc Health Care 1990;11:472–9.

[23] Chandra RK. Reduced secretory antibody response to live attenuated measles and poliovirus vaccines in malnourished children. BMJ 1975;2(5971):583–5.

[24] Bahl R, Bhandari N, Kant S, et al. Effect of vitamin A administered at Expanded Program on Immunization contacts on antibody response to oral polio vaccine. Eur J Clin Nutr 2002;56: 321–5.

[25] el-Gamal Y, Aly RH, Hossny E, et al. Response of Egyptian infants with protein calorie malnutrition to hepatitis B vaccination. J Trop Pediatr 1996;42:144–5.

[26] Fawzi WW, Msamanga GI, Spiegelman D, et al. A randomized trial of multivitamin supplements and HIV disease progression and mortality. N Engl J Med 2004;351:23–32.

[27] Sylvia MJ, Barnett ED, Maloney SA, et al. Comparison of a new rapid ImmunoDot method vs. standard ELISA testing for antibody to varicella, measles, rubella, tetanus and diphtheria in refugees [abstract 1059]. Presented at the 42nd Annual Meeting of the Infectious Diseases Society of America. Boston, September 30–October 3, 2004.

[28] Hostetter MK, Iverson S, Thomas W, et al. Medical evaluation of internationally adopted children. N Engl J Med 1991;325:479–85.

[29] Johnson DE, Miller LC, Iverson S, et al. The health of children adopted from Romania. JAMA 1992;268:3446–51.

[30] Albers LH, Johnson DE, Hostetter MK, et al. Health of children adopted from the former Soviet Union and Eastern Europe: comparison with preadoptive medical records. JAMA 1997;278: 922–4.

[31] Miller LC, Hendrie NW. Health of children adopted from China. Pediatrics 2000;105:e76.

[32] Saiman L, Aronson J, Zhou J, et al. Prevalence of infectious diseases among internationally adopted children. Pediatrics 2001;108:608–12.

[33] Staat MA. Infectious disease issues in internationally adopted children. Pediatr Infect Dis J 2002;21:257–8.

[34] Centers for Disease Control and Prevention. Reported tuberculosis in the United States, 2003. Atlanta, GA: US Department of Health and Human Services, Centers for Disease Control and Prevention; 2004. Available at: http://www.cdc.gov/nchstp/tb/surv/surv2003/default.htm. July 10, 2005.

[35] Centers for Disease Control and Prevention. Recommendations for prevention and control of tuberculosis among foreign-born persons: report of the working group on tuberculosis among foreign-born persons. MMWR Morb Mortal Wkly Rep 1998;47:1–16.

[36] Centers for Disease Control and Prevention, Division of Tuberculosis Elimination. Testing for TB disease and infection: tuberculin skin testing. In: Core curriculum on tuberculosis. Atlanta, GA: US Department of Health and Human Services, Centers for Disease Control and Prevention; 2000. Available at: http://www.cdc.gov/nchstp/tb/pubs/corecurr/Chapter4/Chapter_4_Skin_Testing.htm. Accessed July 10, 2005.

[37] American Academy of Pediatrics. Tuberculosis. In: Pickering L, editor. 2003 Red book: report of the Committee on Infectious Diseases. Elk Grove Village, IL: American Academy of Pediatrics; 2003. p. 642–60.

[38] Lifschitz M. The value of the tuberculin skin test as a screening test for tuberculosis among BCG-vaccinated children. Pediatrics 1965;36:624–7.

[39] Jasmer RM, Nahid P, Hopewell PC. Latent tuberculosis infection. N Engl J Med 2002;347: 1860–6.

[40] Ferebee SH. Controlled chemoprophylaxis trials in tuberculosis: a general review. Bibl Tuberc 1970;26:28–106.

[41] Comstock GW, Ferebee SH. How much isoniazid is needed for prophylaxis? Am Rev Respir Dis 1970;101:780–2.

[42] Anonymous. Targeted tuberculin testing and treatment of latent tuberculosis infection. Am J Respir Crit Care Med 2000;161(Suppl):S221–47.

[43] Pediatric Tuberculosis Collaborative Group. Targeted tuberculin skin testing and treatment of latent tuberculosis infection in children and adolescents. Pediatrics 2004;114(Suppl):1175–201.

[44] Miller LC. Tuberculosis. In: Miller LC, editor. The handbook of international adoption. New York: Oxford University Press; 2005. p. 215–29.

[45] Vernon TM, Wright RA, Kohler PF, et al. Hepatitis A and B in the family unit. Nonparenteral transmission by asymptomatic children. JAMA 1976;235:2829–31.

[46] Zwiener RJ, Fielman BA, Squires Jr RH. Chronic hepatitis B in adopted Romanian children. J Pediatr 1992;121:572–4.

[47] Miller LC. Hepatitis B. In: Miller LC, editor. The handbook of international adoption. New York: Oxford University Press; 2005. p. 230–42.

[48] Lange WR, Warnock-Eckhart E. Selected infectious disease risks in international adoptees. Pediatr Infect Dis J 1987;6:447–50.

[49] Macariola DR, Daniels D, Staat MA. Intestinal parasites in an international adoptee. Infect Med 2002;January:13.

[50] Drugs for parasitic infections. Med Lett Drugs Ther 2004. Available at: http://www.medletter.com/freedocs/parasitic.pdf. Accessed July 10, 2005.

[51] Centers for Disease Control and Prevention, National Center for Infectious Diseases, Division of Parasitic Diseases. DPDx: laboratory identification of parasites of public health concern. Available at: http://www.dpd.cdc.gov/dpdx/Default.htm. Accessed July 10, 2005.

[52] Miller LC. Intestinal parasites and other enteric infections. In: Miller LC, editor. The handbook of international adoption. New York: Oxford University Press; 2005. p. 251–64.

[53] Centers for Disease Control and Prevention. Multiresistant Salmonella and other infections in adopted infants from India. MMWR Morb Mortal Wkly Rep 1982;31:285–7.

[54] Helms M, Simonsen J, Olsen KEP, et al. Adverse health events associated with antimicrobial drug resistance in *Campylobacter* species: a registry-based cohort study. Clin Infect Dis 2005; 191:1050–5.

[55] Drumm B, Koletzko S, Oderda G. *Helicobacter pylori* infection in children: a consensus statement. European Paediatric Task Force on *Helicobacter pylori*. J Pediatr Gastroenterol Nutr 2000;30:207–13.

[56] Rothenbacher D, Inceoglu J, Bode G, et al. Acquisition of *Helicobacter pylori* infection in a high-risk population occurs within the first 2 years of life. J Pediatr 2000;136:744–8.

[57] American Academy of Pediatrics. *Helicobacter pylori* infections. In: Pickering L, editor. 2003 Red book: report of the Committee on Infectious Diseases. Elk Grove Village, IL: American Academy of Pediatrics; 2003. p. 304–5.

[58] *Helicobacter* pylori. In: Miller LC, editor. The handbook of international adoption. New York: Oxford University Press; 2005. p. 286–91.

[59] Miller LC, Tichonova L, Borisenko K, Ward H, et al. Epidemics of syphilis in the Russian Federation: trends, origins, and priorities for control. Lancet 1997;350:210–3.

[60] Chen XS, Gong XD, Liang GJ, et al. Epidemiologic trends of sexually transmitted diseases in China. Sex Transm Dis 2000;27:138–42.

[61] American Academy of Pediatrics. Syphilis. In: Pickering L, editor. 2003 Red book: report of the Committee on Infectious Diseases. Elk Grove Village, IL: American Academy of Pediatrics; 2003. p. 595–607.

[62] Aronson J. HIV in internationally adopted children. Washington, DC: Joint Council for International Children's Services; 2002.

[63] American Academy of Pediatrics. Human immunodeficiency virus infection. In: Pickering L, editor. 2003 Red book: report of the Committee on Infectious Diseases. Elk Grove Village, IL: American Academy of Pediatrics; 2003. p. 360–82.

[64] American Academy of Pediatrics. Hepatitis C. In: Pickering L, editor. 2003 Red book: report of the Committee on Infectious Diseases. Elk Grove Village, IL: American Academy of Pediatrics; 2003. p. 336–40.

[65] Centers for Disease Control and Prevention. Guidelines for laboratory testing and result reporting of antibody to hepatitis C virus. MMWR Morb Mortal Wkly Rep 2003;52(RR-3):1–13.

[66] Emerick K. Treatment of hepatitis C in children. Pediatr Infect Dis J 2004;23:257–8.

[67] Adler SP. Molecular epidemiology of cytomegalovirus: viral transmission among children attending a day care center, their parents, and caretakers. J Pediatr 1988;112:366–72.

[68] Hostetter MK. Internationally adopted children and cytomegalovirus. Pediatrics 1989;84:937–8.

[69] Fein H, Naseem S, Witte DP, et al. Tungiasis in North America: a report of 2 cases in internationally adopted children. J Pediatr 2001;139:744–6.

[70] Redman JC. *Pneumocystis carinii* pneumonia in an adopted Vietnamese infant. A case of diffuse, fulminant disease, with recovery. JAMA 1974;230:1561–3.

[71] American Academy of Pediatrics. Hepatitis B. In: Pickering L, editor. 2003 Red book: report of the Committee on Infectious Diseases. Elk Grove Village, IL: American Academy of Pediatrics; 2003. p. 318–36.

[72] American Academy of Pediatrics. Pertussis. In: Pickering L, editor. 2003 Red book: report of the

Committee on Infectious Diseases. Elk Grove Village, IL: American Academy of Pediatrics; 2003. p. 472–86.

[73] American Academy of Pediatrics. Mumps. In: Pickering L, editor. 2003 Red book: report of the Committee on Infectious Diseases. Elk Grove Village, IL: American Academy of Pediatrics; 2003. p. 440–3.

[74] American Academy of Pediatrics. Rubella. In: Pickering L, editor. 2003 Red book: report of the Committee on Infectious Diseases. Elk Grove Village, IL: American Academy of Pediatrics; 2003. p. 536–41.

[75] Christiansen D, Barnett ED. Comparison of varicella history with presence of varicella antibody in refugees. Vaccine 2004;22:4233–7.

PEDIATRIC CLINICS

OF NORTH AMERICA

ELSEVIER
SAUNDERS

Pediatr Clin N Am 52 (2005) 1311–1330

Immediate Behavioral and Developmental Considerations for Internationally Adopted Children Transitioning to Families

Laurie C. Miller, MD

*Department of Pediatrics, International Adoption Clinic, Tufts University School of Medicine,
The Floating Hospital for Children–New England Medical Center,
Box 286 NEMC 750 Washington Street, Boston, MA 02111, USA*

When Robert and Betty decided to adopt, they never imagined that their journey would take them 8000 miles from home to a small industrialized city in a remote region of Russia. "Except for one trip to Europe, we'd never been out of the US before." The legal requirements for foreigners adopting Russian children in the region necessitated two trips for the couple. On the first trip, they had the opportunity to meet their 11-month-old child, Anton, and to spend several hours playing with him in the director's office. They videotaped every moment they had with Anton. Otherwise, their time was occupied with meetings with lawyers and agency representatives and lots of paperwork needed to permit the legal adoption of the child to take place. Six weeks later, they returned to collect their son and to finalize the court proceedings. This time, the trip was easier, because everything was familiar. They knew that there were friendly people waiting at the end of their journey, and most importantly, they would be able to reunite with their son. They had looked at their videotape of their time with Anton "hundreds of times," and had prepared his room in their house. They came fully prepared with a suitcase full of cute outfits received as baby shower gifts, toys, and lots of baby gear. Excited and giddy, they entered the orphanage director's office and presented her with several gifts. Moments

This article was supported in part by the Jacqueline Munroe Noonan Foundation and National Institutes of Health R21DAD18095.

E-mail address: lmiller1@tufts-nemc.org

later, Anton was brought in by one of his caregivers. He solemnly looked at all the excited adults in the room and burst into tears, burying his head in his caregiver's shoulder.

This is just one of many ways in which new adoptive parents encounter their children. For some, the first time they meet their child is the day of the court proceedings to finalize the adoption in the child's birth country. For others, adoptive parenthood begins at the end of a jet way as their child, escorted from his or her country of origin, is entrusted to them. Although the parents have had months or even years to prepare for these moments, little preparation is possible for the infants and young toddlers who are adopted. As described in elsewhere in this issue (see the article by Johnson), many children have lived in difficult circumstances before their adoptive placement. Most were born to mothers who did not receive prenatal care [1]. Some were exposed prenatally to drugs, alcohol, smoking, or sexually transmitted diseases (syphilis most commonly). Many experienced neglect or suboptimal care, malnutrition, infectious diseases, and other medical problems [2–9]. At the time of adoption, growth and developmental delays are common, along with disorders of sensory and emotional regulation and "orphanage behaviors" (self-comfort and/or self-soothing behaviors) [10–15]. These factors all conspire to make the initial transition of the child to his new adoptive family potentially difficult.

Many children and their parents weather this amazing change easily and readily move ahead together in their lives together as a family. Understandably, however, others experience some difficulties during the transition. It is common for children to display some emotional or behavioral issues during this time, which are often related to eating, sleeping, bathing, diapering, or playing.

In this article, the immediate behavioral and developmental issues of newly adopted children after placement are discussed. Because there has been little systematic evaluation published about these issues, most of this discussion is based on clinical and research experience in the International Adoption Clinic at the New England Medical Center, which as been assisting families before, during, and after adoption since 1988. Some strategies that we have found helpful to ease the transition for the parents and the child are also reviewed.

The transition of a new child into the family may be divided into several phases (Table 1). First is the actual moment when the child is placed into the physical care of the new adoptive parent(s). Next is the period of initial adjustment, usually while the parent(s) are still in the child's birth country finalizing the adoption and necessary legal requirements to allow the child to travel to the United States. The third phase is the trip back to the United States with the child. The final part of the transition period is the adjustment of the child and family into a routine in their home together. As indicated previously, some families whose children are escorted to the United States (South Korea and, occasionally, Guatemala and India) plunge directly into the final phase. Most families, however, travel to meet and bring home their children. Some families travel "blindly," that is, with no information about the child before arrival in the birth country. For example, parents who adopt from Ukraine typically identify their

Table 1
Usual transition arrangements in common birth countries of internationally adopted children coming to the United States

Country	Transition	Time in child's country of origin[a]
China	Children are brought to the hotel or another public place by orphanage workers to meet the parents. Children who have been in foster care are removed from their foster families and brought to the hotel; some spend days or weeks in the orphanage "in preparation" for placement with adoptive parents.	~2–3 weeks
Russia	Parents meet children in the baby home, usually in the director's office or playroom. A familiar caregiver may stay a few moments to help the child acclimate.	~2–3 weeks spread over two visits
Guatemala	Parents come to orphanage and meet the child in the director's office, playroom, or nursery room. Children in foster care may be brought by their foster family or the lawyer arranging the adoption to the adoptive parents' hotel. Occasionally, adoptive parents are permitted to visit the child several months before the adoption is finalized.	~3–5 days
Kazakhstan	A lengthy residency requirement for adoptive parents allows gradual transition. Parents meet the child in the orphanage, and, over several weeks, spend more time in different environments with the child.	3 weeks
Ukraine	Parents identify the child from an official list provided and then meet the child at the orphanage.	3–7 weeks
South Korea	Child is usually escorted to United States. Some parents travel to receive the child.	4–7 days

[a] See http://www.travel.gov.

children in-country without previous information. Parents who make two trips (most regions of Russia and, until it closed recently to foreign adoptions, Vietnam) have a brief opportunity to get acquainted with their child on the first trip. The time interval between trips is often lengthy, however, and young children usually do not remember a previous short visit. Not surprisingly, there are stark differences during the transition depending on the age of the child. Because the average age at arrival for newly adopted children from other countries is approximately 22 months (our data, as stated previously), this article focuses on young toddlers. Specific concerns for older and younger children are discussed elsewhere in this article.

First moments of transition

The moment of the transition of the child to the new adoptive family is emotional and dramatic. Everything about the child's life changes at that moment: name, nationality, language, religion (for many), culture, opportunities, and status

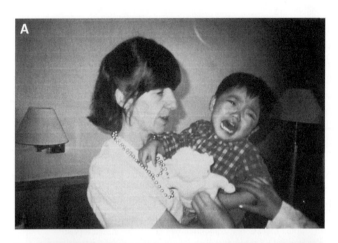

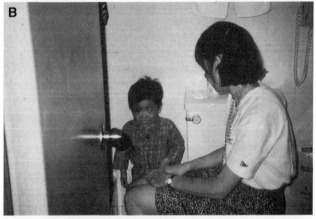

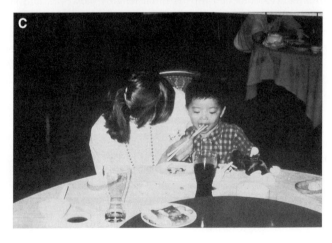

(Fig. 1). Children leave all that is familiar, including beloved caregivers, friends, routines, food, bed, toys, room, smells, and even climate. Literally, children leave with only the clothes they are wearing. Although adoption is perhaps the most loving of human acts, it must be recognized that from the child's point of view, it is equivalent to a kidnapping. Although parents have viewed photographs and videotapes and have planned and thought about the adoption for months, most children are usually too young for any realistic preparation.

It is not surprising, therefore, that many parents report problems at the time of their child's acute transition. Depending on their innate temperament, developmental stage, and previous life experiences, children may present as withdrawn, distraught, or social and engaging when meeting their new parents. For example, parents who recently adopted from China described the first few days with their new daughter: "She seemed totally withdrawn and passive for the first three days with us. She wouldn't make eye contact, barely ate, and moaned in her sleep." Other parents say, "He didn't stop crying for hours. I felt so helpless that I couldn't console him. Finally he took a Cheerio and gave a small, brave smile." Many parents mistakenly consider their child's desperate clinging as "instant attachment": "As soon as the orphanage director handed her to me, she hugged me and didn't let go for 3 days." Other parents may erroneously interpret the withdrawal of their new child as "autism": "He rocked his head from side to side for 20 minutes before falling asleep, and wouldn't snuggle with me." One family adopting from India reported, "Daniel wouldn't smile or make eye contact with us. He seemed completely blank—we felt something was seriously wrong. Then, in the restaurant he got a look at the waitress, and started to smile and coo. We felt she must have reminded him of the young women caregivers he had in the orphanage. We can barely imagine how strange and different we must have looked to him." Others believe (perhaps correctly) that their children are sedated before the transition (although stress can produce similar behaviors): "She slept for 18 hours the first day with us, then woke up, took one look at us, and started to wail." In China, children often take lengthy bus rides to the (five-star) hotel where their new parents wait. Some are cared for by unfamiliar caregivers on this journey to their new lives. Some children in China reside in foster care before adoption, but direct transition from the foster family to the adoptive family is rarely arranged. Rather, an official or orphanage caregiver brings the child from the foster family to the adoptive family. At times, children are removed from their foster families hours or days before the transition and temporarily placed

Fig. 1. The first few moments of transition may be difficult. (*A*) Child being passed from her caregiver to her new adoptive mother. The caregiver tries to offer a toy for comfort. (*B*) Several hours later, the child looks terrified. The adoptive mother wisely did not undress her new daughter. This would have been seen as an invasion of privacy and, furthermore, would have removed the only familiar vestiges from the child's life—her clothes. (*C*) Later that day, the child is calmer and accepts food from her new adoptive mother. Note the same clothing on the child. (*From* Miller LC. Handbook of international adoption medicine. New York: Oxford University Press; 2005. p. 140; with permission.)

into an orphanage—an additional trauma and loss during this vulnerable time. One mother wrote an anguished e-mail from China:

> Hello everyone,
>   I am in China now. I have had little Sara, age 2½, for 2 days now. What a 2 days it has been. I am exhausted. When I first saw Sara, I called out "Leilei" which is her nickname. She responded to me, came over, and started sharing her little bag of treats she had with her. I was pleasantly surprised! She didn't cry at all. She began laughing, running around, picked up my pen and papers, and started writing. I said to myself, "OK, she wants to sign the adoption paperwork right now and get going!" She imitates adults very well and is extremely clever. She's also very cute I might add. By the time we left, she let me pick her up. After we got back to the hotel, she began to realize that all this fun and games is not just an afternoon out, but something different. She began crying for her foster mother. The crying became intense. Then she started tantrums. I have no experience with tantrums so I was startled. At night, she cried and cried until she wore herself out. Yesterday and today, she was OK at most of the meals and on the bus as we proceeded to do the paperwork and other adoption requirements. But as soon as we get back to the room, she throws herself on the floor, bangs on the pillows, points to the door, and calls for mama (her foster mother). This is gut-wrenching. I never knew a child could cry so dramatically for so many hours straight. Tonight I had to literally wrestle her on the bed so that she wouldn't go to the door. She needed to sleep because she wouldn't take a nap. Instead, she screamed and cried. She handed me her shoes and jacket to coax me into going out the door to look for her foster mother. She even started cleaning the room up in an attempt to make things all set so we could leave the room. Needless to say, I am physically and mentally drained. I expected grieving from her. But this is so hard. She is also very stubborn and persistent. Please, if you know how to handle tantrums, please give me advice. I appreciate everyone's prayers too. This is going to be a long journey for this child to heal from her grieving and eventually bond with us. Please tell me what to do. I just don't know how to handle this.

Parents adopting from Guatemala often have the opportunity to meet their child's foster parents in a relaxed setting over several hours. This understandably eases the transition for the child. Some children are brought by the lawyer arranging the adoption to the hotel, preventing the adoptive parents from meeting the foster families. Parents adopting from orphanages may have a short visit there before leaving with the child the same day. Occasionally, parents adopting from Guatemala are permitted to visit the children some months before the adoption is finalized.

Adoption of young infants

Few young infants (< 6 months of age) are placed for international adoption in 2005, although this number is increasing with the growing recognition of the adverse effects of institutionalization on children. Young infants seem to make the transition to their new adoptive families much more readily than older children. Although young infants may become distressed with all the changes in their lives, they generally adjust more quickly to their new situation and more easily accept comfort from their new adoptive parents.

Adoption of older children

Preparation of older children for international adoption is vitally important to the success and ease of the first few days with their adoptive family—and likely beyond. Although a child's level of understanding varies with age, it is important for older children themselves to express a wish to be adopted and a willingness to leave their birth country. Older children are more able to understand in advance the losses that occur with adoption. They are also likely to be more frustrated at their inability to communicate and to be sadder at the loss of their friends. (A number of children in our clinic talked so incessantly and anxiously about friends left behind in the orphanage that their adoptive parents later returned to the orphanage to adopt these other children as well.)

Older children who have lived in difficult family situations before institutionalization may have understandable anxieties about again being placed in a family. Some of these children have thrived in the safety and security of the orphanage and fear that their new family may be like their birth family. New adoptive parents commonly report that these older children may become distraught or angry if they observe any alcohol consumption, perhaps assuming that the adoptive parents are going to react as their birth parents did.

Easing the transition

Some adoption agencies can assist with strategies to help children of any age with the transition. It is sometimes possible for adoptive parents to send packages to the orphanage or foster family in advance of their arrival. Families who travel twice to complete their adoption can leave a package after the first trip. Packages containing photograph albums of the adoptive family and their house, neighborhood, and pets can help children to prepare for their new lives. Items should be labeled in the local language so that caregivers can share this information with the child. Laminated photographs of family members can be attached to the child's crib or affixed to a special small pillow. Parents should then wear the same clothing as they do in the photographs when they first meet their new child. Some families send tape recorders (with appropriate voltage adaptors) and cassettes of their voices talking and singing. Toys or blankets sent before adoption can accompany a child as he or she travels to the new home. Duplicate sets of all items sent in advance should be kept in case of loss. It is also helpful for families to take as many photographs as possible of their child's caregivers, room, and roommates, because this is of great interest to children later.

Time together before returning home

As families leave the orphanage with their child, it may be the child's first experience off the grounds of the institution. For many, it may be the first car trip, and motion sickness is quite common. Even more striking, for some children, departure from the orphanage is their first experience outdoors. Many parents poignantly describe their child's fascination with the sky, trees, clouds, and sun. Families usually spend several days to weeks at an apartment or hotel while finalizing the adoption and fulfilling all needed legal requirements. This time together can be fraught with difficulties but may also be a special time during which the new family can develop some early attachments without the distractions of home and the fatigue of jet lag. Some families seek to circumvent this "waiting period," but most find it valuable and worthwhile. During these early days together, most parents try to abide by the orphanage schedule to provide some consistency for the child; however, this is not always possible or desirable.

Life in a small hotel room with a toddler can be challenging. Having some basic snacks, books, and toys available is helpful. Child-proofing the space is essential; many children have no experience with free exploration and no awareness of potential hazards [16]. During these early days, simple activities may be problematic.

Feeding

Determining what and how the child eats may be a challenge for first-time parents. Many young children from orphanages have never eaten solid food or been fed from a spoon. Orphanages commonly feed children from bottles with large holes cut in the nipples to speed feeding times. Consequently, children work hard using their pharyngeal muscles during feeding to prevent choking rather than exercising the muscles of mastication. Making this adjustment can be difficult and time-consuming (and may require the help of an occupational or speech therapist after return home). New textures and tastes can also be challenging for newly adopted children [13,14]. Parents may become anxious about their ability to feed their child properly, especially if the child is malnourished, as many newly adopted children are [2,4–7,12,17–20].

Many parents wonder if it is necessary to bring food for the child from the United States. Traveling with large amounts of baby food is not necessary; local equivalents are usually readily available. Parents should be reassured that their child has subsisted on locally available foods and can continue to do so until returned to the United States. Parents may wish to travel with powdered formula, however. They should be instructed to use bottled or boiled water to make up the formula solution. Milk-based formula is usually well tolerated; children nearly always receive milk or milk-based formulas in the orphanages. Some children have transient lactose intolerance related to intestinal (usually parasitic) infections. Occasionally, parents may wish to purchase the locally used formula and use this for the initial meals. Most children can be switched rapidly to a new

(American) formula. In some cases, children may have received dilute formula or been fed on a schedule that was manageable for the orphanage rather than appropriate for the child.

Bathing

Aversive reactions to bathing are also common. Bathing in the orphanage may consist of a quick plunge into cold water, followed by a rough towel-dry. Children thus learn that bathing is an unpleasant experience. It takes a surprising amount of time for children to recognize that bath time can be pleasant. Slow introduction to bathing may be less distressing for some children.

Toilet training, bowel function, and diapering

Many children are said to be "potty trained." Young children in orphanages often spend considerable time "on the potty"; but when this practice is discontinued, diapers are needed. For parents with busy schedules of court hearings, embassy visits, and other required activities, it is best to assume that the child is not trained. Bowel disturbances are frequent in the early days of the transition. Some children develop constipation, whereas others have diarrhea. Changes in diet, activity, and emotional upset may all contribute to these symptoms. Persistent bowel abnormalities (especially diarrhea) often reflect intestinal parasitic infection. Careful hand washing after diaper changes should be emphasized. Children may be drinking or eating less than is typical in the first few days after adoption and may have constipation as well. Surprisingly often, children become distraught when placed supine for diaper changes. For some, this positioning probably recalls being placed back in a crib alone and losing adult attention. With time, this distress usually lessens.

Sleep

Surprisingly, sleep problems are not prominent in the first few days after adoption. Most children usually sleep well in the same room (and occasionally bed) with the parent(s). Emotional exhaustion may aid the child and the parents to sleep. Sleep difficulties frequently emerge after arrival home and are related to changes in sleeping environments, time zones, and increased expectations of interpersonal interactions with adults.

Play

Play is often difficult during these early days. Children may be overwhelmed by the richness and variety of experiences they have suddenly encountered. Attention spans may be brief and scattered. Children may have had extremely limited play experiences with little or no concept of interactive play with a toy or a person; prior orphanage play may have centered on acquiring a desired toy and preventing others from taking it away. Interactive and imaginative play is infrequent until children learn to trust that their toys and adult attention remain available.

Developmental delays

Parents may note some obvious developmental delays that may change quickly during the first few days or weeks, such as the child unable to roll over who learns to sit within days. Some children indeed make rapid progress of this nature, whereas others may have temporarily regressed in their developmental abilities but then rapidly regain those skills. Discrepancies may exist between developmental skills reported before adoption and those observed by parents on meeting a child. More substantive delays are discussed elsewhere in this article. Withdrawn self-stimulatory behaviors may persist during this phase of adjustment. In contrast, some children exhibit surprising improvement from the time the parents met them on the initial visit. The Norwegian researcher Andersen [21] suggests that care may improve after a child has been assigned to an adoptive family. The child acquires the social status and qualities of the adoptive family and is now viewed in a more favorable light by the caregivers.

Health

Prospective parents worry how to manage health problems of their new child in the early days after adoption. If they are still in the city in which the child resided, the orphanage physicians remain available to give medical advice. For children in foster care (eg, in Guatemala), the pediatrician who has been providing well-child care may be contacted. Facilitators may have medical contacts, and large international hotels often have physicians on call. The US embassy or consulate also has names of (usually bilingual) physicians in the area and can assist with emergencies. An additional resource is the American Academy of Pediatrics directory, which lists international members by city and country of residence. Providing these names to traveling parents in advance may sometimes be reassuring. It is also comforting to adopting parents to be able to contact their child's American physician by phone or e-mail, and setting this up before travel is helpful.

Many parents request their pediatrician to prescribe medications to take with them on the trip. Although these medications are usually not needed, it can be reassuring to have them available (Box 1).

In actuality, most children usually remain healthy throughout the adoption process, with the exception of minor respiratory symptoms. Adopting parents may themselves become ill, however [22,23]. Parents should carefully prepare themselves in advance for the rigors of an adoption trip. The physical and emotional demands of the trip, along with uncertain hygiene, often contribute to health problems for traveling parents. Consultation with a travel medicine clinic in advance of the trip is recommended so that necessary vaccines can be ad-

---

Box 1. Basic supplies for traveling parents (adjust as appropriate for child's age)

Adhesive plasters
Alcohol wipes
Antibacterial wipes
Antibiotic ointment
Antihistamine
Antipyretic
Diaper rash cream
Decongestant
Dosage syringe
Insect repellent
Nasal aspirator
Oral antibiotic (eg, amoxicillin, azithromycin, cefixime)
Pedialyte (Abbott, Abbott Park, Illinois)
Permethrin
Sunscreen
Sodium optic drops
Thermometer
Vaseline
Waterless soap gel

Adapted from Borchers DA. Helpful medical items to take to China for your child. Available at: http://fwcc.org/medicalitems.html. Accessed February 15, 2004.

---

ministered and basic travel advice reviewed (http://www.istm.org, http://www.cdc.gov/travel) [24–26].

Trip home

Most children make the trip home to the United States uneventfully. The rigors of air travel, including confinement to an airplane seat, jet lag, dehydration, unfamiliar food, and fatigue, combined with the emotional intensity of an adoption, can make travel exceptionally stressful, however. It is not surprising that many children have prolonged crying during the trip. New adoptive parents must be prepared for the difficulties their child may experience during this trip. Requests for bulkhead seats when traveling with young infants, ample supplies of toys and games for toddlers and older children, and availability of snacks and lots of diapers can make the trip more manageable. Facilitators should explain some basics about air travel to older children in their birth language so that they are prepared. Picture books can be helpful. Helpful resources on air travel with children are available on the Internet (http://www.flyingwithkids.com/).

Settling in at home

The adjustment of the new adoptive family continues after return home. Children usually recover from the physical rigors of the trip before parents do. Eating and sleeping issues quickly become prominent, however, and additional behavioral concerns may also arise. Attachment between parent and child also becomes strengthened. Relationships with siblings (and sometimes a parent) who did not travel must be established. Some parents may need to return to work relatively soon after return, delaying attachment and other adjustments (see section on parental leave). The child's true developmental capabilities become more apparent during this time. Each of these topics is discussed in this section.

Eating

In addition to the feeding difficulties related to solids described previously, which may take time and the help of an occupational or speech therapist to resolve, many other problems related to eating become apparent after arrival home. Some children are "ravenous" or "insatiable"; parents frequently describe their child's appetite as "like a truck driver." Some stuff their cheeks with food (which may relate to previous food shortage or to oral-motor sensation seeking) [14]. Some children become extremely agitated and anxious when placed in a high chair before food is ready. Malnourished children are understandably hungry and are responding appropriately, because they have lived with hunger and the need to compete with others for food. It takes time to understand that they now have unrestricted access to food. It is helpful to offer unlimited food to these children and to offer more after they have consumed all they want. Showing children the full refrigerator and cupboards ("This is your milk, here is your cereal, this is your juice, these are your crackers. If you want anything, just ask Mama or Papa and we will give it to you") can be very reassuring, especially to children who have resided in orphanages where food has just appeared after being prepared in a kitchen that most of the children never see. Most children respond to this with smiles and incredulity, but after a few days, they settle into a more normal and less frenzied mealtime. Rarely, children gorge until they vomit, but this usually diminishes rapidly after adoption. For children who have had no previous opportunity to regulate their own food intake, meeting their new family may be the beginning of learning to request food and responding to satiety for the first time.

Some children hoard or hide food. Parents report finding food hidden in pockets, on shelves, or under pillows. These children usually have suffered from hunger and other privations. Sometimes, it is helpful to provide these children with their private "stash" of food in a special container and to let them know that it can be replenished on request at any time. Leaving food out and available (eg, fruit basket, snacks) reinforces the message that food is plentiful and readily available. Some children are comforted by carrying small amounts of food with them at all times.

Other children have surprisingly poor appetites and may rarely, if ever, request food. Some parents note that their children not only never seem hungry but do not seem to enjoy food. Although these children do not have sensory or physical impairments that interfere with mastication, swallowing, or digestion, it seems as though some of the normal regulatory mechanisms related to hunger and satiety are deranged. One speculation is that this is a reaction to the rote orphanage schedules of feeding; children who are forced to eat even if not hungry and are not fed if they are hungry may develop such unusual responses. Intestinal infections or delayed gastric emptying may also contribute to this finding. Gradually, as children become accustomed to family meals and associate eating with pleasurable social relations, these behaviors tend to lessen.

Young children may still enjoy their bottles for some time after arrival home; there is generally no rush to wean children to toddler ("sippy") cups. The bottle may be comforting for several months as well as providing needed exercise for oral-facial muscles of mastication and speech. Some children may progress from using their bottle directly to using a straw or an open cup.

A number of children refuse milk. Some prefer kefir or yogurt-type drinks (or buttermilk), which probably taste more familiar. These can be prepared or purchased in the United States and gradually mixed with increasing amounts of milk. Alternatively, flavorings (chocolate or strawberry) may be added to milk until the child becomes accustomed to the taste.

Sleeping

Sleep disturbances are extremely common among newly arrived international adoptees (and their parents). The duration of time required to recover from jet lag is often underestimated (usual estimates are 1–2 days for each time zone crossed) [27]. The transition of the child to the new sleeping arrangements in the adoptive home is more problematic. Difficulties arise with the timing, duration, location, and quality of sleep.

Unlike typical behaviorally based sleep problems common in infants and toddlers, new adoptees are struggling with enormous life changes, insecurity, losses, and attachment to a new family rather than with behavioral manipulations and bad bedtime habits. Thus, recommendations for managing sleep disturbances must account for these differences. In her book, *Toddler Adoption: The Weaver's Craft*, Mary Hopkins-Best [28] writes: "Always assume that a request for parental contact and comforting represents a need for a toddler struggling to develop attachment and meet that need on demand, day or night. Parents need to reframe their thoughts about getting up at night with a new toddler as a wonderful opportunity to build attachment rather than a dreaded chore." Some examples of the variety of sleep problems commonly encountered are provided.

Case 1

Abigail was a happy vigorous 14-month-old during the day. When it came time to put her to bed at night or for naps, she became agitated and upset. She would cry anxiously the second her parents tried to leave her, even if she seemed to be completely asleep. Bedtime became an ordeal for Abigail and her parents. They were unable to devise a ritual to help her separate from them to sleep. She would waken every 2 hours and scream frantically until they came to soothe her. "She really sounds panicked" reported her mother. Abigail became fearful of being alone in her bedroom and refused to nap there. She would fight her urge to sleep.

The interpretation of this case scenario is that Abigail is struggling with all the transitions in her life and truly needs to be comforted during the night, when she feels especially vulnerable. Sleeping in her parents' room or, preferably, having an adult in her room may ease this transition for Abigail. As she feels more secure in her new environment, her parents can gradually help her learn to sleep independently. Most new arrivals have never slept in a room alone. Quickly responding to Abigail's cries while using the minimum interactions necessary to soothe her at night (talking minimally, or patting rather than removing her from her crib and feeding her) is helpful to avoid beginning bad habits that need to be addressed later.

Case 2

Thomas, an 18-month-old child, was extremely active and busy and loved to cruise around the house and play. When taken in for a nap, he became combative and agitated, however. When placed in his crib, he held onto the railing and rocked his body so hard that the crib moved 3 ft away from the wall. He stopped screaming the minute his mother came in and gave a big smile, holding out his toy to her. Exhausted, he fell into a deep sleep in his car seat later that day while his mother was doing errands.

The interpretation of this case scenario is that Thomas is in the "sponge" phase; he is so eager to learn and explore that he figures he cannot "waste time" by taking a nap. These babies usually settle down into a good sleep pattern after an initial explosion of developmental catch-up. Until then, naps may not happen; however, quiet games, singing, or rocking in a darkened room with a parent may help the baby to "recharge" for the next part of his day. Planned excursions in the car around nap time also help; the restraint of the car seat and white noise of the traffic can be helpful soporifics.

Case 3

Amanda, adopted from foster care in Guatemala, just turned 2 years old. She is a happy-go-lucky toddler during the day. During the night, she awakens with heart-rending sobs that go on and on even while her parents try to comfort her. "She calls out 'Mama, Mama' but shakes her head 'No' when I say 'I'm right here'," says her mother.

The interpretation of this case scenario is that Amanda is probably mourning her foster mother. Mourning or grieving often becomes apparent during sleep time. The depth of Amanda's feelings is a reflection of the strong attachment she had to her foster mother. Her adoptive mother can tell her that she understands how much Amanda may miss her Guatemalan foster mom, and this also lets Amanda know that someone recognizes and empathizes with her loss.

Developmental delays

Developmental delays at the time of international adoption are common and have been documented in children arriving from virtually all countries [2–5, 9–11,17–19,29]. One study of 129 internationally adopted children from 22 countries showed that developmental abilities at arrival correlated with adequacy of growth before adoption [12]. Little is yet known about the long-term developmental outcomes of internationally adopted children who arrive with delays. Although physicians are taught to react aggressively to abnormal findings, "wait and see" is sometimes a useful approach to understanding developmental delays within the first few weeks after arrival. Motor delays usually improve relatively quickly, whereas language and cognitive skills take longer to progress. Invasive diagnostic tests, although important, need not be obtained immediately on arrival (except under unusual circumstances). The trauma of these tests should not be underestimated in a fragile child who has recently been adopted. Although not all cases have such a happy ending, the following case is instructive.

The telephone rang with a call from the referring pediatrician.

> You're going to be seeing Alfred this afternoon. He's a 12-month-old from Russia. I don't know what happened to him. I reviewed the preadoptive videotape with his parents when he was 9 months old and he looked great: happy, interactive, and sociable. When they went to get him, they learned that he'd been hospitalized for pneumonia for 1 month. They just got home on Saturday; I saw him in the office on Monday. I'm really worried about him. He won't make eye contact, he doesn't make any sounds, and he is barely able to sit. He stares incessantly at his hand, and flicks his fingers. I'm sure he's autistic. I've set up appointments for him to see pediatric neurology, a developmental pediatrician, get a cranial MRI, and to start applied behavioral analysis therapy. I gave him four vaccines, drew five vials of blood, and placed a tuberculin skin test. We sent him for a chest radiograph too. Oh, we couldn't get a urine sample, so I did a suprapubic tap.

When Alfred appeared in the office, he was tiny and frail. He clung anxiously to his parents and refused to meet my gaze. "He's so much better than he was on Monday," his parents claimed. "He can sit and crawl now, and he doesn't stare so much at his hand. Do you think he's all right"? During our visit, Alfred certainly seemed fragile and delayed. After awhile, however, he began to seek my gaze shyly and to engage with toys and with his parents. We decided to postpone all his appointments, let the family go home and relax and recover from the exhaustion of their trip and all the new adjustments, and speak by telephone in a week. "He's doing so much better, doctor!" his mother told me. "He's pulling to stand, and he even laughed today when I was making faces at him." A return appointment was set up for the following week. Alfred already looked like a new boy. He was giggling and smiling, and frequently checking in with his mom. Although still delayed, he started to display some curiosity and to interact. Three months later, 15-month-old Alfred has mild language delays and is joyful and happy.

Community-based resources are available to support children's development as they transition and adjust to their new families and schools. Early intervention (birth to 3 years of age) programs can be helpful for developmentally delayed children and their (often inexperienced) parents. Older children are entitled to receive needed support services via the public school system. Virtually all international adoptees qualify for these services because of their "at-risk" backgrounds and the need to learn a new language.

Orphanage behaviors

After arrival home, "orphanage behaviors" sometimes become apparent. These behaviors are usually self-soothing and provide sensory input. Many types are seen. Most commonly, children rock on their hands and knees or using the trunk while seated. Various types of swaying or "bobbing" motions are sometimes habitual, as are head-banging, head-shaking, and head-bopping. Some children display dissociative behaviors, such as hand-staring or flapping; staring at lights, fans, or shadows; or seeming to be "in a trance." Some children are aggressive to themselves or others, with frequent biting, hitting, or scratching. Many have high pain thresholds, showing little distress with obviously painful injuries. Others seem to be seeking particular sensory inputs by intently smelling objects or scrutinizing objects closely. Other commonly observed sensory-stimulating activities include hair-twirling, ear-pulling, and bruxism [19].

These behaviors are most commonly seen at times of stress or boredom or when a child is tired. For most children, these behaviors disappear within a few days or weeks; occasionally, they persist as habits. For children with obvious sensory-seeking behaviors, parents can try to provide ample sensory inputs (eg, by rocking the child in a rocking chair, the child's need for this sensation may be met). Children with persistence of these behaviors should be assessed for other signs of neurologic, developmental, emotional, or behavioral disturbances, however, and the quality of the parent and child attachment should be evaluated. Some behaviors may continue in some otherwise well-adjusted, high-functioning, happy children.

Parental leave

Pediatricians should discuss realistic expectations about parental leave during a preadoption visit. Children found to be more delayed than expected on arrival to the United States usually benefit from extended time with their new parent(s), and deferment of group care may advisable. Many parents think that their child "was used to having children around" and believe that the child misses that environment. Under most circumstances, the advantages provided by a single, attentive, loving adult usually override the benefits of group care for young infants and toddlers.

Sibling adjustments

The addition of a new child to the family is stressful for other siblings, whether the new child arrives by birth or adoption. Preparation of older siblings is key. Cognitive understanding, age, and temperament all contribute to a child's adjustment to his new sibling. School-aged children and teens usually adjust well to the arrival of a new sibling. Younger "only" children may have more difficulty. In contrast to the arrival of a newborn, the sudden appearance of a determined and mobile toddler can be especially challenging for a preschooler who thought he wanted a younger sister. This can be especially difficult for the doted-on only child who is still distressed from being left alone with Grandma when Mom and Dad went to China for 3 weeks. Suddenly, a younger sister is tearing up his Lego constructions. Mom and Dad may feel guilty for leaving him and may themselves be dealing with "postadoption remorse." If the new little sister is displaying any problems, the adjustment can become distressing for the whole family.

In general, children who travel with their parents to get the new sibling make an easier adjustment to the new arrival. Seeing the process firsthand, understanding where their new sibling has come from, and not having to be separated from parents can be helpful for the older child(ren) in the family. If older children are brought on the adoption trip, it is advisable to bring an extra adult to assist. The number of adults should be equal to or, preferably, outnumber the number of children, including the new adoptee.

Parent adjustment

Postadoption depression
Magazines and books are filled with happy stories about international adoption. Most new adoptive parents are thrilled and delighted with their new children. Some parents experience postadoption depression or remorse, however [28]. This usually remains unspoken, because adoptive parents feel shame or embarrassment that they are not immediately happy with their new child after all that was necessary to complete the adoption. Postadoption depression may arise from many sources. The child may have unexpected medical, developmental, or behavioral problems that seem overwhelming. Adjustment to the realities of parenthood, sleep deprivation, and difficulties in attachment may all contribute to postadoption depression. Adoptive parents are exceedingly reluctant to discuss this unless directly questioned. An open-ended question ("Is the adoption ev-

erything you expected? Is everything going as you imagined"?) allows parents to express some of their ambivalent feelings.

Attachment

Attachment between parents and children develops over time, coincident with physical proximity and providing care to the child. Feeling love for the child and wishing to care for the child are early stages of attachment, which deepen with time. The myth of "instant attachment" has already been discussed. Parents should be reassured that it is normal not to feel attached to a birth or adopted child right away. Spending time together and providing for a child's basic needs (eg, feeding, bathing, diapering, putting to bed) are the basic building blocks of attachment. These activities should be reserved for parents. Well-meaning relatives and friends who wish to help the new parents should do so by offering to perform household chores rather than child care. It is important for parents to be the source of this care insofar as possible in the early weeks after adoption. Children who have had multiple caregivers and gone through this major life transition need to be reassured by this routine and to understand that the parent(s) can be relied on to provide this care.

Older child adoptions

Approximately 10% of international adoptees are adopted after the age of 5 years. These children have had heterogeneous experiences before adoptive placement. Some have experienced time with their birth families: this can range from loving and attentive care to severely neglectful or abusive care. Other children have resided in prolonged institutional care but could not be placed for adoption because of legal, medical, or other considerations. Children with prolonged experience of adversity may have considerable language and cognitive delays. Some have learned many negative behaviors in the orphanage and may take longer to transition successfully to their new adoptive families. Appropriate school placement for these older children should be carefully considered; preacademic and social skills should be carefully assessed.

Adoption questions

Older children may have a good understanding of the adoption process and may retain many memories of their lives before adoption. Processing these memories is part of their adjustment phase; depending on the age and emotional awareness of the child, it can occur within the first few weeks or months after arrival and remains with them for life. For example, 8-year-old Michael wrote this note (in English) to his birth mother, Irina, a few months after arriving in Massachusetts. He had lived with Irina until approximately 10 months before his adoption, when he was removed because of neglect. "Hello Irina. It's Sergei. I'm Michael now. It's been a long time since I saw you. I miss you." Younger children are also processing memories but may be unable to verbalize them. Bad dreams, unexpected reactions to strangers or environments (reminding them of someone or something), sudden tears, moodiness, irritability, distractibility, grieving, or sadness may all reflect this task.

Anniversaries

The adoption adjustment is a lifelong and dynamic process [30]. A calendar can be helpful in commemorating the date the child met his new family, his adoption, and in promoting understanding of the meaning of adoption and family. Some families celebrate "gotcha day," the anniversary of the date the child joined the family. This can evolve over time to reflect the child's understanding of and questions about the meaning of adoption. Once the child has been home a year, the calendar starts to repeat and the child has a store of memories of the regular rituals and events of the year (eg, "Remember last year on Valentine's Day when we decorated special cookies"?). Many parents report that their child's sense of belonging seems to solidify as the cycle of the year begins again and they understand the permanence of their new lives with their families. Another important date is when the time point is passed that the child has been part of the family longer than he was in his birth country. Some parents believe that this point marks the end of the "transition" phase.

Acknowledgments

The children and families attending the International Adoption Clinic at New England Medical Center are appreciated for all they have taught us over the years. The assistance and support of Wilma Chan, Kathleen Comfort, and Linda Tirella are gratefully acknowledged.

References

[1] Shaginian N. The influence of psychological and social factors on pregnancy and abandoned newborns. Presented at the Joint Council of International Children's Services. Washington, DC, April 10, 2002.

[2] Jenista JA, Chapman D. Medical problems of foreign-born adopted children. Am J Dis Child 1987;141(3):298–302.

[3] Johnson DE, Miller LC, Iverson S, et al. The health of children adopted from Romania [see comments]. JAMA 1992;268(24):3446–51.

[4] Miller LC, Hendrie NW. Health of children adopted from China. Pediatrics 2000;105(6):e76.

[5] Albers LH, Johnson DE, Hostetter MK, et al. Health of children adopted from the former Soviet Union and Eastern Europe. Comparison with preadoptive medical records. JAMA 1997; 278(11):922–4.

[6] Bureau JJ, Maurage C, Bremond M, et al. [Children of foreign origin adopted in France. Analysis of 68 cases during 12 years at the University Hospital Center of Tours] (see comments). Arch Pediatr 1999;6(10):1053–8 [in French].

[7] Nicholson AJ, Francis BM, Mulholland EK, et al. Health screening of international adoptees. Evaluation of a hospital based clinic [see comments]. Med J Aust 1992;156(6):377–9.

[8] Saiman L, Aronson J, Zhou J, et al. Prevalence of infectious diseases among internationally adopted children. Pediatrics 2001;108(3):608–12.

[9] Smith-Garcia T, Brown JS. The health of children adopted from India. J Community Health 1989;14(4):227–41.

[10] Rutter M. Developmental catchup and delay, following adoption after severe global early privation. J Child Psychol Psychiatry 1998;39:465–76.

[11] Rutter M, Andersen-Wood L, Beckett C, et al. Quasi-autistic patterns following severe global privation. J Child Psychol Psychiatry 1999;40:537–49.

[12] Miller LC, Kiernan MT, Mathers MI, et al. Developmental and nutritional status of internationally adopted children. Arch Pediatr Adolesc Med 1995;149(1):40–4.

[13] Cermak S, Groza V. Sensory processing problems in post-institutionalized children: implications for social workers. Child Adolesc Social Work J 1998;15(1):5–37.

[14] Cermak SA, Daunhauer LA. Sensory processing in the post-institutionalized child. Am J Occup Ther 1997;51(7):500–7.

[15] Faber S. Behavioral sequelae of orphanage life. Pediatr Ann 2000;29(4):242–8.

[16] Hostetter MK. Epidemiology of travel-related morbidity and mortality in children. Pediatr Rev 1999;20(7):228–33.

[17] Jenista JA. Medical issues in international adoption. Pediatric Annals 2000;29.

[18] Miller LC. Initial assessment of growth, development, and the effects of institutionalization in internationally adopted children. Pediatr Ann 2000;29(4):224–32.

[19] Miller LC. Handbook of international adoption medicine. New York: Oxford University Press; 2005.

[20] Aronson J. Medical evaluation and infectious considerations on arrival. Pediatr Ann 2000; 29(4):218–23.

[21] Andersen TM. Social implications for institutionalised children. In: Rygvold A-L, Dalen M, Saetersdal B, editors. Mine—yours—ours and theirs. Oslo: University of Oslo; 1999. p. 118–33.

[22] Chen LH, Barnett ED, Wilson ME. Preventing infectious diseases during and after international adoption. Ann Intern Med 2003;139(5 Pt 1):371–8.

[23] Ryan ET, Wilson ME, Kain KC. Illness after international travel. N Engl J Med 2002;347: 505–16.

[24] World Health Organization. International travel and health. Available at: http://www.who.int/ith/. Accessed February 15, 2004.

[25] Centers for Disease Control and Prevention. The yellow book. Health information for international travel. Available at: http://www.cdc.gov/travel/yb/. Accessed February 15, 2004.

[26] Center for Disease Control and Prevention. Health information for the international traveller, 2001–2002. Atlanta: US Department of Health and Human Services, Public Health Service; 2001.

[27] Rose SR. International travel health guide. Northampton, MA: Travel Medicine; 2001.

[28] Hopkins-Best M. Toddler adoption: the weaver's craft. Indianapolis, IN: Perspectives Press; 1997.

[29] Benoit TC, Jocelyn LJ, Moddemann DM, et al. Romanian adoption. The Manitoba experience. Arch Pediatr Adolesc Med 1996;150(12):1278–82.

[30] Brodzinsky DM, Schecter MD, Henig RM. Being adopted. New York: Anchor Books; 1993.

ELSEVIER
SAUNDERS

PEDIATRIC CLINICS
OF NORTH AMERICA

Pediatr Clin N Am 52 (2005) 1331–1349

Health Care in the First Year After International Adoption

Elaine E. Schulte, MD, MPH[a],*, Sarah H. Springer, MD[b,c]

[a]International Adoption Program, Department of Pediatrics, MC-88, Albany Medical College,
Albany, NY 12208, USA
[b]American Academy of Pediatrics Section on Adoption and Foster Care,
141 Northwest Point Boulevard, Elk Grove, IL 60007-1098, USA
[c]Medical Director, International Adoption Health Services of Western Pennsylvania,
Pediatric Alliance, PC, 4070 Beechwood Boulevard, Pittsburgh, PA 15217, USA

If the child has no acute medical issues, an office visit is recommended within 4 to 6 weeks after the initial visit, regardless of the child's age. At minimum, this allows the provider to review all postadoption laboratory work, confirm the initiation and time line for catch-up of immunizations, and, probably most importantly, obtain more specific information from parents about the child's experiences in his new home. At this time, most parents are able to provide more detailed information about the child's developmental, behavioral, and transitional progress.

This article is divided into areas focusing on addressing specific medical decisions and supporting families as they transition a new child into their family. Although some data exist to guide the provider, there is little scientific evidence on the most efficient and cost-effective scheme for postadoption care; therefore, most of the information presented here is based on the combined clinical experiences of the authors and other colleagues in the adoption medicine field.

* Corresponding author.
E-mail address: Schulte@mail.amc.edu (E.E. Schulte).

0031-3955/05/$ – see front matter © 2005 Elsevier Inc. All rights reserved.
doi:10.1016/j.pcl.2005.06.012   *pediatric.theclinics.com*

Transitional issues for children and their families

Contextual considerations: attention to transitions, grieving, and healthy attachment

Providers caring for newly adopted children should remember and respect the tremendous transitions that the child and his or her family are experiencing. Even though we know that gaining a permanent family provides a child with innumerable long-term advantages, at the time of transition into a new family, culture, and country, the child experiences the loss of everything previously familiar to him or her. Even extremely young infants are aware of sudden changes in their environment, including sights, sounds, tastes, smells, and human interactions. Older children may feel as if they were dropped onto another planet and may react with any number of developmental, behavioral, or emotional concerns. A child's response to these life changes may be puzzling or extremely challenging to the new parents, who had fallen in love with that same child who seemed delightful in his or her previous environment.

If given the opportunity to meet with families before their international adoption, providers can assist families in preparing to support their child's transition as described elsewhere in this issue (see the article by Miller). The opportunity to prepare the child for the transition associated with adoption is usually not available; the content and extent of information provided to the child are often limited and unknown to the parents. Providing parents with an understanding of the child's experience and with specific coping strategies can be helpful, however.

Most international adoptions involve long-distance traveling, which can be overwhelming to adults and children alike. For the child, it may be the first time he or she has left the confines of an institutional care setting or small town. Airplanes, trains, buses, cars, big cities, escalators, and other technology are likely all new, and even frightening, to the child. Add to that 24 or more hours of traveling across multiple time zones, and, clearly, most children can be expected to be exhausted physically and emotionally by the time they arrive at their new homes.

Primary care providers can assist children to settle in by helping families to prepare low-key arrivals with quiet time at home with the new family for at least the first several weeks. Although there are usually many friends and family members eager to welcome a new child home, the airport is not the time for a gathering of dozens of noisy well wishers. Adoptive parents should plan time off from usual activities, limit visitors to small groups and short stays of those who are likely to be important to the child (eg, grandparents and other close relatives, close family friends) and commit to just "be at home" getting to know the child while allowing him or her to get to know them. Some children settle into their new homes and families quickly, whereas others take longer to adjust. Families should plan ahead to have as much time available and flexibility as possible in meeting their particular child's transition needs. Providers may be called on to write letters for parenting leave from work. This time is easily justified as necessary for attachment and bonding, the key determinants of the child's and family's long-term emotional health.

Because most internationally adopted children speak and understand a language different from that of their parents, communicating with the new family member is a critical consideration. Although communication with infants is mostly nonverbal, toddlers, preschoolers, and older children (and their new parents) may struggle with language barriers. Adopting parents should learn at least a few key phrases in the child's native language before adopting. Families can usually meet their child's basic needs by trial and error without a translator, but it is difficult for the child to share his or her fears, feelings, and questions about all the changes he or she is living through if he or she cannot communicate more deeply. Thus, parents of school-aged children should arrange for a translator to be available for at least several weeks after the child arrives home. Caution is warranted when working with translators as well, however. As with the use of translators and cultural interpreters in all medical settings, communication should be with the assistance of a translator who is professionally trained to provide communication as free of bias as possible. Families enlisting the support of a translator should realize that children with a history of adoption may perceive a person speaking their first language as a potential sign that they are going to be returning to the country where they were born. Translators are essential when addressing topics that may be perceived as threatening, such as hospital admission, surgery, or a parent's expected prolonged absence.

Grief and loss

Unfortunately, transitions from an orphanage or foster care to an adoptive family are not always planned with adequate preparation or consideration of the child's emotional needs. Even when transition planning is optimal, most children experience grief over the loss of significant caregivers, peers, siblings, and the "home" that was familiar to them before adoption. Infants and toddlers who are grieving may be cranky and irritable for no apparent reason and may sometimes cry inconsolably. Older children may be profoundly sad, quiet, withdrawn, angry, aggressive, or defiant. Children may worry about caregivers, birth family, or orphanage friends, wondering if they are safe or if those persons are concerned about the child's new life. Some children feel guilty for having left caregivers, peers, parents, or siblings behind.

Although the child's grief evokes sadness in the new parents and may contribute to difficult behaviors during the adoption trip home, grief is an emotionally healthy response to loss. A child's feelings of grief generally suggest that the child has had at least one significant previous interpersonal relationship. As parents comfort the child, he or she gradually transfers that psychologic attachment to his or her new parents, laying down a foundation for a solid future parent-child relationship. Parents can help children through this process by sharing pictures of the loved ones, allowing and encouraging letters or telephone calls when possible, and providing language support to allow the child to talk about his or her feelings. Grieving typically lasts just days or weeks for extremely young children but may be a process that takes many months or years for older children. Many years after adoption, children and adults may continue to grieve for the memories and loss of important people in their lives. Most children work through their feelings informally as they complete a life book, talk with older adoptees, or read and discuss books about the variety of adoption experiences. Sometimes, professional counseling is helpful with a therapist experienced with issues of grief, loss, and attachment [1,2]. Parents should be encouraged to be flexible in their approach as they support their child's development of his or her own adoption story. Even as the child grieves over important losses, the parents and the child are adjusting to each other while struggling to build a new interpersonal relationship. This "attachment" is a special and enduring relationship between a child and a significant person or persons, involving deep feelings of trust, pleasure, and security. Healthy parent-child attachment develops after many cycles of an infant having needs met by a loving, reliable, and nurturing caregiver who is emotionally attuned to the infant's needs. Attachment provides an internal working model for the infant to understand self, other people, and the world at large [3]. The process of developing attachment stimulates biochemical and cellular changes in the brain, laying down cellular pathways on which later cognitive functioning and interpersonal skills rely (see the article by Weitzman and Albers elsewhere in this issue).

Children who spend their infancy and early childhood residing in child welfare institutions do not usually experience individual emotionally attuned care. They are thus at risk for alterations in their attachment behaviors and in their neurobiology. This can have profound effects on their later social, emotional, and cognitive functioning. The internal working model that a child develops as the result of institutional caretaking is not one of safety, security, and trust but rather one that says, "it's every kid for himself or herself." Children with a history of institutional care learn to entertain themselves, comfort themselves, and meet their own basic needs at an early age (see the article by Weitzman and Albers elsewhere in this issue).

When a parent adopts a child who has spent most of his or her early life in an institution, the primary care provider can help the parents to adjust their responses and learn techniques to promote healthy new behaviors and parent-child attachment. Parents may find it easiest to think of their newly adopted child as "a psychologic newborn in an older child's body" and then to reorient their interactions with the child to promote the development of strong attachment. In practice, this means the parents may find themselves treating the child as if he or she were much younger psychologically, for example, rocking a school-aged child before bedtime or playing peek-a-boo with a kindergartener. Parents should plan to have as much quiet time at home alone with the child as possible and should aim to be the only one(s) to meet their child's physical and emotional needs. The child thus learns to trust the parent as the source of safety and nourishment.

New adoptive parents may be impressed by a child's self-sufficiency, "brave-ness" when hurt, or ability to entertain himself or herself for extended pe-riods. They should be careful to intervene, however, making sure the child sees that the parent is the active provider of food, comfort, and entertainment. These activities support the child's ability to use the parent as a secure base in the world. Parents should mirror the child's emotional state and join the child in whatever activity he or she pursues, working to have the child develop pleasure in sharing his or her experiences with the parent [4].

Some children respond to the efforts of their new parents readily and begin to develop the foundations of strong attachments quickly, whereas others are much more threatened by their new parents' attempts to connect. When children resist their parents' offers of support, parents can use activities that the child does enjoy to create opportunities for small moments of connection building on these over time. Most children love "rough housing" play, and parents can engage their children in play where their body positions promote eye contact between themselves and the child. Most children enjoy swinging; parents can push the child from the front, establishing closeness and eye contact briefly with each forward movement of the swing. Games of peek-a-boo and hide-and-seek can create and repeat joyful moments of the parent and child finding each other, and older children may enjoy similar pleasures by playing catch, ping-pong, tennis, and other reciprocal games.

Primary care providers should attend to and monitor for signs of strong at-tachment developing between adopted children and their new parents. If children struggle to grant the status of "secure base" to their new parents within a few months of the adoption, some families may require ongoing work with therapists experienced in addressing attachment disturbances in a family systems context (see the article by Nalven elsewhere in this issue).

Transition to starting daycare or school

Once a child has developed a comprehension of his or her new world and is beginning to use the new parent(s) as a secure base from which to explore it, or, more commonly, when parents simply must return to work, the child can be transitioned into other caregiving settings. The child should be introduced gradually to the new caregivers, with the parent and child visiting together several times before the child is left alone. Initial stays without the parent should be short (approximately 30 minutes) and gradually increased to include a meal and nap time. Transition objects and photographs of the parent(s) and child together (in a child-safe photograph album, key chain, or the like) can help the child to realize that the parents are going to return and that this is not the whole world changing yet again. Caregivers must be made aware that this child may have greater transition needs than children who have been with their parents since birth. Most children do adjust to childcare arrangements within a few months, but some struggle with insecurities and separation anxiety for years, often related to past experiences with separation and loss. When anxieties are severe or limit a child's ability to function, professional counseling with a therapist experienced in adoption and childhood trauma can be helpful.

One of the questions parents may ask at follow-up visits involves the risks, benefits, and timing of daycare placement. There is no research that has examined the outcome of the timing of childcare placement after international adoption. Daycare poses the typical infection risks to these children. Additionally, it is thought that young children acquire language skills most appropriately when working with an adult (parent) on a one-to-one basis rather than in a classroom of toddlers who are all learning language skills. For parents who must return to work, it is advised that they find a small group setting, with high standards for infection control, for their child. Children who have lived in institutional settings may find it easier to attend daycare or school rather than be in a more intimate family setting. In this case, children may be better supported to develop healthy attachment relationships with their family and other primary caretakers if they are cared for at home by a nanny or attend a small family-based daycare facility.

The child may have continued attachment concerns over time. Generally, internationally adopted children transition to daycare settings similar to nonadopted children. For the child who has not bonded well with the parent, delay in daycare placement would be recommended. In addition, parents by adoption, like those by birth, are at risk for postadoptive depression or other difficulties in adjusting to their role in parenting their child. Primary care providers may find that community-based support groups or mental health services may be indicated for parents as well.

School entry

Entering school shortly after international adoption presents a particular challenge, because children may not have had any formal schooling in their country of origin. Language and academic skills may not be appropriate for the level of classroom functioning expected of a child their age. Parents are understandably eager to have their new children attending school at an age-appropriate level, but some children need to start in a lower grade to learn basic academic skills. Some children are ready to begin school shortly after joining their new families, whereas others need more time at home, learning to be a member of a family, before they are ready to venture out into the world.

Ideally, parents and schools should work together to plan a gradual introduction to the school, with visits and half-day attendance until the child is ready for full-time attendance. All children should have second language support arranged before starting school, which should last until parents, teachers, and the child think that he or she has completely learned the new language—typically, at least several years. Children older than kindergarten or first-grade age may benefit from a sliding grade level placement, starting out in a lower grade to allow for basic academic catch-up and language learning but finishing the year with a class one or more levels higher, as achievement permits and age-appropriate social needs dictate. Careful attention should be paid to academic struggles, because children who have experienced severe deprivation in the past are at high risk for learning and cognitive disabilities (see the articles by Nalven and Weitzman and Albers elsewhere in this issue).

For children adopted at school age, involvement in an English as a second language (ESL) program should be considered with the following caveats. ESL programs in the United States are primarily designed to support the educational progress of children maintaining their native language (L1) while learning to converse and learn in a second language (typically English.) Internationally adopted children are often unskilled in their native languages, however, and are losing their native language while acquiring their new primary language. As a result, ESL services may be useful to support children's adjustment to a new school setting, but these services alone cannot identify or remediate any fundamental speech and language delays. For older children, an initial speech evaluation after adoption by a speech or language pathologist fluent in the child's birth language is ideal. If this is not possible, a skilled bilingual interpreter should assist in speech evaluation. Speech and language difficulties with articulation, grammar, and language processing are best identified in the birth language (see the articles by Dole, Nalven, and Weitzman and Albers elsewhere in this issue) [5].

Federal law mandates that all children older than 3 years of age are required to have an educational assessment in their primary language. Ideally, this is completed through and paid for by the school system, although parents may need to be involved in identifying an appropriate translator through local agencies, refugee support groups, universities, or professional translating services (see the article by Dole elsewhere in this issue).

Daily routines

Eating

Most internationally adopted children are malnourished at the time of adoption, with as many as 68% falling more than 2 standard deviations from the mean on one or more parameters of growth [5–7]. Most children have not had access to appropriate quality and quantity nutrition before adoption, often eating food of marginal nutritional value on a schedule unrelated to their hunger and without the option to eat when they are hungry. Most children learn adaptive behaviors under such circumstances, such as eating as much as they can whenever the opportunity arises and eating quickly before food is taken away by caretakers or other children. When these same children move into the care of parents who can provide plenty of food, this previously adaptive behavior can be alarming, and many new adoptive parents are extremely concerned about the huge volumes of food that their children eat and the rapid pace of the child's eating. They worry that the child may become ill and that he or she may become obese over time.

The recommended approach to this feeding behavior is to let the child have access to as much healthy food as he or she wants as often as he or she wants it.

Children need to learn that they are now in a situation where there is enough food and what it feels like to be satiated; many children have never felt this sensation and do not associate it with a reason to stop eating. They learn that they can trust the new parent(s) to provide food in ample volume and frequency and that they can stop eating when they feel satiated, because there is more available later. To develop good long-term eating habits, the child needs to learn to regulate his or her own intake, knowing that he or she can eat when hungry and can stop when full. If parents continue to restrict the child's intake, the child may continue to feel the need to "hurry up and eat more before Mom takes it away," and the long-term habit of eating whenever there is the opportunity may continue. When allowed to eat freely, most young children begin to trust that their parents are going to provide food and slow down their intake within several months of joining the family.

Older children and children who have had to be completely self-sufficient (eg, children who have previously lived on the streets or without any adult caretakers) may hoard food even when parents do not restrict their dietary intake. It is important for new parents to realize that this was an adaptive behavior that helped the child to survive before adoption; they should not punish the child for behaving in this way. It is helpful to have plenty of healthy (and nonmessy) foods always readily available to the child, such as bowls of fruit or pretzels on tables throughout the house. Some children benefit from having a backpack with healthy snacks that they can carry with them whenever they wish. Parents may need to work to gain the cooperation of schools and other caregivers with this plan. Most children begin to trust their new parents within several months of having plentiful food; however, occasionally, it may take many months, or even years, for some children to trust their parents to provide food. Professional counseling with a therapist experienced in childhood trauma and deprivation can be helpful if a child's eating does not normalize within several months of joining his or her new family.

Although most new internationally adopted children eat huge amounts of food, some struggle with eating. Some children may be sensitive to tastes or textures that they perceive as unpleasant. Others have oral-motor coordination problems and have difficulty in chewing or swallowing. Both of these difficulties may be related to feeding practices typical of many institutional care settings. In many orphanages around the world, infants are fed with propped bottles, often with large holes cut in the nipple to accommodate porridge flowing out of the bottle. Children eat while lying supine in bed, trying to gulp quickly to keep from choking on the thick sludge. Older infants and toddlers are often fed the same porridge from a bowl with a large serving spoon used to shovel the cereal from the bowl directly to the child's mouth. Children are frequently gagged by the spoon and must keep gulping so as not to choke. Eating in an orphanage is rarely pleasant or social, because caregivers, who often have 20 or more children to feed, simply do not have the time to feed children slowly or playfully. Any of these experiences can cause the child to develop poorly coordinated suck and swallow reflexes or severe tactile defensiveness in the mouth and on the face.

For most children, gentle and loving feeding practices overcome these struggles within a few weeks. Parents should use a small soft spoon to feed the child and start with foods with textures and tastes that the child finds acceptable. Many parents find that foods similar to those a child received before adoption are a good starting point, even if these are things that would usually be fed to a much younger child. The texture and variety of foods can gradually be increased as the child is able and willing to tolerate the change. Gentle but firm (not tickly) touch on the face and hands during mealtime and at other times can help the child to learn to be more tolerant of different sensations in and around the mouth. Additional oromotor activities, such as hand play in dry beans, rice, water, pudding, or whipped cream, may be helpful in allowing the child to explore new textures. Learning to trust new parents to provide nourishment is a basic component of healthy psychologic attachment of the child to his or her parents. Feeding a child also provides a parent with a basic feeling of competency in his or her new role.

When parents are extremely anxious about feeding their new child or when a child continues to be resistant to eating even after several weeks, referral for evaluation and ongoing consultation with a professional feeding therapist is recommended. This can prevent the development of a maladaptive "feeding war" in addition to the child's already selective eating.

Bathing and toileting

Many young children, even those less than 1 year of age, are said to be "toilet trained" when living in an orphanage. Like eating, toileting follows a routine in institutional settings. As a group, children are made to sit on small potties after meals and are not allowed to leave until all have voided or moved their bowels. The child is not yet really in control of his bowel or bladder function during this "training." Parents should expect to have children in diapers after adoption until the usual time that children are able to control and plan ahead for their toileting functions, generally around 2½ to 3 years of age.

Even children who truly have gained mastery of their bowel and bladder control often regress in these skills as a manifestation of stress associated with the many transitions related to their adoption. It is important for parents to realize that this "regression" is a common childhood response and that they should not punish the child for urine or stool "accidents." Older children may have been punished in the past for nocturnal enuresis and may try to hide wet clothes or bedding. In this situation, parents need to be supportive rather than punitive and help the child to realize that he or she simply needs to change the sheets. Occasionally, toileting struggles are the result of organic causes, but most are related to stress and resolve with time.

Baths in orphanages are often unpleasant, involving a fast functional hosing off with hot or cold water rather than a fun playtime for the child. As a result, many newly adopted children vigorously protest bath time. Parents may need to clean the child with sponge baths at first and gradually desensitize the child to water with activities like playing in a bowl or sink full of lukewarm water, playing together in a wading pool, or bathing with the child. For young children, hosting a "bath party," where the child can watch other young children have fun with bath toys and bubbles in the tub, is often quite successful in helping the child to learn to enjoy bath time.

Sleep

Newborns learn to sleep for extended periods by gaining neurologic maturity, increasing the interval between feeding times, and experiencing many cycles of having their needs met by consistent, loving, and nurturing caregivers. Children adopted beyond infancy may not have developed good sleep habits or may lose previous good habits in response to transitioning to a new family, time zone, culture, and daily routine. Children may have never slept alone or in a quiet or dark room. Unfortunately, some children may have experienced abuse or other trauma during the nighttime, making bedtime a particularly challenging time. Many children with a history of trauma have sleep onset and maintenance difficulties regardless of the timing of their negative experiences.

To sleep peacefully throughout the night, all children must feel safe and secure, be able to get themselves back to sleep if they wake at night, and trust that their parents are there to protect them. Just as for a newborn, this only occurs after the child experiences many cycles of having his or her needs met by the same loving, nurturing, and consistent caregivers. Fatigue and anxiety can combine to leave a child emotionally vulnerable; parents can help their child to make tremendous gains in attachment and sleeping by being there for him or her as a comforting presence. "Cry it out" techniques are counterproductive for newly adopted children who do not yet trust that their parents are still going to be there. Such an approach may simply reinforce a child's impression, learned in an orphanage, that he or she is "in this life alone." Instead, parents should be physically and emotionally present at the minimal level that the child needs to feel safe and secure, gradually weaning themselves out of the child's bedtime routine. Initially, it may be helpful for parents to sleep in the child's room, gradually removing themselves over the first several months that the child is home. Making sure that the child falls asleep in his or her own bed during this process can ensure that the child can eventually fall asleep peacefully on his or her own in his or her own room and sleep through the night without difficulty.

Postadoptive behaviors

Sensory behaviors

Sensory seeking or avoidance is frequently reported in children after international adoption. It is unclear what the actual incidence of "sensory integration" difficulties is in the adopted population, at least partly because opinions about the validity of the diagnosis vary widely among professionals. Children with sensory processing difficulties are described as those who have sensory over- or under-responsivity; they may be sensory seeking or have sensory discrimination dysfunction or dyspraxia. Occupational therapists with specific training in this area can assist with the diagnosis and management. Children who exhibit self-stimulating behaviors, such as rocking or head banging, do not necessarily have a sensory processing disorder. These behaviors typically abate with time, although they may never totally disappear.

Autistic-like behaviors

Most infants in institutional care spend their days lying in a crib, devoid of toys, visual or auditory stimulation, or movement. More importantly, the children experience limited human interaction, with little or none of what they receive through the individualized, emotionally attuned, nurturing interactions that we know stimulate infant growth and development. Toddlers and preschoolers often are allowed to play in beautifully equipped playrooms with adults watching but not interacting socially. As a result, institutionalized children have to come up with ways to amuse themselves. Many develop repetitive motion behaviors that provide some sensory input, are self-soothing, and are a distraction from total boredom. These may take on many forms, but commonly include rocking, hand play (flapping, light and shadow play with fingers), head banging, and mastur-bation. These are adaptive behaviors in the orphanage environment but look quite alarming to new adoptive parents (and to their health care providers) when seen on preadoptive videotapes or when the child moves into a family setting.

For most newly adopted children, the frequency and intensity of these autistic-like behaviors diminish rapidly over the first several months in the new family as life becomes more stimulating and nurturing. Many children revert to these self-soothing behaviors, however, when they are stressed, tired, or bored. Parents can learn to interpret these cues and respond appropriately. Many children continue to use these repetitive motions to get themselves to sleep, sometimes for months or even years after adoption. These are akin to the many other sleep association habits that adults and children alike use and should not alarm parents or pedia-tricians as long as the child is appropriately developing other social, emotional, and interpersonal skills.

Children who do not respond to nurturing and emotionally attuned parenting, who would rather continue to self-stimulate than to interact with the world, need a full developmental and behavioral evaluation. Such children may be "truly autistic," as are some children in any large cohort, or may have "institutional autism" (or "reactive attachment disorder with autistic features (see the article by Weitzman and Albers elsewhere in this issue). Regardless of the final diagnosis, all these children can benefit from early referral to intensive therapy programs designed to treat autism.

Medical visit considerations

As described elsewhere in this volume (see the article by Barnett), primary care providers should conduct a thorough postadoption physical examination and ensure that routine postadoption screening laboratory tests and immunizations have been completed. Diagnoses raised before adoption, including possible rickets, hip dysplasia, congenital heart disease, or retinopathy of prematurity, may require confirmation or further assessment. Any scars, neurocutaneous abnormalities, or birth marks, including Mongolian spots, should be documented in the medical record.

Before adoption, parents may be most concerned about potential medical concerns for their child; however, these are the issues most readily assessed and treated after adoption. All children screened before adoption for infectious diseases, such as HIV, syphilis, or hepatitis B, require repeat screening for these infections. In addition, complete blood cell counts should be scrutinized for possible evidence of anemia, thalassemia, or hemoglobinopathies. Elevated lead levels have been reported after international adoption, and routine immediate postadoptive screening for lead exposure is extremely important to ensure that adequate dietary, and perhaps medical, interventions are offered if indicated.

All internationally adopted children should be screened and monitored for possible hearing, vision, growth, and developmental difficulties given their prenatal and preadoptive experiences. The following recommendations and rationale for screening for these concerns and referral for additional medical consultation in this population of children are described.

Hearing

At each visit, the primary care provider should ask parents about hearing concerns, being careful to differentiate what the child responds to (eg, telephone ringing, door bell, dog barking in the other room) without using a visual prompt. One study described 3.8% of international adoptees with hearing loss [8].

Regardless of a child's adoption history, the presence of permanent or recurrent transient hearing loss during the first years of life has the potential to compromise a child's speech and language acquisition. All internationally adopted children who are slow to acquire language skills should have a hearing assessment. The age of the child and the degree of the speech and language delay determine the timing of the assessment. Most adoption providers agree that evaluation and intervention should be provided sooner rather than later (within weeks rather than months).

Conductive and sensorineural hearing loss occur at increased rates in internationally adopted children. The lack of a detailed family history or accurate past medical history may not allow determination of a specific cause of hearing impairment. Children may have a history of frequent upper respiratory tract infections; chronic otitis media; use of ototoxic topical medications; or congenital bacterial, viral, protozoal, or spirochetal infections. Screening for certain infections (eg, cytomegalovirus [CMV], herpes, parvovirus B-19, toxoplasmosis, syphilis) is usually not definitive but may offer some explanation for parents. High-resolution CT or MRI may be indicated to delineate possible abnormal ear anatomy. In addition, a pediatric otolaryngologist can be helpful in further eluci-dating an underlying cause of hearing loss.

Hearing can be assessed using a variety of methodologies, depending on the age of the child and his or her willingness to cooperate. Children less than 3 years of age should be referred to a reliable hearing center, where they may undergo otoacoustic emission testing, auditory brain stem response, behavioral observa-tion audiometry, or visual reinforcement audiometry. Most experienced exam-iners use behavioral measures to assess the hearing of children as young as 6 months. Children 3 years of age or older can be screened in the primary care provider's office, depending on the child's ability to cooperate. Occasionally, language barriers mandate testing typically used for younger children. Any questionable test results should mandate referral to a hearing center.

Vision

Parents should be questioned about their child's vision at every office visit, and an eye examination should be completed at each visit for at least the first year. Many visual problems are noticed by the parents long before they are apparent in the clinical setting. Common concerns include crossed eyes and light sensitivity. Many children of Asian descent as well as some children from Eastern Europe have widely spaced eyes with flat nasal bridges. One eye may appear to disappear behind the labial fold ("pseudostrabismus"). The most useful test of alignment is the cover test. At any age, a person with misaligned eyes focuses with the stronger eye, allowing the weaker eye to drift. Some children, especially those who are quite young, cannot cooperate for reliable cover testing. In these cases, the corneal light reflex can be used. If the eyes are straight, the reflection of the light falls near the center of each pupil while the child is fixing on an object directly in front of him or her [9]. Because previously institutionalized children are more likely to have strabismus (occurring in 10%–25% of internationally adopted children), all previously institutionalized international adoptees should be examined by a pediatric ophthalmologist within the first few months after arrival [8,10,11].

Prenatal substance exposure

Ongoing evaluation for fetal alcohol syndrome (FAS) and alcohol-related neurodevelopmental disorder (ARNDD) should be conducted for any interna-tionally adopted child, particularly for those whose birth mothers were reported to have used alcohol during pregnancy. Providers must remember that as children grow, the phenotypic facial features can evolve and may be more or less suggestive of prenatal alcohol exposure (see the article by Davies and Bledsoe elsewhere in this issue). Learning and behavioral problems attributable to mater-nal alcohol use may become more apparent as children grow older. One early suggestion of alcohol exposure is poor catch-up growth in the microcephalic infant or child. These children may also demonstrate weak verbal development and increased impulsivity. If suspicions of FAS or ARNDD arise, referral to a specialty center is indicated. Confirmation of a diagnosis of prenatal alcohol exposure may be quite difficult given a child's lack of history, but providers should be vigilant about this possibility over time, because additional information or new physical examination findings may become evident (see the article by Bledsoe and Davies elsewhere in this issue).

Growth monitoring

Most children grow rapidly during the first months in their new home, crossing percentiles on the height, weight, and head circumference curves until they have an approximation of their genetic potential. Because we do not usually have parental height data, it is difficult to determine whether children are truly capable of regaining all their growth potential. Most children begin to follow a curve within 2 standard deviations of the mean, using the National Center for Health Statistics (NCHS) growth charts, within 9 to 12 months after arrival. Some children, however, particularly older children who endured malnutrition and deprivation for longer, may continue to show catch-up growth for years after adoption. With the exception of the rare child who was well nourished at arrival and continues to grow appropriately along the same curve, a child who is not exhibiting catch-up growth after international adoption should be evaluated for other conditions that might cause growth failure, such as tuberculosis or FAS (see the article by Mason elsewhere in this issue).

Routine developmental screening

Data over the last 15 years have consistently suggested that between 50% and 90% of internationally adopted children have a developmental delay on meeting their new family [5–7,10,12,13]. Delays in gross motor, fine motor, cognition, and language are all common [6]. The degree of recovery seems to be more dependent on the duration of time spent in an institution than on the age at adoption [13]. The likelihood of long-term developmental, behavioral, or academic problems increases with the age at adoption (D.E. Johnson, MD, PhD, International Adoption Project, unpublished data, 2002). Delays in specific areas of development may be partially or completely reversible after adoption; numerous authors have suggested that the rate of development exceeds the rate of normal development over a period of years, with such catch-up development continuing for an indefinite period [5,13–15]. The degree of reversibility, especially for children with severe delays, and the constraints to full recovery are unknown [5].

The primary care provider should remember that developmental and behavioral issues may have multiple causes, including genetic predisposition, prenatal exposures, and individual experiences with early neglect or abuse. Because each child's experience is unique, it is impossible to predict a child's long-term outcome at the initial meeting (see the article by Nalven and Albers elsewhere in this issue).

After a child's adoption, primary care providers should perform a baseline screening of development at the first visit and repeat screenings at follow-up visits, at least two to three times during the first year home and then at least semiannually, depending on the severity of the delay. Providers may be most familiar with the Denver II Developmental Screening Test [16]. This screening test relies on children's past typical experiences and exposures, most of which an institutionalized child has not had, and requires more time than is typically available during a routine primary care visit. More recently available measures include the parents' evaluations of developmental status (PEDS) and the pediatric symptom checklist (PSC). Both instruments have high sensitivity and specificity and are easy to administer in the office. They rely on parent input; thus, they may not be as accurate on the first visit, given the parent's unfamiliarity with the child's skills. The PEDS (www.pedstest.com) is designed for children aged 0 to 8 years. The PSC (www.psc.partners.org) is a behavior screening tool designed for any child 4 years of age or older, and the 35-question form can be downloaded from the web site.

Developmental delay: when to refer to early intervention

The decision to refer to an early intervention (EI) program or to the school district because of developmental delays should not be a difficult one, because most children qualify for services and parents are typically quite motivated to support their child's ongoing development. Almost 90% of children who have spent more than 1 year in an institution are delayed in at least one area of development at the time of arrival in their new families [12]. Prior studies of growth and cognitive development have determined that after adoption, many institutionalized children make developmental gains faster than the normal maturational curve [17,18]. It is impossible to predict which children are going to catch up and which children are going to have ongoing needs, however. For this reason, it is recommended that providers refer children for evaluation and treatment of developmental delays sooner rather than later. Occasionally, parents or an EI program or school district wants to take a "wait and see" approach. Providers may need to intervene on the child's behalf should a local development program or school district elect not to provide services.

After the postadoption screening, primary care providers should carefully review development progression, with an emphasis on speech and language acquisition. This is critical because communication difficulties are significantly related to behavioral concerns. Not all infants and toddlers develop English according to the same language acquisition trends that are seen in their non-adopted English-speaking peers. Glennen and Masters [19] have created criteria

Table 1
Criteria for referral for speech and language services

Age at adoption	Suggested referral criteria
0–12 months	Refer as if primary English speaker
13–18 months	Refer if not producing 50 words or 2 word phrases at 24 months
19–24 months	Refer if not using English by 24 months, 50 words at 28 months, or 2 word phrases at 28–30 months
25–30 months	Refer if not using English within several weeks at home or if not speaking 50 English words or 2 word phrases by 31 months

Data from Glennen S, Masters MG. Typical and atypical language development in infants and toddlers adopted from Eastern Europe. Am J Speech Lang Pathol 2002;11:417–33.

for referral for speech and languages services (Table 1) based primarily on language production, age at adoption, and time elapsed since adoption.

Age uncertainty and determination

Although many internationally adopted children are born in hospitals or have a reliable birth history, there are children for whom a true birth date is unknown. Sometimes, children were born at home with no official recording of the birth. More commonly, children come into care after having been abandoned, usually on the streets or at the door of an orphanage, police station, or hospital. In China, virtually all the children who are available for international adoption have been abandoned as infants because of the country's "one child" law (and most of these children are girls because of the centuries old cultural preference for a male child). An infant is sometimes found with a note specifying his or her birthday; however, more often, an estimated date is assigned. Older children may know their age or birthday. The growth and developmental delays associated with malnutrition and neglect often make children appear younger than their chronologic age; thus, age estimates before or shortly after arrival into the institution are often an underestimate of the child's true age. Younger ages are sometimes intentionally assigned because of the belief that is more difficult to find adoptive homes for older children.

As reviewed previously (see the article by Mason elsewhere in this issue), most children have growth and developmental delays at the time of adoption. The degree of delay can be quite alarming to parents (and primary care providers), and when there is an assigned birth date, parents frequently assume that the child must truly be significantly younger. Most children, however, begin to make rapid gains in growth and development within days or weeks of joining a family and continue to catch up for months (or even years for older children) after their arrival.

It is therefore rarely, if ever, advisable to make decisions about changing a child's birthday until at least a year after the adoption, when catch-up growth and development can be taken into account. Bone age testing is not helpful any earlier than this, because malnutrition and deprivation delay bone age just as they affect other areas of a child's development. It is only after malnutrition and other stressors have resolved that a bone age film may be helpful. In addition, the standard deviation for a bone age assessment is typically at least several months in either direction, making it a useful test only for children for whom the birthday might be off by many months or years.

Most often, concerns about age discrepancies resolve as children catch up in growth and development. When significant concerns persist a year or more after adoption, it may be reasonable to consider legally changing a child's birth date. Before making such a change, parents and pediatricians should carefully consider what might be gained or lost for the child involved. For children with significant developmental disabilities, a later birthday (ie, making the child younger) may provide the child with more time to receive educational support but may inadvertently deny the child services, because his or her performance is then closer to his or her stated age. A child who is quite small and socially immature might fit in better with school classmates of a younger age. Children who may appear emotionally and physically younger than their reported age may enter puberty well before their classmates. Perhaps most importantly, a child whose birthday was changed after adoption may later feel a profound sense of loss for that piece of his or her original identity. Documents at the time of adoption require a date of birth, and that has become a part of his or her identity, even if not factually correct. For children for whom there is not likely to be identifying information to allow them to reconnect with birth families, that original birthday, although assigned, may be the only remnant of the child's original identity. Because there is no way to know which young children may find this to be profoundly important later in their lives, parents should think carefully before changing this piece of their child's history. Many professionals involved with this population of children suggest that changing a birth date is indicated only if the date is going to changed by 1 year at least, preferably retaining the originally stated month and date of birth. If the decision is made to change a child's birth date, this may involve significant costs as well as requiring documentation for court proceedings from a range of professionals (eg, medical, psychological, dental) supporting this decision.

Referrals to medical consultants

It is not uncommon to see many diagnoses and unusual terminology on some adoptive referrals. For example, physicians in other countries often use ultrasound imaging to examine numerous organs, leading to diagnostic interpretations that may not be based on US pediatric standards. If there is a question of pathologic findings on examination or by history, referral to a subspecialist is warranted. Common situations include the child suspected to have congenital heart disease or neurologic abnormalities or the child with an infectious disease that poses risks to family members. Timing of these referrals should balance the urgency of a child's medical needs with the transition needs of the child. Obviously, a child is better able to handle the stress of medical care after developing some trust that the new parents are going to provide comfort and protection. Even with repeated physical examinations without pathologic findings and normal laboratory results, the provider may still wish to refer the child to the sub-specialist if only to relieve parental anxiety.

Timing of elective surgery

Timing of elective surgery is ultimately at the discretion of the surgeon. As with any type of surgery, the risks and benefits of the procedure as well as those of anesthesia need to be explained to the parent. Many surgeons prefer that a child be at least 6 months of age or weigh 20 lb before performing any type of elective surgery. The most common type of elective surgery that an internationally adopted child may face is circumcision. For the older adopted child, it is recommended that the procedure be explained to the child in the language he or she is most comfortable with. Truly elective procedures should be deferred until at least several months after arrival (the longer the better) to allow the child to be comforted as much as possible by his parents during the perioperative period.

References

[1] Zeitlin SV. Grief and bereavement. Prim Care 2001;28(2):415–25.
[2] Committee on Psychosocial Aspects of Child and Family Health, American Academy of Pediatrics. The pediatrician and childhood bereavement. Pediatrics 2000;105(2):445–7.
[3] Ainsworth MD. Object relations, dependency, and attachment: a theoretical review of the infant-mother relationship. Child Dev 1969;40(4):969–1025.
[4] Wieder S, Greenspan SI. Climbing the symbolic ladder in the DIR model through floor time/interactive play. Autism 2003;7(4):425–35.
[5] Miller LC, Kiernana MT, Mathers MI, et al. Developmental and nutritional status of internationally adopted children. Arch Pediatr Adolesc Med 1995;149:40–4.
[6] Miller LC, Hendrie N. Health of children adopted from China. Pediatrics 2000;105(6):E76.
[7] Albers LH, Johnson DE, Hostetter MK, et al. Health of children adopted from the former Soviet Union and Eastern Europe. Comparison with preadoptive medical records. JAMA 1997;278(11):922–4.
[8] Johnson DE. Long-term medical issues in international adoptees. Pediatr Ann 2000;29(4):234–41.
[9] Simon JW, Calhoun JH. A child's eyes; a guide to pediatric primary care. Gainesville, FL: Triad Publishing Company; 1998.
[10] Johnson DE, Albers L, Iverson S, et al. Health status of Eastern European orphans referred for adoption. Pediatr Res 1996;39(4 Pt 2):134A.
[11] Spitz R. The first year of life: A psychoanalytic study of normal and deviant development of object relations. New York: International Universities Press; 1965.
[12] Johnson DE, Dole K. International adoptions: implications for early intervention. Infants Young Child 1999;11(4):34–45.
[13] Ames EW. The development of Romanian orphanage children adopted into Canada. Burnaby (BC): Simon Fraser University; 1997. p. 1–138.
[14] Benoit TC, Jocelyn LJ, Moddemann DM, et al. Romanian adoption: the Manitoba experience. Arch Pediatr Adolesc Med 1996;150:1278–82.

[15] O'Connor TG, Rutter M, Beckett C, et al for the English and Romanian Adoptees Study Team. The effects of global severe privation on cognitive competence: extension and longitudinal follow-up. Child Dev 2000;71(2):376–90.
[16] Frankenburg WK, Dodds JB, Archer P, et al. Denver II developmental screening manual. Denver, CO: Developmental Materials; 1990.
[17] Aronson J, Johnson D, Melnikova M, et al. Catch-up brain growth in children adopted form Eastern Europe and Russia. Presented at the Ambulatory Pediatric Association Annual Conference. San Francisco, CA, May 1–4, 1999.
[18] Morison S, Ames E, Chisholm K. The development of children adopted from Romanian orphanages. Merrill Palmer Q 1995;41:411–30.
[19] Glennen S, Masters MG. Typical and atypical language development in infants and toddlers adopted from Eastern Europe. Am J Speech Lang Pathol 2002;11:417–33.

ELSEVIER
SAUNDERS

PEDIATRIC CLINICS
OF NORTH AMERICA

Pediatr Clin N Am 52 (2005) 1351–1368

Long-Term Growth and Puberty Concerns in International Adoptees

Patrick Mason, MD, PhD[a,b,*], Christine Narad, APRN, BC[a]

[a]*International Adoption Center, Inova Fairfax Hospital for Children, 8505 Arlington Boulevard,
Suite 100, Fairfax, VA 22031, USA*
[b]*Northern Virginia Endocrinologists, Fairfax, VA, USA*

As the number of children adopted internationally grows, we are beginning to understand better the multitude of issues with which they present when joining their new families. Studies continue to implicate the preadoption environment as one of the major causes for observed impairments. On arrival, children seem to be at risk for a wide variety of medical and developmental abnormalities. Problems like parasitic infections, untreated medical conditions, rickets, inadequate immunizations, and speech and motor delays are far more common in children placed for adoption than in most patients cared for by pediatricians in North America. One of the most common and consistent abnormalities seen on arrival is poor growth. The cause of this growth failure is not known but is likely varied. The child's health care team must be aware of the potential causes and be prepared to work with the family to ensure adequate catch-up growth. In this review, we discuss the growth failure observed in international adoptees, focusing on children who have spent time in orphanage settings. Catch-up potential, contributing issues, and possible mechanisms are explored. In addition, we discuss the phenomenon of early puberty and its relation to prearrival growth failure and postarrival catch-up.

* Corresponding author. International Adoption Center, Inova Fairfax Hospital for Children, 8505 Arlington Boulevard, Suite 100, Fairfax, VA 22031.
E-mail address: international.adoption@inova.com (P. Mason).

Environmental influences of growth

Growth is a fundamental theme for children and one that health care practitioners follow closely. A child's ability to grow to his or her full potential seems to be related to many issues, including genetics, nutrition, medical conditions, pre- and postnatal exposures, and the hormonal milieu, to name but a few. The environment in which a child lives is known to influence growth rate and, ultimately, growth outcome, and much has been written regarding the impact of poverty, war, and malnutrition [1–3].

The influence of deprivation and neglect on growth has been extensively studied recently, although the impact of adverse living conditions on growth has been known for centuries. In the 1200s, King Frederick II of Sicily unintentionally performed the first studies on the effects of early deprivation during an effort to learn whether an "innate" language of human beings existed. To determine this, he isolated infants to see if they developed spontaneous language. These infants not only failed to develop language but failed to grow and died quickly because of the lack of attention [4]. More contemporary, and less apocryphal, reports continue to document the fact that children living in institutionalized settings failing to meet their basic needs generally have poor growth and high mortality rates [4–6]. Spitz [7,8] reported that without consistent attention, children living in foundling homes exhibited poor growth and development as well as a high mortality rate despite evidence of adequate nutrition. Talbot and colleagues [9] noted a strong correlation between poor growth and a high incidence of abandonment, neglect, and maternal psychopathologic findings and also found significant growth improvement in a subset of children after a psychologic intervention program was initiated for the family.

Another well-known account of growth failure in an institutional setting was reported by Widdowson [10]. She followed the children in two German orphanages run by two different women. One was a caring and loving woman who was attentive to the needs of the children, whereas the second was a dominating and unpleasant woman. Despite similar food rations, the children under the care of the loving woman grew better than did those cared for by the unpleasant matron. After 6 months, the women were reassigned to each other's orphanages and the strict woman was given increased rations. Despite this, the children under her care who had previously been growing well had a decreased growth rate. The children who were then under the care of the loving woman grew better, despite smaller rations of food and their past poor growth.

Growth after international adoption

Although a worldwide estimate that 226 million children less than 5 years of age experience growth stunting [1], in the past, the likelihood of a typical pediatric practitioner encountering such a child was rare. This changed after the

Christmas Day execution of Nicola and Elena Ceausescu in 1989. After the Romanian revolution and the subsequent publicity surrounding the children housed in deplorable conditions in orphanages, large numbers of families from the West went to Romania to adopt children. The breakup of the former Soviet Union and the relaxation of adoption rules in China also led to the adoption of a growing number of institutionalized children by North American and Western European families. Now, for the first time, physicians and practitioners who care for children are seeing increasing numbers of children presenting with a history of chronic abuse, neglect, or care that fails to meet the basic necessities of life. As our experience grows, we are beginning to understand the impact that this environmental neglect has on the health, development, and growth of children.

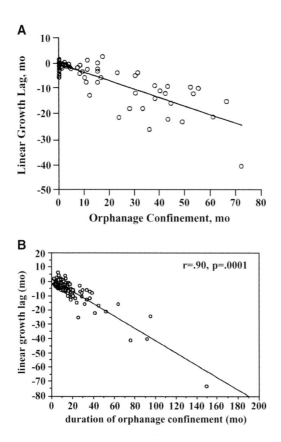

Fig. 1. (*A*) Effect of orphanage confinement on linear growth (linear growth lag = height, age = chronologic age) ($r = -0.79$, $P < .001$, $y = -1.05 - 0.32x$ [x = length of orphanage confinement in months]). (*From* Johnson DE, Miller LC, Iverson S, et al. The health of children adopted from Romania. JAMA 1992;268(24):3449; with permission.) (*B*) Linear growth in months is inversely proportional to the duration of orphanage confinement for 192 Chinese adoptees (*From* Miller LC, Hendrie NW. Health of children adopted from China. Pediatrics 2000;105(6):E76; with permission.)

Johnson and coworkers [11] first reported on growth impairment in children adopted from Eastern European orphanages. They found evidence of growth failure in 34% of the children adopted from Romania on arrival in the United States. They also noted that the orphanage environment had an ongoing effect on the physical growth of the child: height z scores decreased as the length of institutionalization increased. They estimated that a child loses roughly 1 month of growth in height for every 2.6 months that he or she lives in an orphanage ($r = -0.79$; Fig. 1A). Miller and Hendrie [12] noted a similar correlation between growth failure and the duration of institutionalization in girls adopted from China, with a deviation of 1 month of height from mean age levels for each 2.86 months spent in an orphanage ($r = 0.90$, $P = .001$; see Fig. 1B). Although the validity of such relations in predicting the extent of growth stunting is debated, these studies do point out the cumulative influence that these environments may exert on the growing young child.

Benoit and colleagues [13] found that of the children they examined from Romania, 32% were below the fifth percentile for height, 36% for weight, and 45% for head circumference. Rutter [14] evaluated 111 children less than 2 years of age. He found that the mean height z score was approximately -2, the mean weight z score was -2.37, and the mean head circumference was z score was -2.14. Miller and coworkers [15] examined 129 children recently adopted into the United States and found significant stunting: a mean height z score of -1.36, mean weight z score of -0.76, and mean head circumference z score of -1.03. Groze and Ileana [16] studied 475 adopted families who responded to a questionnaire and found that 72% of children were below normal in weight and 80% were below normal in height at the time of arrival in their adoptive families (Table 1).

Table 1
Review of postarrival anthropometric measurements for internationally adopted children

Studies	Weight z score	Height z score	Head circumference z score
Johnson and colleagues, 1992 [11] Romania, N = 65	−1.10	−1.68	−1.06
Miller and colleagues, 1995 [15] 22 countries, N = 129	−0.76	−1.36	−1.03
Johnson and colleagues, 1996 [93] Russia, N = 210	−1.71	−2.09	−1.15
Albers and colleagues, 1997 [94] Eastern Europe, N = 56	−1.05	−1.41	−1.25
Rutter, 1998 [14]	−2.2 ± 2.4	−2.3 ± 1.7	− 2.2 ± 1.3
Johnson and colleagues, 1999 [95] Romania, N = 59	−3.56 ± 2.0	−2.47 ± 1.29	−2.08 ± 1.53
Johnson, 2000 [34]	−1.62 ± 1.49	−1.25 ± 1.15	−1.36 ± 1.3
Miller and Hendrie, 2000 [12] China, N = 192	−1.17	−1.51	−1.43
Mason and colleagues, 2000 [36] Eastern Europe, N = 339	−1.67	−2.03	—

Psychosocial short stature: a possible mechanism

The cause of poor growth in these children is likely multifactorial and includes issues like prematurity, intrauterine growth failure (IUGR), genetics, prenatal drug and alcohol exposures, nutritional deficiencies, and medical illnesses. The phenomenon of poor growth in children living in neglectful and deprived conditions is not, however, limited to Eastern European orphanages. Children living in western societies who are raised in abusive and neglectful homes demonstrate similar growth failure. The nomenclature for this condition has varied throughout the years, but it is now commonly termed *psychosocial short stature* (PSS) [17]. By understanding the multiple presentations and possible mechanisms behind PSS, we can better understand the root causes of the institutional short stature seen in our adopted population and better tailor treatments to ensure catch-up growth.

PSS is a failure in growth that occurs in association with emotional deprivation or psychologic harassment, for which there is no other explanation [17]. Several distinct subtypes have been described that pertain to children residing in institutional care settings. The first pattern (type I) occurs in infants under stress or deprivation. Babies characteristically demonstrate poor growth and decreased appetite but show normal growth hormone (GH) response [17]. This growth failure may be related to the absence of touch and consequent underuse of calories for growth [18].

The second pattern (type II) is seen in older children living in stressful or deprived environments. In these children, stature is affected more than weight and bizarre behaviors, including abnormal food rituals and hyperphagia, are commonly encountered [19,20]. This form of growth failure seems to be attributable to reversible GH deficiency [19,20]. When children are removed from these situations and placed in caring and nurturing environments, there is a return to normal GH secretion and evidence of catch-up growth. Miller and colleagues [21] demonstrated the reversible nature of the GH insufficiency in a child whose GH profile normalized after his removal from the stressful environment. Improvement in GH release seems to occur through an increase in GH pulse amplitude with no change in pulse frequency [22,23]. A subset of older children has now also been described (type III); unlike most of the children with the older type of PSS (type IIA), these children present with anorexia, more symmetric growth failure (height and weight), and a more normal GH response to provocative testing [24,25]. Children adopted from international orphanages have been shown to demonstrate each of these growth patterns on arrival, suggesting that the stunting seen in many adopted children may be consistent with PSS.

One of the hallmarks of PSS is the reversible nature of growth failure when the child is removed from the adverse environment. King and Taitz [26] reported on the catch-up growth of children after abuse. At the time of the initial assessment, all the children had evidence of poor growth (mean height z score of -1.32). Those children removed and placed in long-term foster care had the most marked increase in growth: more than 55% of the children increased by more than one point compared with only 11% of those who remained in their original homes. Wyatt and coworkers [27] examined 45 preschoolers after the children were placed in foster care. They found an above-average increase in height velocity and an increase in the mean height z score of 0.61. Colombo and colleagues [28] also noted a greater increase in the growth of previously malnourished children who were placed in adoptive homes compared with those who remained in their original home or were institutionalized. Gohlke and coworkers [29] recently found that children with PSS who were removed from their adverse environment improved in height velocity and height SD. Additionally, most showed improved GH concentrations; only 18% of the children studied seemed to have irreversible GH deficiency after their care transition.

To make the argument that the observed growth failure in adopted institutionalized children is similar to that in children with PSS reported from North America and Western Europe, significant catch-up growth must be observed. Two studies [30,31] examined the growth of 240 female Korean orphans adopted into the United States. These studies showed that all the girls had evidence of growth improvement, with a correlation between the extent of catch-up and the age of the child at adoption. Johnson and colleagues [32] reported a mean growth velocity z score of +5.5 for children adopted from Romania. Job and Quelquejay [33] followed four siblings from Colombia adopted into France and found that despite the fact that all four were stunted on arrival, each child had spontaneous catch-up of more than 2 SDs. Benoit and coworkers [13] observed that all the children adopted at younger than 6 months of age and 87% of those adopted at older than 6 months of age had caught up within 1 year after adoption. Despite significant growth stunting on arrival, Rutter [14] found catch-up in weight and height for most children in a cohort of Romanian adoptees; at follow-up, only 1% of the children had a height less than the third percentile. A child's ability to return to age norms may be related to several factors, including age at placement and the extent of stunting on arrival. Johnson [34] reported that catch-up to age norms had been achieved by 78% of the Romanian children who had been adopted before 18 months of age. Older children demonstrated a similar height velocity at adoption; however, because of the greater deficit at arrival, they failed to catch up fully within the period of observation [34].

We surveyed 339 families who had adopted children from Eastern Europe [35] and asked for the growth parameters of the children at birth, adoption, and follow-up. Our results confirmed the results of previous studies, demonstrating stunted growth before adoption, with the mean height z score falling from -0.14 at birth to -2.03 at the time of adoption (mean age at adoption = 3.66 years; see Table 1). Our adoptive families reported a significant catch-up in their child's growth, to -0.69 at the time of the survey (mean age = 8.0 years, average of 4.33 years spent with their US family). Linear regression analysis revealed that the age and height at the time of adoption were negative predictors of growth, whereas body mass index (BMI) was a positive predictor. The three variables accounted for 57% of the variance ($r^2 = 0.57$, $P = .001$).

It is apparent that children adopted from institutional settings in Eastern Europe and China have evidence of growth failure, which seems to relate directly to the duration of time these children spent in the orphanage setting. It is likely that a multitude of factors contributes to this "institutional short stature." Although there is compelling evidence to suggest that adopted children are likely experiencing PSS, this has not yet been fully confirmed. Furthermore, the exact environmental mechanisms that influence the child's GH secretion and ultimately influence his or her ability to grow have not yet been determined. Numerous theories have been proposed to understand the cause of PSS. Green and colleagues [36] suggested that nutritional factors are unlikely to play a role because of the rapidity of hormonal changes. Changes in sleep patterns have also been proposed as a cause of other forms of GH abnormalities [37,38]. Children with PSS have been shown to exhibit unusual sleep patterns that may lead to abnormal GH secretion [39], because maximal GH release occurs during sleep [40]. Children who remain in stressful environments not only fail to show the expected improvement in spontaneous GH production but fail to grow in response to administration of GH [41,42]. This suggests that the cause of growth failure seen in children who live in stressful environments cannot be attributed completely to insufficient spontaneous GH release but may also be related to induced GH insensitivity.

Stress as an influence on growth?

The poor growth and developmental abnormalities seen in institutionalized children might be mediated through the hypothalamic-pituitary-adrenal (HPA) "stress" axis, which has clearly been shown to have a significant impact on the body's growth response. This system could be one of the key links between the external environment and the observed changes in the child at adoption. By understanding this system, we may be able to understand better the causes and, ultimately, the prevention of the underlying abnormalities.

Numerous animal studies have shown that lifelong changes in an organism's responsiveness to stress can be controlled through early life experiences. Using animal handling models [43,44] and animal models of prenatal maternal stress, alcohol consumption, and malnutrition [45,46], investigators have demonstrated that one can influence development of the HPA axis, creating abnormal levels of stress hormones. These abnormal levels of the stress hormone have been shown to correlate with poor cognitive [47] and emotional functioning [48,49] and with poor growth. Numerous experiments with rodents have demonstrated the ability of acute stressors to increase the HPA axis hormone levels, along with a concomitant decrease in GH levels [50–54]. Researchers are elucidating the mechanisms through which stress influences GH, but several studies have shown an inverse correlation between the stress-induced HPA hormones and release of GH [55–59].

Similar to the findings in animals, we have seen that children who experienced adverse events early in their lives seem to be at risk to develop an abnormal stress response later in life [60–64]. Early childhood development in an orphanage has been shown to affect the development of the HPA axis adversely. Carlson and Earls [65] showed that children living in orphanages with a poor quality of care had lower baseline morning cortisol levels and abnormally elevated noon and afternoon values compared with children living in enriched environments. In our studies of children living in Romanian orphanages, we demonstrated a significant elevation in cortisol responses to stressful stimuli [66]. Compared with US controls, children living in these orphanages had significantly higher cortisol levels (measured before and after a physical examination and blood draw) [67]. We also noted that the institutionalized children had evidence of significant growth stunting; mean heights noted for the girls and boys were -4.76 and -4.13 SDs below the mean for age, respectively. We also found that stunted growth correlated with cortisol values ($r = -0.187$, $P = .029$), suggesting that the HPA axis may be a link between environmental influences and physical and developmental responses.

We know that when a child is removed from an adverse environment, catch-up growth is a fundamental component of recovery. Less is known about whether the observed growth changes after adoption correlate with a change in the HPA axis of the child after he or she has lived in a nurturing family or whether these adverse changes are lifelong, as is the case for animals. Gunnar and coworkers [68] evaluated children from Romania 6.5 years after their adoptions and found that a subset of children who were older at the time of adoption still had significantly higher cortisol values than did children who spent less time in an orphanage. Ongoing studies are currently examining whether responsiveness of the HPA axis occurs after adoption and whether these changes correlate with the child's ability to grow.

Long-term impact of growth: precocious puberty?

Growth delay seems to be an almost universal finding in adopted post-institutionalized children. There seems to be a strong correlation between the extent of growth failure and the time a child spent in an orphanage. Although the mechanisms for growth loss have yet to be fully elucidated, they may share components with psychosocial growth failure. As pediatric practitioners begin to care for these children, we can confidently counsel the new families regarding the likelihood of catch-up growth. Growth improvements do not always occur but are common enough that we often advise parents to delay having their children evaluated for poor growth for at least 3 to 6 months after arrival in anticipation of this expected improvement. If an increase in growth velocity has not occurred by 6 months after adoption, a referral to a pediatric endocrinologist is likely warranted. Although the observed increase in growth velocity is the general rule, long-term outcome data regarding the postinstitutionalized child are not available.

Unfortunately, rapid growth changes may come at a price, especially for girls. Several studies and anecdotal accounts from parents have suggested that internationally adopted girls may be at risk for early puberty, which may ultimately affect final adult height. Adolfsson and Westphal [69] initially described girls adopted from India and Bangladesh who had evidence of early puberty. All the girls studied were small at arrival (-2.1 SDs). They noted pronounced post-adoption catch-up growth in these children (improvement of 3.2 SDs). Among the girls who manifested early puberty, four had begun menstruation by the age of 7.6 years, which led to the suggestion that early puberty was related to the increased metabolic activity exhibited during catch-up growth.

Proos and colleagues [70] later reported that girls from India who were adopted by Swedish families also experienced puberty significantly earlier than Swedish and Indian control groups. Most girls had evidence of malnutrition on their arrival in Sweden, but after adoption, most had a significant improvement in growth. Bourguignon and coworkers [71] found similar results, reporting that several internationally adopted children, including one boy, had evidence of early puberty and that the timing of puberty may be related to catch-up growth. Baron and colleagues [72] suggested a correlation between the risk of early puberty and the extent of catch-up growth in 13 children adopted into France. In contrast to these reports, Job and Quelquejay [33] studied four children adopted from a single family and showed no relation between catch-up growth and precocious puberty.

Virdis and colleagues [73] described 19 girls adopted from developing countries who were referred for precocious puberty. In this study, all the girls had demonstrated signs of puberty by the age of 6.9 years. Girls who were older at the time of adoption showed evidence of greater malnutrition and had the greatest delay in bone age. At 1 year after adoption, these differences were no longer observed. In several of the girls, puberty was medically delayed using gonadotropin-releasing hormone agonist (GnRHa), which demonstrated a slowing in their bone age advancement and, ultimately, a greater predicted final height. The nontreated girls had a rapid advancement through puberty, with a corresponding rapid change in bone age that resulted in heights less than predicted. Researchers concluded that the rapid completion of puberty resulted in an overall negative impact on final adult height.

The concern regarding early puberty and its impact on ultimate adult height in adopted children led Mul and coworkers [74] to examine the benefits of GH therapy for girls undergoing pharmacologic delay of puberty. They reported that the addition of GH in adopted girls undergoing hormonal delay with GnRHa resulted in a greater height velocity and increased predicted adult height compared with those receiving GnRHa alone. This finding differs from that of Tuvemo and colleagues [75], who found little enhancement to final height with GnRHa, GH, or both. Several fundamental differences existed between the two studies, including the duration of treatment and the method of predicting height before treatment, which would have an impact on interpretation of the results. Further studies are needed to determine the normal course and ultimate final adult heights for children placed through intercountry adoption. Furthermore, the use of GH to augment height gain after delay of puberty needs additional evaluation.

Most studies to date have examined the predictors of precocious puberty in small numbers of children. Few large studies exist that examine the frequency of early puberty in internationally adopted children. Baron and coworkers [72] surveyed 99 French families and found that by parental report, precocious puberty was noted in 44.9% of the girls and 8.6% of the boys. In our survey of children adopted from Eastern Europe [35], 30% of the girls' families reported any signs of early puberty. No boys were reported with early puberty. The mean age for breast development in our survey was 8.8 ± 2.5 years, and pubic hair was first reported at an average age of 9.1 ± 2.3 years. By most accounts, this is nearly normal and would not likely meet the criteria for early puberty. The concerning finding was that menarche occurred at a mean age of 10.5 ± 2.6 years, as opposed to a mean of 12.88 ± 1.2 years reported for girls born in the United States [76]. This suggests that the duration of time between breast budding and menarche was less than 2 years, which differs from the 2.9 years reported for many US-born children [76]. The accelerated speed with which the girls progressed through puberty was similar to that reported by Virdis and colleagues [73]. The trend of rapidly progressing puberty may be of greater concern for the young girl and her family than the actual age of onset for breast budding.

There clearly are some limitations in interpreting the data to date. Sampling and recall bias may be influencing the results. The cross-sectional nature of our data limits the conclusions that can be drawn concerning any specific child. Preliminary analysis of the data from the University of Minnesota International Adoption Project, which collected data from 55% of the children adopted to the State of Minnesota between 1990 and 1998, suggests a similar trend toward early and rapidly progressing puberty (Dana Johnson, MD, PhD, personal communication, 2005). Among the 126 girls for whom complete data for the onset of breast, pubic hair, and menarche was reported, there is evidence of rapid completion of puberty. Mean age for the onset of breast budding was 10.49 years (95% confidence interval: 10.0–11.0), that for pubic hair development was 10.58 years (95% confidence interval: 10.3–11.8), and that for menarche was 11.1 years (95% confidence interval: 10.8–11.3). Analysis and review of these data need to be completed before a true assessment can be made, but the data do continue to suggest a trend toward rapid completion of puberty in internationally adopted girls. Early and accelerated puberty may further compound the "differences" felt by the young girl in her new environment and could "further aggravate the psychological problems associated with both early puberty and adoption" [73]. This potential additional risk for girls warrants further investigation. As discussed previously, the timing of menarche in adopted girls occurs early by US standards. Our own review of the expected age of menarche in the countries from which most children have been adopted (Fig. 2) revealed that the girls who are demonstrating early puberty after adoption are doing so not

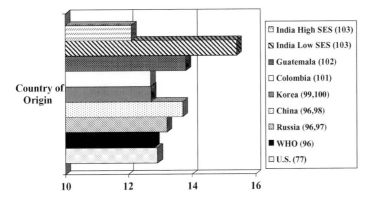

Fig. 2. Mean age of menarche in countries of adoption. The mean age of menarche is reported for several countries from which most children are adopted and is compared with US mean values. SES, socioeconomic status; WHO, World Health Organization.

only early by US standards but by the standards in their birth countries. Clearly, a genetic norm for this early puberty is unlikely [96–103].

Much is known about the risk of early puberty for girls adopted internationally, but precocious puberty in boys seems to be much less common. Bourguignon and coworkers [71] noted early puberty in a single boy. Baron and colleagues [72] reported that of the 99 French families surveyed, early puberty was reported in 44.9% of the girls (49 girls) compared with only 8.6% of the boys (3 of 35 boys surveyed). No other studies have been reported that describe early puberty in boys. The cause of this female predominance for early puberty is not fully understood. It may be an extension of the significantly higher rates of idiopathic central precocious puberty seen in girls in general. Other causes of early puberty specific to the population of adopted girls cannot be excluded. As further studies elucidate the basis of early puberty in girls, the differential expression of puberty between boys and girls in this population may become apparent.

What is truly "early" puberty for internationally adopted children?

The current data examining the onset and progression of puberty in girls after adoption suggest that the mean age at thelarche or adrenarche may not seem truly early by US standards, whereas menarche does seem to be occurring early. There is, however, great controversy as to the definition of "normal" as well as "early" with regard to pubertal timing. Data collected in the 1960s regarding nonadopted girls had suggested that thelarche typically occurred at 11.2 ± 1.0 years and menarche occurred, on average, at 13.5 ± 1.0 years [77]. Menarche in North America had been reported to occur somewhat earlier, at a mean age of 12.7 years [78]. Within the past decade, many US physicians and parents have noted an earlier trend for thelarche and perhaps menarche. This impression was validated in a study reported by Herman-Giddens and coworkers [76], who found that the breast development occurred at the mean age of 10.0 ± 1.8 years and that menarche occurred at the mean age of 12.9 ± 1.2 years (Table 2). This was similar to the Third National Health and Nutrition Examination Survey (NHANES III) study [79] findings, which reported a mean menarcheal age of 12.7 years. Given the earlier observed timing of physical changes, the relatively larger SDs, and numerous issues raised about the methodologies used in the various studies, what is normal and what would then constitute early puberty [80–83] have come into question. The cause of this trend to earlier puberty is not clearly established and likely is attributable to multiple factors. Improved genetics, environmental factors and exposures, health, and nutrition [84,85] all are likely to have had a significant positive impact (for a full review, see the article by Parent and colleagues [86]).

What then is the cause of early puberty in internationally adopted girls, and how common is early puberty in this group? The relative risk for a girl adopted internationally is not known, and the data are limited in the studies that have been conducted to date. The relative risk of early puberty for children in their new countries seems higher, in general, than for native-born children. Girls adopted internationally into Belgium seemed to be at an 80 times increased risk for early puberty compared with girls born in Belgium [87]. In Denmark, Teilmann and coworkers [88] estimated the rate of early puberty to be 20 times higher in adopted girls than in native Danish girls.

The rate for this increased risk has yet to be calculated for children adopted into the United States. Our study is the only one to date reporting early puberty in adopted children. Our survey of 193 girls found that 30% (57 of 193 girls) were reported by their family to have early breast bud development and that 12% (23 of 193 total girls) had menarche by mean age of 10.5 ± 2.6 years. The low number of reports from the United States may reflect a negative referral bias, given the described controversy surrounding our definition of normal, and thus the early age of puberty in the United States. The completion of the International Adoption Project at the University of Minnesota is likely to add to findings about the US experience.

The question remains, however, regarding the cause of the observed early rates of puberty for adopted girls. Multiple factors are likely to play a role. Improved

Table 2

Review of pubertal timing in girls after international adoption compared with reference populations [76,77]

Study	Marshall and Tanner [77]	Herman-Giddens and colleagues [76]	Proos and colleagues [70]	Baron and colleagues [72]	Mason and colleagues [35]	Johnson (personal communication, 2005)
Subjects	192	15,439 (white)	107	30	193	126
Breast	11.2 ± 1.0	10.0 ± 1.8			8.8 ± 2.5	10.5
Menarche	13.5 ± 1.0	12.9 ± 1.2	11.6	11.3	10.5 ± 2.6	11.1

nutrition and rapid growth changes have been implicated [69–72]. Other influences are also likely to play a role. The impact of early deprivation and stress may influence this risk of early puberty. The HPA stress axis has been shown to have an impact on the timing of puberty in animal models and clinical cases [89–92]. Reports have demonstrated the influence of early life on the HPA axis of adopted children in an orphanage setting [65,68]; thus, this factor may also play a role. The report of Krstevska-Konstantinova and colleagues [87] calls into question the relation between early puberty and deprivation because they found that children who migrated into Belgium with their families also had an increased rate of early puberty. These researchers did not, however, measure cortisol values or the response of the HPA axis to stress, so it still is possible that this axis has an impact on early puberty. Other factors (eg, environmental toxins, endocrine disrupters) could perhaps explain the relation between the child's environment and his or her risk of early and rapid pubertal changes [86]. Further multicenter studies are needed to understand better not only the relative risk of early puberty but the possible cause of these changes.

Summary

We are beginning to understand the consequences of an adopted child's early environment on subsequent growth and puberty. On arrival to their new family, international adoptees are frequently much smaller than their age-matched peers. The influences and mechanisms responsible for institutional short stature have yet to be fully elucidated, but there are likely many. Most children show significant and rapid growth catch-up, which makes a more detailed evaluation by a physician unnecessary for many children. The hormonal mechanisms that govern these changes are unknown at present but may be similar to those previously reported for PSS. In girls, growth acceleration may come at the price of early puberty, which may be associated with acceleration of the pubertal process, leading to early menarche and premature cessation of bone elongation. The physical changes associated with puberty may cause further stress for the affected child and her adopted family. In deciding to intervene, the health care practitioner must consider not only the influence of the child's early puberty on the final adult height but the impact on the child's current emotional and developmental status. At the present time, the long-term benefit of pharmacologic intervention to delay puberty or to enhance growth has yet to be fully elucidated and further studies are needed to determine whether this approach offers any advantages for the child. As families in the West adopt more children from abroad, there is increased need for specialized medical services to evaluate and treat these children. Many adopted children quickly overcome the impact of their early environment and demonstrate rapid growth and development improvements. Health care providers must be aware of these potential problems so as to address and anticipate the postadoption medical issues or problems that may develop. It is only with future research that we can understand the cause of such issues and help to alleviate the difficulties that new parents and children must overcome as they become a family.

References

[1] UNICEF. The state of the world's children 1998. New York: Oxford University Press; 1998.
[2] Waterlow JC. Post-neonatal mortality in the Third World. Lancet 1988;2(8623):1303.
[3] Martorell R, Mendoza F, Castillo R. Poverty and stature in children, vol. 14. New York: Raven Press; 1988.
[4] Gardner L. Deprivation dwarfism. Sci Am 1972;227:76–82.
[5] Chapin H. A plan of dealing with atrophic infants and children. Arch Pediatr 1908;25:491–6.
[6] Chapin H. Are institutions for infants necessary? JAMA 1915;64:1–3.
[7] Spitz R. Hospitalism, an inquiry into the genesis of psychiatric conditions in early childhood. Psychoanalytical Study of Children 1945;1:53–74.
[8] Spitz R. Hospitalism, a follow-up report. Psychoanalytical Study of Children 1946;2:113–7.
[9] Talbot NBSE, Burke BS, Lindemann E, et al. Dwarfism in healthy children: its possible relation to emotional, nutritional and endocrine disturbances. N Engl J Med 1947;236:783–9.
[10] Widdowson E. Mental contentment and physical growth. Lancet 1951;1:1316–8.
[11] Johnson DE, Miller LC, Iverson S, et al. The health of children adopted from Romania. JAMA 1992;268(24):3446–51.
[12] Miller LC, Hendrie NW. Health of children adopted from China. Pediatrics 2000;105(6):e76.
[13] Benoit TC, Jocelyn LJ, Moddemann DM, et al. Romanian adoption. The Manitoba experience. Arch Pediatr Adolesc Med 1996;150(12):1278–82.
[14] Rutter M. Developmental catch-up and deficit following adoption after severe global early privation. English and Romanian Adoptees (ERA) Study Team. J Child Psychol Psychiatry 1998;39(4):465–76.
[15] Miller LC, Kiernan MT, Mathers MI, et al. Developmental and nutritional status of internationally adopted children. Arch Pediatr Adolesc Med 1995;149:40–4.
[16] Groze V, Ileana D. A follow-up study of adopted children from Romania. Child Adolesc Social Work J 1996;13(6):541–65.
[17] Blizzard RM, Bulatovic A. Syndromes of psychosocial short stature. In: Lifshitz F, editor. Pediatric endocrinology. 3rd edition. New York: Marcel Dekker; 1996. p. 83–93.
[18] Field T. Massage therapy for infants. J Dev Behav Pediatr 1995;16:105–11.
[19] Powell GF, Brasel JA, Blizzard RM. Emotional deprivation and growth retardation simulating idiopathic hypopituitarism. I. Clinical evaluation of the syndrome. N Engl J Med 1967;276(23):1271–8.
[20] Powell GF, Brasel JA, Raiti S, et al. Emotional deprivation and growth retardation simulating idiopathic hypopituitarism. II. Endocrinologic evaluation of the syndrome. N Engl J Med 1967;276(23):1279–83.
[21] Miller JD, Tannenbaum GS, Colle E, et al. Daytime pulsatile growth hormone secretion during childhood and adolescence. J Clin Endocrinol Metab 1982;55(5):989–94.
[22] Albanese A, Hamill G, Jones J, et al. Reversibility of physiological growth hormone secretion in children with psychosocial dwarfism. Clin Endocrinol (Oxf) 1994;40(5):687–92.
[23] Stanhope R, Adlard P, Hamill G, et al. Physiological growth hormone (GH) secretion during the recovery from psychosocial dwarfism: a case report. Clin Endocrinol (Oxf) 1988;28(4):335–9.
[24] Skuse D, Albanese A, Stanhope R, et al. A new stress-related syndrome of growth failure and hyperphagia in children, associated with reversibility of growth-hormone insufficiency. Lancet 1996;348(9024):353–8.
[25] Gohlke BC, Frazer FL, Stanhope R. Body mass index and segmental proportion in children with different subtypes of psychosocial short stature. Eur J Pediatr 2002;161(5):250–4.

[26] King JM, Taitz LS. Catch up growth following abuse. Arch Dis Child 1985;60(12):1152−4.

[27] Wyatt DT, Simms MD, Horwitz SM. Widespread growth retardation and variable growth recovery in foster children in the first year after initial placement. Arch Pediatr Adolesc Med 1997;151(8):813−6.

[28] Colombo M, de la Parra A, Lopez I. Intellectual and physical outcome of children undernourished in early life is influenced by later environmental conditions. Dev Med Child Neurol 1992;34(7):611−22.

[29] Gohlke BC, Frazer FL, Stanhope R. Growth hormone secretion and long-term growth data in children with psychosocial short stature treated by different changes in environment. J Pediatr Endocrinol Metab 2004;17(4):637−43.

[30] Winick M, Meyer KK, Harris RC. Malnutrition and environmental enrichment by early adoption. Science 1975;190(4220):1173−5.

[31] Lien NM, Meyer KK, Winick M. Early malnutrition and "late" adoption: a study of their effects on the development of Korean orphans adopted into American families. Am J Clin Nutr 1977;30(10):1734−9.

[32] Johnson D, Miller L, Iverson S, et al. Post-placement catch-up growth in Romanian orphans with psychosocial short stature. Pediatr Res 1993;33:89A.

[33] Job JC, Quelquejay C. Growth and puberty in a fostered kindred. Eur J Pediatr 1994;153(9):642−5.

[34] Johnson DE. Long-term medical issues in international adoptees. Pediatr Ann 2000;29(4):234−41.

[35] Mason P, Narad C, Jester T, Parks J. A survey of growth and development in the internationally adopted child. Pediatr Res 2000;47:209A.

[36] Green WH, Campbell M, David R. Psychosocial dwarfism: a critical review of the evidence. J Am Acad Child Psychiatry 1984;23(1):39−48.

[37] Guilhaume A, Benoit O, Gourmelen M, et al. Relationship between sleep stage IV deficit and reversible HGH deficiency in psychosocial dwarfism. Pediatr Res 1982;16:299−303.

[38] Wolff G, Money J. Relationship between sleep and growth in patients with reversible somatotropin deficiency (psychosocial dwarfism). Psychol Med 1973;3:18−27.

[39] Mouridsen S, Nielsen S. Reversible somatotropin deficiency (psychosocial dwarfism) presenting as conduct disorder and growth hormone deficiency. Develop Med Child Neuro 1990;32:1087−104.

[40] Sassin JF, Parker DC, Mace JW, et al. Human growth hormone release: relation to slow-wave sleep and sleep-walking cycles. Science 1969;165(892):513−5.

[41] Frasier SD, Rallison ML. Growth retardation and emotional deprivation: relative resistance to treatment with human growth hormone. J Pediatr 1972;80(4):603−9.

[42] Tanner JM. Resistance to exogenous human growth hormone in psychosocial short stature (emotional deprivation). J Pediatr 1973;82(1):171−2.

[43] Levin S. Infantile experience and resistance to physiological stress. Science 1957;126:405−6.

[44] Meaney MJ, Aitken DH, van Berkel C, et al. Effect of neonatal handling on age-related impairments associated with the hippocampus. Science 1988;239(4841 Pt 1):766−8.

[45] Ogilvie KM, Rivier C. Prenatal alcohol exposure results in hyperactivity of the hypothalamic-pituitary-adrenal axis of the offspring: modulation by fostering at birth and postnatal handling. Alcohol Clin Exp Res 1997;21(3):424−9.

[46] Clarke AS, Wittwer DJ, Abbott DH, Schneider ML. Long-term effects of prenatal stress on HPA axis activity in juvenile rhesus monkeys. Dev Psychobiol 1994;27(5):257−69.

[47] Lupien SJ, McEwen BS. The acute effects of corticosteroids on cognition: integration of animal and human model studies. Brain Res Brain Res Rev 1997;24(1):1−27.

[48] de Haan M, Gunnar MR, Tout K, et al. Familiar and novel contexts yield different associations between cortisol and behavior among 2-year-old children. Dev Psychobiol 1998;33(1):93−101.

[49] Schmidt LA, Fox NA, Rubin KH, et al. Behavioral and neuroendocrine responses in shy children. Dev Psychobiol 1997;30(2):127−40.

[50] Armario A, Lopez-Calderon A, Jolin R, et al. Sensitivity of anterior pituitary hormones to graded levels of psychological stress. Life Sci 1986;39:471–5.

[51] Kokka N, Garcia JF, George R, et al. Growth hormone and ACTH secretion: evidence for an inverse relationship in rats. Endocrinology 1972;90(3):735–43.

[52] Brown GM, Martin JB. Corticosterone, prolactin, and growth hormone responses to handling and new environment in the rat. Psychosom Med 1974;36(3):241–7.

[53] Armario A, Castellanos JM, Balasch J. Adaptation of anterior pituitary hormones to chronic noise stress in male rats. Behav Neural Biol 1984;41(1):71–6.

[54] Schalch S, Reichlin S. Plasma growth hormone concentration in the rat determined by radioimmunoassay: influence of sex, pregnancy, lactation, anesthesia, hypophysectomy and extracellular pituitary transplants. Endocrinology 1966;79:275–80.

[55] Kuhn CM, Pauk J, Schanberg SM. Endocrine responses to mother-infant separation in developing rats. Dev Psychobiol 1990;23(5):395–410.

[56] Rivier CV, Vale W. Involvement of corticotropin-releasing factor and somatostatin in stress-induced inhibition of growth hormone secretion in the rat. Endocrinology 1985;117(6): 2478–82.

[57] Smith EL, Coplan JD, Trost RC, et al. Neurobiological alterations in adult nonhuman primates exposed to unpredictable early rearing. Relevance to posttraumatic stress disorder. Ann NY Acad Sci 1997;821:545–8.

[58] Barbarino A, Corsello SM, Della Casa S, et al. Corticotropin-releasing hormone inhibition of growth hormone-releasing hormone-induced growth hormone release in man. J Clin Endocrinol Metab 1990;71(5):1368–74.

[59] Barinaga M, Bilezikjian LM, Vale WW, et al. Independent effects of growth hormone releasing factor on growth hormone release and gene transcription. Nature 1985;314(6008):279–81.

[60] Elizinga B, Schmahl C, Vermetten E, et al. Higher cortisol levels following exposure to traumatic reminders in abuse related PTSD. Neuropsychopharmocology 2003;28:1656–65.

[61] Gunnar MR, Brodersen L, Nachmias M, et al. Stress reactivity and attachment security. Dev Psychobiol 1996;29(3):191–204.

[62] Nachmias M, Gunnar M, Mangelsdorf S, et al. Behavioral inhibition and stress reactivity: the moderating role of attachment security. Child Dev 1996;67(2):508–22.

[63] Halligan SL, Herbert J, Goodyer IM, et al. Exposure to postnatal depression predicts elevated cortisol in adolescent offspring. Biol Psychiatry 2004;55(4):376–81.

[64] Brown ES, Varghese FP, McEwen BS. Association of depression with medical illness: does cortisol play a role? Biol Psychiatry 2004;55(1):1–9.

[65] Carlson M, Earls F. Psychological and neuroendocrinological sequelae of early social deprivation in institutionalized children in Romania. Ann NY Acad Sci 1997;807:419–28.

[66] Mason P, Stallings J, Worthman C, et al. The effect of institutionalization on growth and the stress response. Pediatr Res 2000;47:134A.

[67] Wothman CM, Stallings JF. Hormone measures in finger-prick blood spot samples: new field methods for reproductive endocrinology. Am J Phys Anthropol 1997;104:1–21.

[68] Gunnar MR, Morison SJ, Chisholm K, et al. Salivary cortisol levels in children adopted from Romanian orphanages. Dev Psychopathol 2001;13(3):611–28.

[69] Adolfsson S, Westphal O. Early pubertal development in girls adopted from Far-Eastern countries. Pediatr Res 1981;15:82.

[70] Proos LA, Hofvander Y, Tuvemo T. Menarcheal age and growth pattern of Indian girls adopted in Sweden. I. Menarcheal age. Acta Paediatr Scand 1991;80(8–9):852–8.

[71] Bourguignon JP, Gerard A, Alvarez Gonzalez ML, et al. Effects of changes in nutritional conditions on timing of puberty: clinical evidence from adopted children and experimental studies in the male rat. Horm Res 1992;38(Suppl 1):97–105.

[72] Baron S, Battin J, David A, et al. Precocious puberty in children adopted from foreign countries. Arch Pediatr 2000;7(8):809–16.

[73] Virdis R, Street ME, Zampolli M, et al. Precocious puberty in girls adopted from developing countries. Arch Dis Child 1998;78(2):152–4.

[74] Mul D, Oostdijk W, Waelkens JJ, et al. Gonadotrophin releasing hormone agonist treatment with or without recombinant human GH in adopted children with early puberty. Clin Endocrinol (Oxf) 2001;55(1):121–9.

[75] Tuvemo T, Gustafsson J, Proos LA. Growth hormone treatment during suppression of early puberty in adopted girls. Swedish Growth Hormone Advisory Group. Acta Paediatr 1999;88(9):928–32.

[76] Herman-Giddens ME, Slora EJ, Wasserman RC, et al. Secondary sexual characteristics and menses in young girls seen in office practice: a study from the Pediatric Research in Office Settings network. Pediatrics 1997;99(4):505–12.

[77] Marshall WA, Tanner JM. Variations in pattern of pubertal changes in girls. Arch Dis Child 1969;44(235):291–303.

[78] Tanner JM, Davies PS. Clinical longitudinal standards for height and height velocity for North American children. J Pediatr 1985;107(3):317–29.

[79] NHANES III. NHANES III reference manual and reports. Analytic and reporting guidelines. Third National Health and Nutrition Examination Survey (1988–1994). Hyattsville, MD: National Center for Health Statistics, Centers for Disease Control and Prevention; 1997.

[80] Rosenfield RL, Bachrach LK, Chernausek SD, et al. Current age of onset of puberty. Pediatrics 2000;106(3):622–3.

[81] Lee PA, Kulin HE, Guo SS. Age of puberty among girls and the diagnosis of precocious puberty. Pediatrics 2001;107(6):1493.

[82] Kaplowitz PB, Oberfield SE. Reexamination of the age limit for defining when puberty is precocious in girls in the United States: implications for evaluation and treatment. Drug and Therapeutics and Executive Committees of the Lawson Wilkins Pediatric Endocrine Society. Pediatrics 1999;104(4 Pt 1):936–41.

[83] Midyett LK, Moore WV, Jacobson JD. Are pubertal changes in girls before age 8 benign? Pediatrics 2003;111(1):47–51.

[84] Kaplowitz PB, Slora EJ, Wasserman RC, et al. Earlier onset of puberty in girls: relation to increased body mass index and race. Pediatrics 2001;108(2):347–53.

[85] Anderson SE, Dallal GE, Must A. Relative weight and race influence average age at menarche: results from two nationally representative surveys of US girls studied 25 years apart. Pediatrics 2003;111(4 Pt 1):844–50.

[86] Parent AS, Teilmann G, Juul A, et al. The timing of normal puberty and the age limits of sexual precocity: variations around the world, secular trends, and changes after migration. Endocr Rev 2003;24(5):668–93.

[87] Krstevska-Konstantinova M, Charlier C, Craen M, et al. Sexual precocity after immigration from developing countries to Belgium: evidence of previous exposure to organochlorine pesticides. Hum Reprod 2001;16(5):1020–6.

[88] Teilmann G, Main K, Skakkebaek N, et al. High frequency of central precocious puberty in adopted and immigrant children in Denmark. Horm Res 2002;58:135.

[89] Rabin D, Gold PW, Margioris AN, et al. Stress and reproduction: physiologic and pathophysiologic interactions between the stress and reproductive axes. Adv Exp Med Biol 1988;245:377–87.

[90] Rivier C, Rivier J, Vale W. Stress-induced inhibition of reproductive functions: role of endogenous corticotropin-releasing factor. Science 1986;231(4738):607–9.

[91] Magiakou MA, Mastorakos G, Webster E, et al. The hypothalamic-pituitary-adrenal axis and the female reproductive system. Ann NY Acad Sci 1997;816:42–56.

[92] Compagnucci CV, Compagnucci GE, Lomniczi A, et al. Effect of nutritional stress on the hypothalamo-pituitary-gonadal axis in the growing male rat. Neuroimmunomodulation 2002;10(3):153–62.

[93] Johnson D, Albers L, Iverson S, et al. Health status of US adopted Eastern European orphans. Pediatr Res 1996;39:134A.

[94] Albers LH, Johnson DE, Hostetter MK. Health of children adopted from the former Soviet Union and Eastern Europe. Comparison with preadoptive medical records. JAMA 1997; 278(11):922–4.

[95] Johnson D, Aronson J, Federici R, et al. Profound, global growth failure afflicts residents of pediatric neuropsychiatric institutes in Romania. Pediatr Res 1999;45:126A.

[96] Wang Y, Adair L. How does maturity adjustment influence the estimates of overweight prevalence in adolescents from different countries using an international reference? Int J Obes Relat Metab Disord 2001;25(4):550–8.

[97] Iampol'skaia IA. Dynamics of puberty levels in girls of Moscow. Gig Sanit 1997;3:29–30.

[98] Graham MJ, Larsen U, Xu X. Secular trend in age at menarche in China: a case study of two rural counties in Anhui Province. J Biosoc Sci 1999;31(2):257–67.

[99] Kim KH, Spurgeon JH, French KE, et al. Somatic comparisons of South Korean children and youths born and reared in a rural area with the descendants of rural to urban migrants. Am J Hum Biol 2002;14(4):476–85.

[100] Hwang JY, Shin C, Frongillo EA, et al. Secular trend in age at menarche for South Korean women born between 1920 and 1986: the Ansan Study. Ann Hum Biol 2003;30(4):434–42.

[101] Chavarro J, Villamor E, Narvaez J, et al. Socio-demographic predictors of age at menarche in a group of Colombian university women. Ann Hum Biol 2004;31(2):245–57.

[102] Kahn A, Schroeder D, Martorell R, et al. Age at menarche and nutritional supplementation. J Nutr 1995;125(Suppl 4):1090–6.

[103] Rao S, Joshi S, Kanade A. Height velocity, body fat and menarcheal age of Indian girls. Indian Pediatr 1998;35(7):619–28.

PEDIATRIC CLINICS

OF NORTH AMERICA

Pediatr Clin N Am 52 (2005) 1369–1393

ELSEVIER
SAUNDERS

Prenatal Alcohol and Drug Exposures in Adoption

Julian K. Davies, MD[a,b,c],*, Julia M. Bledsoe, MD[a,b,c]

[a]*Division of General Pediatrics, University of Washington School of Medicine, Seattle, WA, USA*
[b]*Center for Adoption Medicine, University of Washington Pediatric Care Center, 4245 Roosevelt Way,
NE, Box 354780, Seattle, WA 98105, USA*
[c]*FAS Diagnostic and Prevention Network, University of Washington, Seattle, WA, USA*

Families choosing to adopt domestically or internationally are faced with the possibility of prenatal substance exposure for their child. Alcohol use, drug use, and exposure to environmental agents by pregnant women can be harmful to the developing fetus, with many known short- and long-term effects on organ development, somatic growth, and neurodevelopment. As more families turn to medical providers for consultation before adoption, the challenge of accurately identifying risk factors for poor medical or cognitive outcomes becomes paramount. Prenatal substance exposure is just one of the important factors in this risk assessment, but it is one that parents frequently have questions about before and after the adoption of their child.

One of the greatest challenges when providing a preadoption medical review is obtaining accurate and complete information on children referred for adoption from different countries. Health care providers in most countries acknowledge the significance of medication and substance use in a pregnant woman. In all countries, including the United States, however, mothers may not have received prenatal care and abstracts from medical records provided for preadoptive review typically lack complete medical histories, exact amounts of the substances used, or the timing of use in a woman's pregnancy. Substance use may also be mistranslated or confused by colloquial terms from specific regions of the United States or other countries. Thus, although accurate data from the pregnancy history are crucial to helping medical professionals assess the risk of adverse neuro-

* Corresponding author. Center for Adoption Medicine, University of Washington Pediatric Care Center, 4245 Roosevelt Way, NE, Box 354780, Seattle, WA 98105.

E-mail address: joolian@u.washington.edu (J.K. Davies).

0031-3955/05/$ – see front matter © 2005 Elsevier Inc. All rights reserved.
doi:10.1016/j.pcl.2005.06.015

developmental outcomes in waiting children, these data are frequently not available at the time of a preadoptive medical review.

Even with prenatal history available, it is extremely difficult to disentangle the consequences of prenatal substance exposure from the frequent comorbidities of prematurity, malnutrition, neglect, abuse, multiple placements, or institutional deprivation as discussed elsewhere in this issue. In addition, prenatal exposure to potentially harmful substances often occurs in the context of social dysfunction: poverty, parental addiction, impaired parenting, and poor access to services. A family history of mental illness or learning disabilities is often present, which can carry additional genetic risk for adoptees. In considering long-term data on outcomes in adopted children, any conclusions must control for these various mitigating factors. Nonetheless, the accurate identification of prenatal substance exposure and use of objective diagnostic techniques for fetal alcohol syndrome can help to clarify the risk of developmental outcomes for adopted children.

This article addresses the major potential prenatal substance exposures for children joining families by adoption or, indeed, by birth: alcohol, opiates, tobacco, marijuana, cocaine, and methamphetamines. For each substance, we review the teratogenicity of the exposure and identify the spectrum of neurodevelopmental issues that can present in children exposed to this substance. Diagnosis of the spectrum of fetal alcohol outcomes is also discussed. When possible, we provide country-specific statistics on exposure risks for adopted children.

General principles of teratology

A teratogenic substance, whether it is a drug like alcohol or thalidomide or an exposure like radiation, is a substance that may have the potential to produce a congenital malformation. The timing of exposure in embryogenesis and dose of the exposure have an impact on whether a prenatal substance exposure leads to a malformation or other neurobehavioral manifestation later in life. Some teratogenic exposures have little risk of causing malformation if the timing and dose are below the teratogenic threshold. For example, radiation exposure is not a risk for cancer if the dose and timing of exposure are minimal. It is also difficult, in many instances, to claim a direct causal link between an exposure and an outcome. The discussion that follows incorporates data gathered from animal and human studies to describe the range of outcomes that may be related to prenatal exposures in adopted children.

Prenatal alcohol exposure

Overview

Fetal alcohol syndrome (FAS) is a permanent birth defect caused by maternal consumption of alcohol during pregnancy. It is a clinically defined syndrome, characterized by growth deficiency, central nervous system (CNS) damage and dysfunction, and a unique cluster of minor facial anomalies [1,2]. Although FAS is the most extreme and recognizable expression of the adverse effects of alcohol on the developing human being, alcohol exposure can cause a range of anomalies and disabilities that fall under the umbrella of fetal alcohol spectrum disorders (FASDs) [3].

FAS has been described in all races and countries. Since its description in the medical literature in the United States in 1973 by Jones and colleagues [4], FAS has remained the leading known cause of preventable mental retardation and developmental disability in the United States [5]. The worldwide incidence of FAS is estimated at 1 to 3 per 1000 live births in epidemiologic studies [6,7]. The incidence in a foster care population in the state of Washington, a higher risk group that may be representative of many children placed for adoption, is 10 per 1000 children [8]. It is estimated that greater than 1% of all children born in the United States may have FASDs [5]. In the United States, a recent Centers for Disease Control and Prevention (CDC) survey revealed that approximately 10% of pregnant women used alcohol and approximately 2% engaged in binge drinking or frequent use of alcohol. Furthermore, more than 50% of women of childbearing age who did not use birth control reported alcohol use, and 12.4% reported binge drinking [9].

Prevalence estimates of FASDs in other countries are unclear, in part, because of disagreements regarding diagnostic criteria for the syndrome. Statistics on risk behaviors for FASDs in other countries are available, however, with country profiles of drinking patterns and trends described in the World Health Organization's "Global Status Report on Alcohol 2004" [10]. It is estimated that at least 30% of women of childbearing age in Russia drink alcohol on a regular basis [7]. Weekly alcohol use among Russian teenagers is up to 54% [11]. In Kazakhstan, the prevalence of drinking among women is lower than in Russia; however, the number of juvenile alcoholics is rapidly increasing, despite the state's effort to curb drinking [10]. China has seen a striking increase in alcohol consumption over the past decades, but social and cultural factors seem to have limited drinking among women. Unfortunately, the trends in youth drinkers and urban centers are becoming more similar to those in Western countries [12,13]. Alcohol consumption among young women in South Korea is also on the rise. It is estimated that the number of female drinkers there has increased by 3% a year since 1995, mostly because of the increased presence of women in the work force. The percentage of Korean college students who have one to three drinks per week is 96.4%, with little difference between the sexes; drinking is viewed as a good way to build social ties [14]. The lifetime prevalence of alcohol use among students in Guatemala City was found to be 26.5% [10].

Mechanism

Alcohol is a known teratogen with a range of impacts on multiple organ systems, including the CNS. During gestation, alcohol exposure damages the architecture, neuronal migration, and synaptogenesis of the developing CNS. The timing and dose of alcohol use during pregnancy are important when considering potential implications for the developing fetus. Children born to women who drink heavily on a regular basis in the first trimester of pregnancy have the greatest risk of CNS damage. The first month of pregnancy is particularly crucial for development of the CNS and the midportion of the face. Unfortunately, this early in pregnancy, many women do not realize that they are pregnant and continue their usual pattern of alcohol ingestion.

Although there is no convincing evidence to date of a "safe" threshold of prenatal alcohol consumption, one major dysmorphology textbook argues that low birth weight (LBW) and "mild" disability can be seen at an exposure of roughly 2 alcoholic drinks per day (lower in recent studies). When 4 to 6 drinks are consumed, additional clinical features become evident. Most of the children who are believed to have the full expression of FAS are born to women consuming 8 to 10 drinks or more per drinking occasion, on a regular if not daily basis, for at least the first trimester. It is estimated that the risk of a "serious problem" in the offspring of chronically alcoholic women ranges from 30% to 50%. The greatest risk is that of mental deficiency as well as a host of learning and behavioral disabilities [15].

Fetal host factors are also important in the development of FASDs. Some fetuses seem to be more susceptible to the adverse effects of alcohol use by the birth mother. For example, fraternal twins have been shown to have markedly different outcomes, even though the amount and timing of their prenatal alcohol exposure are the same. One explanation implicates genetically determined differences in the metabolism of alcohol at the fetal level because of differences in alcohol dehydrogenase activity [16].

Diagnosis

There is not a uniformly agreed on approach to diagnosing FASDs. The two most widely used criteria for the evaluation of children with potential FASD continuum diagnoses are the 1996 Institute of Medicine Criteria [17,18] and the University of Washington criteria, published in 1997 and revised in 2004 [19]. The CDC has also just released new guidelines for diagnosis [20]. All proposed diagnostic methods have in common the desire to define FASD cases more clearly with objective, quantitative, and reproducible methods.

FAS is currently defined as a constellation of the following:

- Growth deficiency
- Cluster of facial anomalies, including a thin upper lip, a smooth philtrum (vertical groove between the nose and upper lip), and small palpebral fissure lengths (PFLs; width of eye openings)
- Evidence of CNS damage or dysfunction
- History of maternal alcohol use during pregnancy

To diagnose the spectrum disability of FAS, all four of these criteria should be examined.

Growth deficiency

In the evaluation of growth deficiency in adopted children, there are two important considerations. Growth deficiency is the least sensitive diagnostic criterion for FAS. In many cases of clear-cut FAS, growth deficiency is not present at the time of diagnosis. In one of the longest running FAS diagnostic clinics in the country, only 40% of children who meet the facial, CNS, and prenatal exposure criteria for FAS are growth deficient (Susan Astley, PhD, University of Washington, unpublished data, 2005). These children are often referred to as having atypical FAS. Growth deficiency is not a *sine qua non* for a diagnosis of FAS.

Also, in the population of children waiting for adoption, many children without FAS are growth deficient on the basis of malnutrition and early childhood deprivation. When looking at growth deficiency as a teratogenic effect of prenatal alcohol exposure, it is important to take into consideration other explanatory factors. As a result, it may be prudent to allow time for postadoption "catch-up growth" before ranking the level of growth deficiency in a newly adopted child.

Facial features

Although growth deficiency is the least sensitive criterion for FAS diagnosis, the three sentinel facial features are the most sensitive and specific. In examining a child for the facial features of FAS, there are several tools to aid in the objective evaluation of the lip, philtrum, and PFLs of children. The subject's upper lip thickness and depth of the philtrum can be assessed and scored with the "Lip-Philtrum Guide" (Fig. 1) as originally described by Astley and Clarren [2]. Philtrum depth is ranked by holding the Lip-Philtrum Guide next to the patient's relaxed face and selecting the picture that best matches the patient's philtrum. Upper lip thickness is measured in the same fashion. A score of 4 or 5 is considered consistent with the thin lip and smooth philtrum characteristic of FAS. If the child is present for evaluation, PFLs can be measured in millimeters with a rigid clear plastic ruler, with the examiner seated in front of the subject. This method of eye measurement is prone to significant error in inexperienced hands, however, based on our clinic's experience, where we compare visual esti-mates with computer-assisted measurements. A more accurate and reproducible method is to use FAS Facial Photographic Analysis Software to aid in assessment of facial features [21]. This image analysis software has been used as a screening and diagnostic tool for a foster care population, where it identified the facial features of FAS with 99% sensitivity and 99% specificity [8].

For use in preadoption evaluations, this software tool is most useful if the photograph being evaluated has an internal measure of scale, which allows the PFLs to be assessed accurately. In general, photographs of children forwarded for

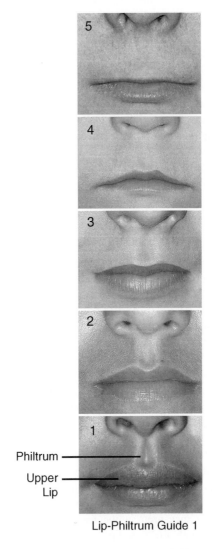

Philtrum

Upper
Lip

Lip-Philtrum Guide 1

Fig. 1. Fetal alcohol syndrome lip—philtrum guide. (Courtesy of S. Astley, PhD, Seattle, WA.)

preadoptive review are not able to be accurately assessed with this software tool unless families have taken the photographs themselves. Before traveling to a child's birth country, parents may be prepared in advance to photograph a child accurately, with an internal measure of scale allowing for later analysis. Our clinic uses an office supply sticker of known width that is placed on the patient's forehead. A close-up photograph should be taken with the patient's unsmiling and relaxed face filling the entire frame. A digital 3-megapixel (or higher resolution) camera is ideal. The lens of the camera should be directly in front of the face (the "Frankfort horizontal plane") to minimize rotation of the face

internal measure of scale

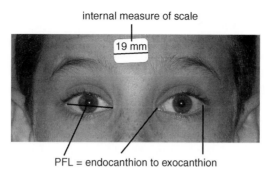

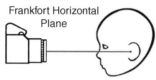

PFL = endocanthion to exocanthion

Frankfort Horizontal
Plane

Fig. 2. Measuring palpebral fissure lengths (PFLs) using an internal measure of scale and the Frankfort horizontal plane. (Courtesy of S. Astley, PhD, Seattle, WA.)

(Fig. 2). This standardized digital frontal facial photograph is used to measure the PFLs, lip, and philtrum accurately [8]. A complete guide for how to obtain and analyze facial photographs with the use of Lip-Philtrum Guides and the FAS Facial Photographic Analysis Software can be found on the University of Washington Fetal Alcohol Syndrome Diagnostic and Prevention Network web site (http://www.fasdpn.org).

The key phenotypic FAS facial features are short PFLs, a smooth philtrum, and a thin upper lip, and the face of FAS requires all three to be present. Other features, such as epicanthal folds, a flat nasal bridge, a short upturned nose, "clown eyebrows" (often associated with microcephaly), or prominent ears, may be seen more often in children with FAS; however, they are not diagnostic because they can be normal developmental or ethnic features, especially in the international adoptee population. There is also evidence that the greater the magnitude of expression of FAS features, the higher is the risk for underlying brain damage [22].

It is far more difficult to assess a child's potential risk of FASDs when the facial features are not extreme. For example, it is possible for an individual who is prenatally exposed to alcohol to have a completely normal facial phenotype. These individuals should still be considered at risk for learning and behavioral problems, which may be as severe as the problems faced by individuals with a FAS facial phenotype. When the FAS facial features are fully present, it is reasonable to conclude that prenatal alcohol exposure had an adverse impact on fetal development. With more normal facial features, however, it is difficult to differentiate the impact of alcohol from that of other genetic and environmental factors.

Central nervous system damage

CNS damage can be determined on the basis of structural malformation (eg, microcephaly or an abnormal brain MRI scan), neurologic disease (eg, seizures), or neuropsychometric data that indicate dysfunction, especially in multiple areas of cognition. Again, it is important to recognize that in the population of adopted children, poor head growth and developmental delay may also be attributable to a range of other causes, including but not limited to prenatal infections, malnutrition, early deprivation, or neurogenetic factors affecting brain growth. A period of catch-up growth and development should be allowed after a child joins his or her family before attributing CNS impairment to prenatal substance exposure. If the underlying cause of the impairment is prenatal alcohol exposure, the impairment persists.

History of maternal alcohol use

Maternal alcohol consumption can be difficult to quantify from adoption records. In all countries, including the United States, the exact amount, type, and timing of alcohol use during pregnancy may be impossible to ascertain.

Typical records include the following statements:

"Parents are registered as alcoholics" (Russia)
"Mother drinks but not to excess" (Kazakhstan)
"Mother drank two bottles of soju (355 mL of 25% liquor) every week until the fourth month of pregnancy" (Korea)

Alcohol use by the birth mother may be simply listed as unknown. When considering potential prenatal alcohol exposure, it is helpful to consider known risk factors frequently comorbid with maternal alcohol use. In studies conducted in the United States, women who give birth to alcohol-affected children have common psychosocial attributes. In general these women:

- Have a history of alcoholism
- Are multiparous
- Are older at the time of an affected pregnancy
- Have a history of mental illness [23]

The presence or absence of these psychosocial factors can be used for alcohol use risk stratification of birth mothers, even in the absence of a specific history in the available records. For example, if a boy born to a 40-year-old multigravida woman with a history of incarceration has a lip and philtrum of grade 4 in photographic evaluation and a borderline head circumference for his age, he should be considered at risk for alcohol-related disability even if no information about alcohol use during pregnancy is available. Because these psychosocial data describing birth mothers of alcohol-affected children were obtained in US studies, extrapolation to women in other countries should be approached with caution. In the absence of similar information from a child's country of origin, however, these data may help to delineate the best estimate of a child's risk for FASDs. Finally, although these comorbid factors should be taken into consideration to assess the risk or probability of prenatal exposure, they cannot be used to serve as evidence when considering an FASD diagnosis.

Outcomes

As a teratogen, alcohol has been implicated in a long list of congenital defects, although our understanding of the actual rates of specific types of malformation has been hampered by lack of diagnostic consensus. Alcohol-exposed children do seem to have higher rates of eye (eg, refractive errors, strabismus, optic nerve hypoplasia), ear (recurrent otitis, conductive and sensorineural hearing loss), cleft palate, cardiac; renal, and orthopedic malformations [24].

The neurodevelopmental outcomes related to prenatal alcohol problems are varied and complex. Each child exposed to alcohol has a different neurobehavioral profile, because the dose and timing of alcohol use in each pregnancy is unique. Each child's genetic makeup and prenatal, postnatal, and postadoptive environments also play a role in his or her outcome. Despite the lack of a specific behavioral phenotype for FAS, the literature does suggest some general patterns of disability. Manifestations of CNS dysfunction may include mental retardation or borderline IQ scores [25], neuromotor deficits, attentional issues and hyperactivity [26], and impaired social and adaptive abilities [27]. Children and adults with prenatal alcohol exposure can have unusual language and communication disabilities, particularly in the arena of social communication [28]. Subtle peripheral nerve damage leading to coordination and sensory integration problems has been described [29]. Prenatal alcohol exposure may also impair "executive functioning," the higher level cognitive functions involved in planning and guiding behavior to achieve a goal in an efficient manner [30]. Importantly, none of these neurodevelopmental patterns are pathognomonic for prenatal alcohol exposure.

These primary neurodevelopmental disabilities can cause significant impairment in an individual's ability to navigate daily activities, school, social relationships, and basic living requirements. These manifestations of FAS can lead to secondary disabilities as affected individuals with an all-too-often "invisible" disability attempt to function in society [25]. Individuals with FASDs are more likely to have a history of educational difficulties, trouble with the law, mental health problems, and substance abuse. Nevertheless, protective factors do exist, and a younger age at diagnosis and higher percentage of life in a stable and nurturing home have been shown to reduce the likelihood of these secondary disabilities [31]. Early diagnosis can help to prevent secondary disabilities by providing early intervention as well as educational and environmental support strategies [26]. Intervention projects to identify protective factors and effective interventions for individuals with prenatal alcohol exposure are currently under way. Excellent handbooks for teachers and parents of children with FASDs are available [32,33].

Children born to alcoholic parents are themselves at risk for alcoholism later in life, regardless of whether or not they have FASDs. Because the disease of alcoholism seems to have a genetic predisposition, children of alcoholic parents should start substance abuse education early, with developmentally appropriate counseling. Adoptive parents should be informed of the risk of alcoholism in their adoptive children so as to facilitate appropriate educational opportunities and to help provide an alcohol-free environment.

Prenatal opiate exposure

Overview

In the United States, 2.3% of pregnancies in the Maternal Lifestyle Study involved heroin or methadone exposure [34]. In international adoption, the most commonly reported prenatal opiate exposure is heroin. Heroin use has made a resurgence in recent years, particularly in Eastern Europe and the former Soviet Union. The United Nations Office for Drug Control and Crime Prevention reported that the number of known heroin addicts rose by 30% in Russia in 1999 and had quadrupled since 1995, with a current prevalence of heroin abuse at 2.1% [11,35]. In Kazakhstan, the prevalence of heroin abuse is estimated at 1.3% [35]. Opiate use is also prevalent in the countries of Southeast Asia and parts of China, particularly near areas where opium is grown and in more urban areas. Although there are no official reports from China, unofficial estimates say that there could be up to 12 million total heroin users [36]. Pregnant women who enter drug treatment programs for addiction receive another opiate, methadone, as a substitute for heroin or opium. Because drug treatment programs are on the rise in Russia and China, prenatal exposure to methadone may also occur [36,37].

Mechanism

Despite the detrimental effects of opiates on the user, including the risk of addiction and exposure to the hazards of intravenous drug use (hepatitis B and C and HIV), opiate exposure to the developing fetus is not considered teratogenic. There is no known congenital malformation associated with prenatal opiate exposure. There have been harmful fetal effects described with heroin and methadone use, however, and infants born to addicted women can suffer withdrawal in the newborn period. Any child referred for international adoption with a maternal history of intravenous drug use should be considered at increased risk for HIV and hepatitis B and C.

Pregnancy

LBW and symmetric intrauterine grown retardation have been reported in the offspring of heroin abusers [38]. Pregnant heroin addicts also have a statistically significant increased risk of preterm delivery. Methadone use seems to have less effect on fetal growth and has not been shown to increase the risk of premature birth. For children born after a pregnancy complicated by opiate use, prenatal growth may be affected by maternal malnutrition and comorbid infections as well as by opiate exposure.

Neonatal abstinence syndrome

Neonatal abstinence syndrome (NAS) has been well described in infants born to opiate-dependent mothers. The symptoms of NAS include CNS symptoms (eg, hyperirritability, tremors, convulsions), gastrointestinal distress, respiratory distress, and autonomic disturbances [39]. It has been reported that the infants of methadone-addicted mothers experience more severe symptoms for a longer time, partly because of the longer half-life of this opiate. Treatment of symptomatic infants generally consists of providing children with a tapering schedule of tincture of opium, morphine, or phenobarbital while monitoring clinical symptoms. During the withdrawal period, infants may dramatically influence normal caretaker interactions because they are often resistant to cuddling or soothing and have a decreased ability to respond normally to auditory or visual stimuli. The long-term impact of these early alterations in socialization may be detrimental, particularly in an orphanage setting, where nurturing caretaking may already be less frequent.

The onset of withdrawal symptoms is usually between 48 and 72 hours after birth. It is highly unlikely that a child born overseas is going to be available for adoption at this point; thus, most families adopting internationally do not directly encounter NAS. Clues to NAS may be present in the preadoption record, however, and should alert families and professionals to the possibility of prenatal opiate exposure and other risks associated with injection drug use in birth mothers (HIV and hepatitis B and C).

Behavior and cognition

In some early studies, concerns about prenatal opiate exposure and poor developmental outcome were described. Reported neurodevelopmental problems included a short attention span, hyperactivity, and sleep disturbances in prenatally exposed children assessed at the age of 12 to 34 months [40]. More recent studies also suggest mild memory and perceptual difficulties in older children, but overall test scores are still within the normal range [41]. In general, it is difficult to differentiate the impact of a poor postnatal environment and prenatal heroin exposure on children's long-term outcome. One study suggests that opiate-exposed children have increased susceptibility to adverse environmental influences compared with nonexposed children [42]. Conversely, a study from Canada suggests that drug-exposed infants adopted out at birth were equivalent to Canadian matched controls in terms of educational achievement and IQ. The adopted children did, however, have increased rates of early adult depression [43].

Prenatal tobacco exposure

Overview

Tobacco smoking during pregnancy is one of the most ubiquitous prenatal exposures. The prevalence of smoking during pregnancy in the United States is estimated by maternal self-report at 11% and is higher in teens (18%) and women with less than 12 years of formal education (27%) [44]. Fortunately, these rates are declining [45]. In Russia, the prevalence was 16% of pregnant women in one study and seems to be increasing [46]. In Kazakhstan, it is estimated that one third of the adult population smokes [47]. In China, the prevalence of tobacco use among pregnant women has been estimated at 2% but is increasing [48], and 60% of nonsmoking pregnant women in Guangzhou had husbands who smoked [49]. The World Health Organization reports that in South Korea, 7% of women smoke tobacco; in Guatemala, 17% of women smoke [47]. True exposure rates are likely to be significantly higher, because parental self-report routinely under-estimates actual exposure. Unfortunately, adoptee tobacco exposure status is often unknown.

Prenatal tobacco exposure has consistently been associated with poor fetal growth and is the single most important cause of LBW in developed countries [50]. Even environmental smoke exposure has been implicated in LBW, fetal death, and preterm delivery [51]. Myriad perinatal complications and child health problems are linked to fetal and childhood smoke exposure. Finally, a growing body of evidence is implicating smoking during pregnancy in a range of adverse behavioral and cognitive outcomes.

Mechanism

Cigarette smoke contains tar, nicotine, and carbon monoxide. Tar contains numerous substances (lead, cyanide, cadmium, and more) known to be harmful to the fetus [52]. Nicotine readily crosses the placenta and distributes freely to the CNS, having direct and indirect effects on neural development [38]. Intrauterine hypoxia, mediated by carbon monoxide and reduced uterine blood flow, is a major mechanism of the growth impairment linked to prenatal tobacco exposure.

Pregnancy

Tobacco smoking during pregnancy has been associated with placenta previa, placental abruption, premature rupture of membranes, preterm birth, intrauterine growth restriction, and sudden infant death syndrome (SIDS) [53]. A dose-dependent association with cleft lip anomalies has also been noted [54].

Tobacco's impact on fetal growth is perhaps the most consistent and concerning, given the range of potential impacts on health and developmental outcomes. Maternal smoking has an impact on fetal growth symmetrically in a dose-related fashion [55] and causes an estimated 5% reduction in relative weight for every pack of cigarettes smoked per day [56]. Because pregnant women who smoke deliver babies weighing 150 to 250 g less than babies of nonsmokers, tobacco smoking essentially doubles the chance of having a LBW baby [57]. Unfortunately, maternal smoking is also associated with a smaller head circumference at birth [58].

Child health

It is difficult to differentiate the impact of prenatal smoking and environmental tobacco smoke on childhood health problems, such as respiratory and ear infections, pulmonary function, asthma, and SIDS. Postnatal smoke exposure increases the incidence of middle ear disease, asthma, wheeze, cough, phlegm production, bronchitis, bronchiolitis, pneumonia, and impaired pulmonary function, and it has also been associated with snoring, adenoidal hypertrophy, tonsillitis, and sore throat [59]. Smoking during pregnancy does cause poor lung growth, affecting pulmonary function in infancy and childhood [60,61], and seems to confer additional risk to postnatal smoke exposures [62].

With respect to tobacco-associated growth impairment, children generally demonstrate "catch-up" with their weight and height percentiles during their first few years of life, with less catch-up noted in head circumference [63,64]. In fact, a trend toward obesity is noted [65].

Behavior and cognition

Dose-effect impacts of prenatal tobacco exposure on behavioral and cognitive outcomes of children have been reported, even after controlling for confounders like socioeconomic status, parental education and mental health, prenatal growth, other prenatal exposures (eg, alcohol), and postnatal disadvantages [66].

Infants born to mothers who smoke tobacco display higher rates of impaired neurobehavior, with reduced habituation, lower arousal, hypertonicity and tremors, sucking difficulties, worse autonomic regulation, and altered cries [67]. Nursery evaluations suggest a withdrawal effect as well [68]. The international adoptee population seems less likely to have these dysregulations repaired by consistent and regulating caregiving while residing in a hospital or orphanage.

There is a consistent association described between prenatal exposure to tobacco and attention deficit hyperactivity disorder (ADHD)–like symptoms [67] and externalizing behavior problems [69,70]. Antisocial traits like disruptive behavior, conduct disorder, and later delinquency have been linked to prenatal tobacco exposure as well [71]. Although these associations are clear, proving the causal relation is challenging, because not all these studies control for confounders, such as prenatal alcohol exposure.

There is a stronger link between prenatal smoking and behavioral outcomes than that described with impaired cognition. Smoking during pregnancy was associated with decreased IQ scores for children by an average of 4 points [72], however, which was prevented by smoking cessation [73]. Other studies are inconsistent but have suggested persistent deficits in auditory-related tasks like verbal memory, language, and auditory processing [74].

It is unclear if these outcomes can be attenuated by nurturing and regulating home environments and to what extent the effects of tobacco interact with other biologic, prenatal, and postnatal risk factors. For internationally adopted children, the potential interaction of these developmental modifiers seems particularly complex, with tobacco-associated risks (eg, LBW and microcephaly, infant neuro-behavior, toddler negativity [75], childhood attention and/or impulse control deficits, antisocial behavior) occurring within a trajectory of caregiving moving from early institutional neglect to later nurturing and stimulating family environments.

Prenatal marijuana exposure

Overview

Marijuana is a popular recreational drug in many parts of the world. In the United States, 22% of high school students have used marijuana in the past month [76]. Estimates of marijuana use during pregnancy vary between 2% in broad surveys using maternal self-report [77] and 20% to 27% in higher risk populations using urine screens [78,79]. In the experience of our international adoption clinic, referrals outside North America have not included reports of prenatal marijuana exposure, but the United Nations Office on Drugs and Crime (UNODC) estimates that the annual prevalence of marijuana use is 3.9% in the Russian Federation, 2.4% in Kazakhstan, 0.3% in China, 0.1% in South Korea, and 3.2% in India [35]. In Guatemala, where the rate of drug consumption among young people is on the rise, marijuana consumption by teenagers is at 4% to 6.7% [80].

Mechanism

The principle psychoactive substance in marijuana, Δ-9-tetrahydrocannabinol (THC), rapidly crosses the placenta and may remain in the body for 30 days before excretion, thus prolonging potential fetal exposure. THC is also secreted in breast milk. Marijuana smoking produces higher levels of carbon monoxide than tobacco [38], which is hypothesized to be a potential mechanism of action of prenatal marijuana exposure's impact on the developing fetus.

Pregnancy

Marijuana use during pregnancy may have a modest effect on prenatal growth, but the results are inconsistent from study to study and diminish when potential cofounders are controlled [81–84]. These effects, if any, are not associated with later growth deficiency, although a few studies have suggested an impact on height [81] as well as persistent negative effects on head circumference in the offspring of heavy marijuana users [63]. This review found no consistent link between prenatal marijuana exposure and other adverse pregnancy outcomes or congenital malformations [85].

Behavior and cognition

Subtle effects of prenatal marijuana exposure on cognition have been observed in two large well-controlled study groups: a predominantly low-risk Ottawa cohort and a higher risk Pittsburgh population. The Ottawa authors argue that although prenatal tobacco exposure is associated with deficits in IQ, impulse control, and other fundamental aspects of performance, prenatal marijuana exposure does not impair IQ or basic visuoperception but influences the application of these skills in problem-solving situations requiring visual integration, analysis, and sustained attention [86]. Marijuana is thus argued to have an impact on higher level executive function and performance in a "top-down" fashion, in contrast to tobacco's "bottom-up" effects [87]. The Pittsburgh study group finds links to inattention and/or impulsivity [88] and subtle deficits in memory and learning [89]. This group also connects prenatal marijuana exposure with academic underachievement, perhaps reflecting less buffering of marijuana's effects by environment in this higher risk population [90].

Prenatal cocaine exposure

Overview

Cocaine has received much attention since the 1980s, when crack cocaine began to plague urban America. Early alarmist predictions about an epidemic of neurologically damaged "crack babies" gave way to guarded optimism with early reports of neurodevelopmental functioning reporting no differences attributable to cocaine exposure. Follow-up studies with more specific measures, however, suggest effects of prenatal cocaine abuse on aspects of neurobehavior and language, as demonstrated with specific developmental tasks.

The rate of prenatal cocaine exposure in the United States ranges from 0.3% to 31% depending on the population surveyed and method of ascertainment [77,78] and was 10% in the ongoing Maternal Lifestyle Study [34]. In our clinic's experience, reports of cocaine exposure in the international adoptee population are quite rare. The UNODC estimates the lifetime prevalence of cocaine consumption to be approximately 2% to 5% in a study of Guatemalan teenagers; in Russia, China, Korea, and other frequent countries of international adoption, the prevalence seems to be much less [35].

Mechanism

Cocaine and its metabolites readily cross the placenta, concentrating in amniotic fluid, and may produce direct neurotoxic effects, disturb monoaminergic (eg, dopamine, norepinephrine, serotonin) pathways, and cause vascular-mediated damage [91].

Pregnancy

⋄The use of cocaine in pregnancy has been associated with a number of obstetric complications, such as stillbirth, placental abruption, premature rupture of membranes, fetal distress, and preterm delivery [92]. Growth restriction is often reported but may require higher levels of exposure and does not seem to persist after birth [93]. There may be a dose-response effect of cocaine on newborn head circumference [94]. Other CNS lesions (eg, stroke, cystic changes, possible seizures), cardiac defects, and genitourinary (GU) anomalies have also been reported, but the few available large, controlled, population-based studies on cocaine exposure and malformations have reached contradictory conclusions [95].

Behavior and cognition

Prenatal cocaine abuse may cause specific neurobehavioral and learning problems, although it is not associated with global cognitive deficits [96,97]. The largest matched cohort study to date found no significant covariate-controlled associations between cocaine exposure and mental, psychomotor, or behavioral functioning through 3 years of age [98]. Infant neurobehavioral abnormalities like irritability or excitability, sleep difficulties, and state regulation difficulty as well as transient neurologic abnormalities like tremor, hypertonia, and extensor posturing have been reported [99,100]. Heavy prenatal cocaine use has been linked to poor memory and information processing in infancy [101]. At 3 years of age, increased fussiness, difficult temperament, and behavior problems were described [102]. Language delay has also been described, with foster or adoptive caregiving described as a promising protective factor [103,104].

Prenatal methamphetamine exposure

Overview

Methamphetamine abuse has increased dramatically in the United States in the past decade, especially in the western and midwestern states [105]. In Russia, cheap imported heroin still prevails, but abuse of home-produced ephedrine-based "vint" and other injectable amphetamines is on the rise and already predominates in certain cities, including Vladivostok and Pskov [106]. Methamphetamine abuse is a significant problem in Southeast Asia as well, with 19% of

Thai female students using methamphetamine in one school-based study [107]. The UNODC reports large increases in methamphetamine production and abuse in China, Singapore, and Thailand [35]. Because methamphetamine is relatively cheap to manufacture from readily available products, "home labs" are becoming increasingly common in many parts of the world. Unfortunately, the chemicals and byproducts involved are highly toxic and flammable.

Methamphetamine is a CNS stimulant that releases large amounts of dopamine, resulting in a sense of euphoria, alertness, and confidence [108]. It can be injected, smoked, snorted, or ingested orally. Prolonged use at high levels results in dependence and erratic behavior [105]. Evidence on the effects of prenatal methamphetamine use is still emerging, but effects on prenatal growth, behavior, and cognition have been described.

Mechanism

Studies of adult methamphetamine abusers have shown potential neurotoxic effects on subcortical brain structures, namely, decreased dopamine transporters, brain metabolism, and perfusion [108]. Although the impact of methamphetamine use during human pregnancy is currently unknown, animal studies have demonstrated neurotoxic effects of amphetamines and remodeling of synaptic morphology in response to prenatal methamphetamine exposure [109]. One study did describe a smaller putamen, globus pallidus, and hippocampus in methamphetamine-exposed children [108].

Pregnancy

Women using methamphetamine during pregnancy may have an increased rate of premature delivery and placental abruption [110]. Methamphetamine use during pregnancy is linked to fetal growth restriction and, occasionally, withdrawal symptoms requiring pharmacologic intervention at birth [111]. Clefting, cardiac anomalies, and fetal growth reduction have been described in infants exposed to amphetamines during pregnancy. These findings have been reproduced in animal studies [112].

Child health

Late effects on child health resulting from prenatal methamphetamine use are unknown. Children who live at or visit methamphetamine home labs face acute health and safety hazards from fires, explosions, and toxic chemical exposures, however. The caregiving environments of methamphetamine users are often characterized by chaos, neglect and abuse, and criminal behavior as well as the presence of firearms, contaminated sharps, and other risks [113].

Behavior and cognition

The scant research describing the outcomes of methamphetamine-exposed children describes possible links with aggressive behavior, peer problems, and hyperactivity [114,115]. A small recent study found that methamphetamine-exposed children scored lower on measures of visual motor integration, attention, verbal memory, and long-term spatial memory [108]. In rats, even low doses of prenatal methamphetamine exposure can alter learning and memory in adulthood [116].

Preadoption consultations case

Baby A

Baby A is waiting in an orphanage in a country overseas. She was born at an estimated 37 weeks of gestation after a reportedly uncomplicated pregnancy with no prenatal care. Apgar scores were reportedly normal. Growth parameters at birth were all reportedly in the fifth percentile at birth. The medical excerpt reports that the birth mother smoked and "used alcohol." There are no other prenatal substance exposures noted.

Baby A was her birth mother's eighth pregnancy and fifth delivery. The birth mother was 36 years of age at the time of delivery. Nothing else is known about the birth mother's mental or physical health or the health or whereabouts of the baby's birth father or siblings.

Baby A came to orphanage care from a hospital at 6 months of age after the parental rights were involuntarily terminated. On arrival at the orphanage, growth deficiency was noted but no other physical abnormalities were detected by the physicians. Her current growth includes height, weight, and occipital frontal circumference (OFC) at the third percentile. Her development is reportedly "adequate" now at 12 months of age. She is crawling, vocalizing, and manipulating objects. She smiles and laughs with familiar caregivers.

Baby B

Baby B is in foster care awaiting adoption. She was born prematurely at 31 weeks of gestation to a 20-year-old mother with a history of narcotic abuse during pregnancy. No alcohol use was noted in the chart. Late prenatal care was received. The birth mother has a history of depression, and the birth father has a history of learning disabilities and attentional problems. He is currently incarcerated. There are no siblings. Baby B's Apgar scores were 5 and 7, and the postnatal course was complicated by "mild" NAS. No other major problems occurred in the newborn period. The infant was discharged to foster care after

4 weeks in the hospital and has been in the same foster home for 12 months. Her growth parameters (height, weight, and OFC) at birth were in the 20th percentile adjusted for prematurity and have remained in that range over time. She is reportedly developing normally for her adjusted age. She also crawls, vocalizes, manipulates, smiles, and laughs.

Case discussions

In both cases, we have children at risk for future learning and behavior problems. This discussion focuses on the considerations during a preadoptive evaluation and when considering overall risk assessment.

Baby A's risks involve alcohol exposure in utero as well as a postnatal history of neglect and suboptimal stimulation while residing in an institutional setting. Although her growth and development are delayed for her stated age, these could be products of her environment rather than the teratogenic effect of alcohol. Without prenatal care documenting growth and development over time, the gestational age described at birth may be erroneous. It is important for the family to obtain as many details as possible about the birth mother's alcohol use, history of other mental or physical health issues, and circumstances surrounding termination of parental rights. Risk factors for heavy alcohol exposure include maternal age and parity. Photographic evaluation of this child's face for FAS is also crucial in helping to predict the risk and potential magnitude of learning and behavioral issues. Finally, the absence of documentation of parental mental or medical illness should not be equated with negative findings, because this information is often not gathered before referral for adoption.

Baby B's risks for long-term learning and behavior issues include prenatal substance exposure. It is important to recognize that when narcotic abuse is listed as the major exposure, there may be alcohol exposure as well. Many drug abusers do not consider drinking alcohol to be their "problem," even if their level of alcohol use could have a significant impact on the developing fetus. Baby B should also have evaluation of her facial features for FAS.

Baby B has had a more stable environment than baby A in these scenarios, and more is known about the family history. Baby B is more overtly at risk for learning and mental health issues, given her reported family history, although Baby A may also have genetic issues that have not been identified or disclosed.

Like Baby A, Baby B's development is also reasonable for her age when adjusted for prematurity. This early development is not a good predictor of long-term cognitive development for either child, however. Difficulties in behavioral regulation, language, memory, problem solving, and higher order thought processes (including "executive functioning") may not appear until later in life. Both children should be followed closely for learning and behavior issues related to prenatal substance exposure, prematurity, postnatal events, and family history. Given the family histories disclosed, both children have their own risk of substance abuse later in life.

Summary

Prenatal alcohol and drug exposures are of significant concern in many domestic and international adoptions. Unfortunately, the rates of these substance exposures are on the rise in many countries of origin. Pregnancy complications, premature birth, prenatal and postnatal growth deficiency, congenital defects, withdrawal syndromes, infant neurobehavioral dysregulation, and complex childhood behavioral and cognitive deficits can all result from such prenatal exposures. This review, and most of the research literature, has examined each of these alcohol and drug exposures one by one. In reality, polysubstance exposure is perhaps more common; however, to date, we have little understanding of how these and other prenatal exposures interact with each other to affect the developing fetus.

For children of adoption, it is sobering to consider how these substance exposures, in combination with other social and biologic risks, may make affected children more vulnerable to the adverse effects of malnutrition, neglect, abuse, multiple placements, or institutionalization. At a minimum, it seems less likely that early neurobehavioral problems can be repaired in such environments. Conversely, adopted children are typically received into loving and nurturing homes with motivated and resourceful parents. This is a remarkable intervention in and of itself, affording children with multiple vulnerabilities the opportunity for catch-up growth and development, formation of stable and secure attachments, early diagnosis of primary disabilities, appropriate services, and prevention of secondary disabilities. The lifelong impact of this caregiving trajectory on the long-term effects of prenatal alcohol and drug exposures remains to be seen.

Acknowledgments

The authors thank Susan Astley, PhD, Lisa Albers, MD, MPH, Cyndi Musar, and Heather Blumer for their assistance.

References

[1] Clarren SK, Smith DW. The fetal alcohol syndrome. N Engl J Med 1978;298(19):1063–7.
[2] Astley SJ, Clarren SK. Diagnosing the full spectrum of fetal alcohol-exposed individuals: introducing the 4-digit diagnostic code. Alcohol Alcohol 2000;35(4):400–10.
[3] Barr HM, Streissguth AP. Identifying maternal self-reported alcohol use associated with fetal alcohol spectrum disorders. Alcohol Clin Exp Res 2001;25(2):283–7.
[4] Jones KL, Smith DW, Ulleland CN, et al. Pattern of malformation in offspring of chronic alcoholic mothers. Lancet 1973;1(7815):1267–71.
[5] Sampson PD, Streissguth AP, Bookstein FL, et al. Incidence of fetal alcohol syndrome and prevalence of alcohol-related neurodevelopmental disorder. Teratology 1997;56(5):317–26.
[6] Stratton K, Howe CJ, Battaglia FC, editors. Fetal alcohol syndrome: diagnosis, epidemiology, prevention, and treatment. Washington, DC: National Academy Press; 1996.

[7] Abel E. The American paradox. In: Fetal alcohol abuse syndrome. New York: Plenum Press; 1998. p. 139–57.

[8] Astley SJ, Stachowiak J, Clarren SK, et al. Application of the fetal alcohol syndrome facial photographic screening tool in a foster care population. J Pediatr 2002;141(5):712–7.

[9] Centers for Disease Control and Prevention. Alcohol consumption among women who are pregnant or who might become pregnant–United States, 2002. MMWR Morb Mortal Wkly Rep 2004;53(50):1178–81.

[10] WHO Department of Mental Health and Substance Abuse. WHO Global Status Report on Alcohol 2004. Available at: http://www.who.int/substance_abuse/publications/global_status_report_2004_overview.pdf. Accessed May 5, 2005.

[11] United Nations Office for Drug Control and Crime Prevention (UNODCCP). Statistics. Vienna, Austria: United Nations Publication; 2002.

[12] Hao W, Chen H, Su Z. China: alcohol today. Addiction 2005;100(6):737–41.

[13] Cochrane J, Chen H, Conigrave KM, et al. Alcohol use in China. Alcohol Alcohol 2003;38(6): 537–42.

[14] Park K. GAPA Bangkok consultation: alcohol in Asia. The Globe 2001;4:30–1.

[15] Jones KL. Smith's recognizable patterns of human malformation. 5th edition. Philadelphia: WB Saunders; 1997.

[16] Stoler JM, Ryan LM, Holmes LB. Alcohol dehydrogenase 2 genotypes, maternal alcohol use, and infant outcome. J Pediatr 2002;141(6):780–5.

[17] Stratton KR, Howe CJ, Frederick C, Battaglia, editors. Fetal alcohol syndrome: diagnosis, epidemiology, prevention, and treatment. Committee to Study Fetal Alcohol Syndrome, Institute of Medicine. Washington, DC: National Academy Press; 1996.

[18] Hoyme HE, May PA, Kalberg WO, et al. A practical clinical approach to diagnosis of fetal alcohol spectrum disorders: clarification of the 1996 institute of medicine criteria. Pediatrics 2005;115(1):39–47.

[19] Astley SJ. Diagnosis of individuals with fetal alcohol spectrum disorders (FASD): the 4-digit diagnostic code. 3rd edition. Seattle, WA: University of Washington Publication Services; 2004.

[20] National Center on Birth Defects and Developmental Disabilities, Centers for Disease Control and Prevention. National Task Force on Fetal Alcohol Syndrome and Fetal Alcohol Effect. Fetal alcohol syndrome: guidelines for referral and diagnosis. Washington, DC: Department of Health and Human Services; 2004.

[21] Astley SJ, Clarren SK. A case definition and photographic screening tool for the facial phenotype of fetal alcohol syndrome. J Pediatr 1996;129(1):33–41.

[22] Astley SJ, Clarren SK. Measuring the facial phenotype of individuals with prenatal alcohol exposure: correlations with brain dysfunction. Alcohol Alcohol 2001;36(2):147–59.

[23] Astley SJ, Bailey D, Talbot C, et al. Fetal alcohol syndrome (FAS) primary prevention through FAS diagnosis: II. A comprehensive profile of 80 birth mothers of children with FAS. Alcohol Alcohol 2000;35(5):509–19.

[24] Martinez-Frias ML, Bermejo E, Rodriguez-Pinilla E, et al. Risk for congenital anomalies associated with different sporadic and daily doses of alcohol consumption during pregnancy: a case-control study. Birth Defects Res A Clin Mol Teratol 2004;70(4):194–200.

[25] Streissguth AP, Kanter J. The challenge of fetal alcohol syndrome: overcoming secondary disabilities. Seattle: University of Washington Press; 1997.

[26] Coles CD, Platzman KA, Raskind-Hood CL, et al. A comparison of children affected by prenatal alcohol exposure and attention deficit, hyperactivity disorder. Alcohol Clin Exp Res 1997;21(1):150–61.

[27] Weinberg NZ. Cognitive and behavioral deficits associated with parental alcohol use. J Am Acad Child Adolesc Psychiatry 1997;36(9):1177–86.

[28] Coggins TE, Friet T, Morgan T. Analysing narrative productions in older school-age children and adolescents with fetal alcohol syndrome: an experimental tool for clinical applications. Clin Linguist Phon 1998;12(3):221–36.

[29] Avaria ML, Mills JL, Kleinsteuber K, et al. Peripheral nerve conduction abnormalities in children exposed to alcohol in utero. J Pediatr 2004;144(3):338–43.

[30] Kodituwakku PW, Kalberg W, May PA. The effects of prenatal alcohol exposure on executive functioning. Alcohol Res Health 2001;25(3):192–8.

[31] Streissguth AP, Bookstein FL, Barr HM, et al. Risk factors for adverse life outcomes in fetal alcohol syndrome and fetal alcohol effects. J Dev Behav Pediatr 2004;25(4):228–38.

[32] Clarren SGB, editor. Teaching students with fetal alcohol spectrum disorder: building strengths, creating hope. Edmonton (AB): Alberta Learning–Special Programs Branch; 2004.

[33] Graefe S, editor. Living with FASD: a guide for parents. 3rd edition. Society of Special Needs Adoptive Parents. Vancover (BC): Groundwork Press; 2003.

[34] Lester BM, El Sohly M, Wright LL, et al. The Maternal Lifestyle Study: drug use by meconium toxicology and maternal self-report. Pediatrics 2001;107(2):309–17.

[35] UNODC Research and Analysis Section. United Nations Office on Drugs and Crime—World Drug Report 2004. Available at: http://www.unodc.org/unodc/world_drug_report.html. Accessed June 10, 2005.

[36] Kulsudjarit K. Drug problem in southeast and southwest Asia. Ann NY Acad Sci 2004; 1025:446–57.

[37] Somlai AM, Kelly JA, Benotsch E, et al. Characteristics and predictors of HIV risk behaviors among injection-drug-using men and women in St. Petersburg, Russia. AIDS Educ Prev 2002; 14(4):295–305.

[38] Chiriboga CA. Fetal alcohol and drug effects. Neurologist 2003;9(6):267–79.

[39] Finnegan LP. Effects of maternal opiate abuse on the newborn. Fed Proc 1985;44(7):2314–7.

[40] Rosen TS, Johnson HL. Long-term effects of prenatal methadone maintenance. NIDA Res Monogr 1985;59:73–83.

[41] Lifschitz MH, Wilson GS. Patterns of growth and development in narcotic-exposed children. NIDA Res Monogr 1991;114:323–39.

[42] Marcus J, Hans SL, Jeremy RJ. A longitudinal study of offspring born to methadone-maintained women. III. Effects of multiple risk factors on development at 4, 8, and 12 months. Am J Drug Alcohol Abuse 1984;10(2):195–207.

[43] Lipman EL, Offord DR, Boyle MH, et al. Follow-up of psychiatric and educational morbidity among adopted children. J Am Acad Child Adolesc Psychiatry 1993;32(5):1007–12.

[44] National Center for Health Statistics. Health. United States, 2004, with chartbook on trends in the health of Americans. Hyattsville, MD: National Center for Health Statistics; 2004.

[45] Hamilton BE, Martin JA, Sutton PD. Births: preliminary data for 2003. Natl Vital Stat Rep 2004;53(9):1–17.

[46] Grjibovski A, Bygren LO, Svartbo B, et al. Housing conditions, perceived stress, smoking, and alcohol: determinants of fetal growth in Northwest Russia. Acta Obstet Gynecol Scand 2004; 83(12):1159–66.

[47] World Health Organization. Tobacco or health. A global status report. Available at: http://www.cdc.gov/tobacco/who/. Accessed June 10, 2005.

[48] Lam SK, To WK, Duthie SJ, et al. The effect of smoking during pregnancy on the incidence of low birth weight among Chinese parturients. Aust NZ J Obstet Gynaecol 1992;32(2):125–8.

[49] Loke AY, Lam TH, Pan SC, et al. Exposure to and actions against passive smoking in non-smoking pregnant women in Guangzhou, China. Acta Obstet Gynecol Scand 2000;79(11): 947–52.

[50] Kramer MS. Intrauterine growth and gestational duration determinants. Pediatrics 1987;80(4): 502–11.

[51] Kharrazi M, DeLorenze GN, Kaufman FL, et al. Environmental tobacco smoke and pregnancy outcome. Epidemiology 2004;15(6):660–70.

[52] Lee MJ. Marihuana and tobacco use in pregnancy. Obstet Gynecol Clin North Am 1998; 25(1):65–83.

[53] Andres RL, Day MC. Perinatal complications associated with maternal tobacco use. Semin Neonatol 2000;5(3):231–41.

[54] Chung KC, Kowalski CP, Kim HM, et al. Maternal cigarette smoking during pregnancy and the risk of having a child with cleft lip/palate. Plast Reconstr Surg 2000;105(2):485–91.

[55] Macmahon B, Alpert M, Salber EJ. Infant weight and parental smoking habits. Am J Epidemiol 1965;82(3):247–61.

[56] Kramer MS, Olivier M, McLean FH, et al. Determinants of fetal growth and body proportionality. Pediatrics 1990;86(1):18–26.

[57] Samet JM. The 1990 report of the Surgeon General: the health benefits of smoking cessation. Am Rev Respir Dis 1990;142(5):993–4.

[58] Kallen K. Maternal smoking during pregnancy and infant head circumference at birth. Early Hum Dev 2000;58(3):197–204.

[59] DiFranza JR, Aligne CA, Weitzman M. Prenatal and postnatal environmental tobacco smoke exposure and children's health. Pediatrics 2004;113(4 Suppl):1007–15.

[60] Stick SM, Burton PR, Gurrin L, et al. Effects of maternal smoking during pregnancy and a family history of asthma on respiratory function in newborn infants. Lancet 1996;348(9034):1060–4.

[61] Gilliland FD, Berhane K, McConnell R, et al. Maternal smoking during pregnancy, environmental tobacco smoke exposure and childhood lung function. Thorax 2000;55(4):271–6.

[62] Jedrychowski W, Flak E. Maternal smoking during pregnancy and postnatal exposure to environmental tobacco smoke as predisposition factors to acute respiratory infections. Environ Health Perspect 1997;105(3):302–6.

[63] Fried PA, Watkinson B, Gray R. Growth from birth to early adolescence in offspring prenatally exposed to cigarettes and marijuana. Neurotoxicol Teratol 1999;21(5):513–25.

[64] Vik T, Jacobsen G, Vatten L, et al. Pre- and post-natal growth in children of women who smoked in pregnancy. Early Hum Dev 1996;45(3):245–55.

[65] Wideroe M, Vik T, Jacobsen G, et al. Does maternal smoking during pregnancy cause childhood overweight? Paediatr Perinat Epidemiol 2003;17(2):171–9.

[66] Weitzman M, Byrd RS, Aligne CA, et al. The effects of tobacco exposure on children's behavioral and cognitive functioning: implications for clinical and public health policy and future research. Neurotoxicol Teratol 2002;24(3):397–406.

[67] Olds D. Tobacco exposure and impaired development: a review of the evidence. MRDD Research Reviews 1997;3:257–69.

[68] Law KL, Stroud LR, LaGasse LL, et al. Smoking during pregnancy and newborn neurobehavior. Pediatrics 2003;111(6 Pt 1):1318–23.

[69] Williams GM, O'Callaghan M, Najman JM, et al. Maternal cigarette smoking and child psychiatric morbidity: a longitudinal study. Pediatrics 1998;102(1):e11.

[70] Fergusson DM, Horwood LJ, Lynskey MT. Maternal smoking before and after pregnancy: effects on behavioral outcomes in middle childhood. Pediatrics 1993;92(6):815–22.

[71] Wakschlag LS, Pickett KE, Cook Jr E, et al. Maternal smoking during pregnancy and severe antisocial behavior in offspring: a review. Am J Public Health 2002;92(6):966–74.

[72] Olds DL, Henderson Jr CR, Tatelbaum R. Intellectual impairment in children of women who smoke cigarettes during pregnancy. Pediatrics 1994;93(2):221–7.

[73] Olds DL, Henderson Jr CR, Tatelbaum R. Prevention of intellectual impairment in children of women who smoke cigarettes during pregnancy. Pediatrics 1994;93(2):228–33.

[74] Fried PA, O'Connell CM, Watkinson B. 60- and 72-month follow-up of children prenatally exposed to marijuana, cigarettes, and alcohol: cognitive and language assessment. J Dev Behav Pediatr 1992;13(6):383–91.

[75] Brook JS, Brook DW, Whiteman M. The influence of maternal smoking during pregnancy on the toddler's negativity. Arch Pediatr Adolesc Med 2000;154(4):381–5.

[76] Grunbaum JA, Kann L, Kinchen S, et al. Youth risk behavior surveillance—United States, 2003. MMWR Surveill Summ 2004;53(2):1–96.

[77] Ebrahim SH, Gfroerer J. Pregnancy-related substance use in the United States during 1996–1998. Obstet Gynecol 2003;101(2):374–9.

[78] Zuckerman B, Frank DA, Hingson R, et al. Effects of maternal marijuana and cocaine use on fetal growth. N Engl J Med 1989;320(12):762–8.

[79] MacGregor SN, Sciarra JC, Keith L, et al. Prevalence of marijuana use during pregnancy. A pilot study. J Reprod Med 1990;35(12):1147–9.

[80] United Nations Office on Drugs and Crime—Guatemala country profile. Available at: http://www.unodc.org/mexico/country_profile_guatemala.html. Accessed June 10, 2005.

[81] Cornelius MD, Goldschmidt L, Day NL, et al. Alcohol, tobacco and marijuana use among pregnant teenagers: 6-year follow-up of offspring growth effects. Neurotoxicol Teratol 2002;24(6):703–10.

[82] Fried PA, James DS, Watkinson B. Growth and pubertal milestones during adolescence in offspring prenatally exposed to cigarettes and marihuana. Neurotoxicol Teratol 2001;23(5):431–6.

[83] Cornelius MD, Taylor PM, Geva D, et al. Prenatal tobacco and marijuana use among adolescents: effects on offspring gestational age, growth, and morphology. Pediatrics 1995;95(5):738–43.

[84] Day NL, Richardson GA, Geva D, et al. Alcohol, marijuana, and tobacco: effects of prenatal exposure on offspring growth and morphology at age six. Alcohol Clin Exp Res 1994;18(4):786–94.

[85] Shiono PH, Klebanoff MA, Nugent RP, et al. The impact of cocaine and marijuana use on low birth weight and preterm birth: a multicenter study. Am J Obstet Gynecol 1995;172(1 Pt 1):19–27.

[86] Fried PA, Watkinson B, Gray R. Differential effects on cognitive functioning in 9- to 12-year olds prenatally exposed to cigarettes and marihuana. Neurotoxicol Teratol 1998;20(3):293–306.

[87] Fried PA. Adolescents prenatally exposed to marijuana: examination of facets of complex behaviors and comparisons with the influence of in utero cigarettes. J Clin Pharmacol 2002;42(11 Suppl):97S–102S.

[88] Goldschmidt L, Day NL, Richardson GA. Effects of prenatal marijuana exposure on child behavior problems at age 10. Neurotoxicol Teratol 2000;22(3):325–36.

[89] Richardson GA, Ryan C, Willford J, et al. Prenatal alcohol and marijuana exposure: effects on neuropsychological outcomes at 10 years. Neurotoxicol Teratol 2002;24(3):309–20.

[90] Goldschmidt L, Richardson GA, Cornelius MD, et al. Prenatal marijuana and alcohol exposure and academic achievement at age 10. Neurotoxicol Teratol 2004;26(4):521–32.

[91] Chiriboga CA. Fetal effects. Neurol Clin 1993;11(3):707–28.

[92] Kain ZN, Mayes LC, Ferris CA, et al. Cocaine-abusing parturients undergoing cesarean section. A cohort study. Anesthesiology 1996;85(5):1028–35.

[93] Nordstrom-Klee B, Delaney-Black V, Covington C, et al. Growth from birth onwards of children prenatally exposed to drugs: a literature review. Neurotoxicol Teratol 2002;24(4):481–8.

[94] Bateman DA, Chiriboga CA. Dose-response effect of cocaine on newborn head circumference. Pediatrics 2000;106(3):E33.

[95] Vidaeff AC, Mastrobattista JM. In utero cocaine exposure: a thorny mix of science and mythology. Am J Perinatol 2003;20(4):165–72.

[96] Wasserman GA, Kline JK, Bateman DA, et al. Prenatal cocaine exposure and school-age intelligence. Drug Alcohol Depend 1998;50(3):203–10.

[97] Singer LT, Minnes S, Short E, et al. Cognitive outcomes of preschool children with prenatal cocaine exposure. Obstet Gynecol Surv 2005;60(1):23–4.

[98] Messinger DS, Bauer CR, Das A, et al. The maternal lifestyle study: cognitive, motor, and behavioral outcomes of cocaine-exposed and opiate-exposed infants through three years of age. Pediatrics 2004;113(6):1677–85.

[99] Tronick EZ, Frank DA, Cabral H, et al. Late dose-response effects of prenatal cocaine exposure on newborn neurobehavioral performance. Pediatrics 1996;98(1):76–83.

[100] Chiriboga CA, Brust JC, Bateman D, et al. Dose-response effect of fetal cocaine exposure on newborn neurologic function. Pediatrics 1999;103(1):79–85.

[101] Jacobson SW, Jacobson JL, Sokol RJ, et al. New evidence for neurobehavioral effects of in utero cocaine exposure. J Pediatr 1996;129(4):581–90.

[102] Richardson GA. Prenatal cocaine exposure. A longitudinal study of development. Ann NY Acad Sci 1998;846:144–52.

[103] Delaney-Black V, Covington C, Templin T, et al. Expressive language development of children exposed to cocaine prenatally: literature review and report of a prospective cohort study. J Commun Disord 2000;33(6):463–80.

[104] Lewis BA, Singer LT, Short EJ, et al. Four-year language outcomes of children exposed to cocaine in utero. Neurotoxicol Teratol 2004;26(5):617–27.

[105] Anglin MD, Burke C, Perrochet B, et al. History of the methamphetamine problem. J Psychoactive Drugs 2000;32(2):137–41.

[106] Rhodes T, Bobrik A, Bobkov E, et al. HIV transmission and HIV prevention associated with injecting drug use in the Russian Federation. Int J Drug Policy 2004;15(1):1–16.

[107] Sattah MV, Supawitkul S, Dondero TJ, et al. Prevalence of and risk factors for methamphetamine use in northern Thai youth: results of an audio-computer-assisted self-interviewing survey with urine testing. Addiction 2002;97(7):801–8.

[108] Chang L, Smith LM, Lopresti C, et al. Smaller subcortical volumes and cognitive deficits in children with prenatal methamphetamine exposure. Psychiatry Res 2004;132(2):95–106.

[109] Weissman AD, Caldecott-Hazard S. Developmental neurotoxicity to methamphetamines. Clin Exp Pharmacol Physiol 1995;22(5):372–4.

[110] Eriksson M, Larsson G, Winbladh B, et al. The influence of amphetamine addiction on pregnancy and the newborn infant. Acta Paediatrica Scandinavica 1978;67(1):95–9.

[111] Smith L, Yonekura ML, Wallace T, et al. Effects of prenatal methamphetamine exposure on fetal growth and drug withdrawal symptoms in infants born at term. J Dev Behav Pediatr 2003; 24(1):17–23.

[112] Plessinger MA. Prenatal exposure to amphetamines. Risks and adverse outcomes in pregnancy. Obstet Gynecol Clin North Am 1998;25(1):119–38.

[113] Swetlow K. Children at clandestine methamphetamine labs: helping meth's youngest victims. Washington, DC: US Department of Justice, Office of Justice Programs, Office for Victims of Crime; 2003.

[114] Billing L, Eriksson M, Jonsson B, et al. The influence of environmental factors on behavioural problems in 8-year-old children exposed to amphetamine during fetal life. Child Abuse Negl 1994;18(1):3–9.

[115] Eriksson M, Billing L, Steneroth G, et al. Health and development of 8-year-old children whose mothers abused amphetamine during pregnancy. Acta Paediatr Scand 1989;78(6):944–9.

[116] Williams MT, Moran MS, Vorhees CV. Behavioral and growth effects induced by low dose methamphetamine administration during the neonatal period in rats. Int J Dev Neurosci 2004; 22(5–6):273–83.

PEDIATRIC CLINICS

OF NORTH AMERICA

Pediatr Clin N Am 52 (2005) 1395–1419

Long-Term Developmental, Behavioral, and Attachment Outcomes After International Adoption

Carol Weitzman, MD[a],*, Lisa Albers, MD, MPH[b]

[a]*Department of Pediatrics, Yale University School of Medicine, 333 Cedar Street, New Haven, CT 06520, USA*
[b]*Developmental Medicine Center, Children's Hospital, 300 Longwood Avenue, Boston, MA 02115, USA*

Children who are adopted internationally typically experience a wide range of life circumstances before joining their families that may have an impact their postadoptive health and development. All children, whether joining their families via adoption or via birth, have individual genetic and environmental strengths and challenges that may support or stress their capacity for healthy cognitive, behavioral, and emotional development over time [1]. Health and living conditions in children's home countries and child welfare systems experienced by internationally adopted children have changed greatly over the past several decades, partially because an increasing number of international adoptees have resided in institutions rather than foster care before their adoption into families. Reflecting the importance of this demographic change, this article highlights the potential impact of children's institutional living on their development, behavior, and attachment after international adoption. Because immediate developmental and behavioral concerns after adoption (see the article by Miller elsewhere in this issue) and an approach to assessment and accessing services for developmental and behavioral concerns (see the articles by Nalven and Dole elsewhere in this issue) are discussed elsewhere in this issue, our discussion focuses on the results of reported long-term follow-up studies

* Corresponding author.
E-mail address: carol.weitzman@yale.edu (C. Weitzman).

pediatric.theclinics.com

examining developmental, behavioral, and attachment outcomes after international adoption.

Impact of institutional care on child development

Although all child welfare institutions are unique, the long-term impact of institutional life on a child's growth and development has been well described for more than a century in many different countries. Delays in or variations from the normal progression of a child's development while residing in an institution have been attributed to multiple factors, including but not limited to malnutrition, emotional neglect via lack of a consistent emotional connection with a caretaker, and lack of developmentally stimulating opportunities or experiences. Prenatal alcohol exposure, lead intoxication, and myriad neurologic or genetic disorders may also cause or contribute to the same children's developmental difficulties. In general, postadoptive improvements of children's developmental skills and behaviors are routinely expected when children leave institutions and join their families. Any child's ongoing developmental or behavioral difficulties after international adoption may represent innate disorders or the irreversible consequences of early life experiences, however.

At the beginning of the twentieth century, child survival while residing in child welfare institutions worldwide significantly improved after innovations in sanitation and medical practices, along with the introduction of commercially available infant formula. In the 1930s and 1940s, as more children survived their infancy and toddler years while living in institutions, concerns were raised about developmental delays for children as the result of stimulus deprivation [2,3]. By the 1950s and 1960s, emphasis was being placed on the irreparable consequences of maternal deprivation in infancy, which was correlated with chronic impairments in multiple areas of functioning unless children entered family environments as infants [4,5]. Importantly, many of these studies were not able to differentiate between the impact of general lack of stimulation while residing in institutional settings and the specific consequences of absence of a child's primary attachment figure. Ascribing all detrimental effects of early institutionalization to maternal deprivation is clearly a gross and inaccurate simplification, however.

Historical and contemporary studies confirm a relationship between length of time and quality of care received while a child resides in an institution and that child's long-term health and development after adoption. Length of time residing in an institution is positively correlated with a child's risk of presenting with developmental, behavioral, and emotional concerns after international adoption [4,6–17]. Quality of care provided in an institution is also correlated with children's postadoptive outcomes, because orphanages associated with improved child health and development outcomes typically provide children with adequate nutrition and health care, a lower child-to-caregiver ratio (3:1 versus 10:1), a lower total number of caregivers over the life of the child, and caregivers who recognize and respond to the distress and vocalizations of children [5]. Unfortunately, most children residing in institutions before international adoption do not experience these preferred institutional conditions.

Gunnar and colleagues [2] have suggested that it is helpful to consider three levels of privation that may have an impact on a child's health and well-being within an institutional setting: (1) basic nutritional, hygiene, and medical needs; (2) stimulation and opportunity to interact with the environment in a way that supports motor, cognitive, language, and social development; and (3) stable interpersonal relationships allowing children to develop an attachment relationship with a consistent caregiver. It is important to realize that although these levels of privation for children may be theoretically described, they are not independent factors in children's real-life experiences. An appreciation of the different levels of support required for optimal child development informs our understanding of the potential challenges for children who reside in institutions during infancy and childhood. For example, provision for a child's basic needs can be observed and reflected in a child's growth parameters, although it is much harder to ensure adequate interpersonal relationships within busy institutional settings. In addition, a child's relatively good growth trajectory while residing in an institution implies an improved likelihood of additional caretaker attention beyond feeding. In actual practice, however, for any child who is adopted from an institution to join their family, the degree of privation suffered before adoption is essentially impossible to determine but may be significant.

Recent international adoptee long-term outcome studies

Studies of child development after international adoption should ideally take into account child-, family-, and geographic-specific variables as they affect children throughout their development from infancy through adulthood. Several critical variables to consider as potential confounders when considering a child's long-term outcome after international adoption include a child's birth family developmental and mental health history; a child's developmental, language, and emotional status at the time of adoption; trajectory of postadoptive development; and family and community services and resources after adoption. Analysis of "child outcomes" should consider easily measured outcomes (eg, developmental level, academic abilities) and long-term functional and emotional measures (eg, employment status, emotional health as an adult) while also considering issues influencing an individual's identity development (eg, adoptee is of same or different race as adoptive family, adoptive country and/or environment provides positive identity experiences for transracially adopted children).

Unfortunately, no single study encompassing preadoptive and family environment variables affecting developmental, school, and emotional outcomes for internationally adopted children has been conducted. Many investigators have examined facets of preadoptive and postadoptive experiences and environments as they have affected children and their families after international adoption. One excellent review was conducted by Professor Marianne Cederblad [17], who was commissioned by the Swedish government to review all available longitudinal studies and case series pertinent to developmental, school, and mental health outcomes for children after international adoption.

After an extensive review of information describing worldwide outcomes of international adoption, Cederblad [17] concluded that children who are internationally adopted have a two to three times greater chance of later school difficulties, psychiatric problems, and relationship difficulties than their non-adopted peers. In general, the older a child is at the time of adoption, the greater is the risk that he or she is going to have psychiatric problems and problems of social adjustment. Although she notes that several studies do not support a significantly greater risk for major developmental and psychiatric concerns after international adoption, sampling bias and validity of outcome measurements may have influenced the conclusions of these studies. She also suggested that a small proportion of the adoptees may show severe symptoms and may be overrepresented in clinical samples, whereas many children who are healthy and develop well are only documented in larger cohort studies. Cederblad [17] concludes her review with a discussion of areas in which research continues to be lacking, including an understanding of specific factors within families and pertinent to an adoptive child's experiences during adolescence and young adulthood.

Although a number of investigators have examined the health and development of children adopted internationally in the past several decades, the results of two key studies are particularly notable. Both are well-designed longitudinal epidemiologic studies examining children adopted from Romania to the United Kingdom and to Canada. These two studies provide the clearest picture of the impact of the most severely depriving conditions of orphanages on child health and development (Table 1):

- The English and Romanian Adoptees (ERA) Study Team compared a random sample of 165 children (including 144 children residing exclusively in institutions before adoption) adopted from Romania into families in the United Kingdom at less than 42 months of age [6–13,18]. Outcomes for this population of children were analyzed by length of institutionalization before adoption: less than 6 months, 6 to 24 months, or 24 to 42 months of institutionalization before adoption. The control group was a sample of 52 children adopted at less than 6 months domestically in the United Kingdom. Follow-up data have been reported for these children up to 6 years of age [8,30,31].
- The Canadian-Romanian study considers the implications of adoption of children from Romanian orphanages (n = 75) by families in British Columbia [14,15]. Analysis of data generally separates children adopted from Romania into those adopted at less than 4 months of age (EA; n = 29,) those adopted from Romania after 8 months of age (RO; n = 46), and comparison children born in Canada and never adopted (CB; n = 46.) Assessment was conducted at time 1 (just less than 1 year with adoptive families) and time 2 (just more than 3 years with adoptive families.)

Table 1
Romanian longitudinal studies

	English and Romanian Adoptees study [6–13]	Canadian study [14,15,30,31]
Type of study	Stratified random sample	Cohort follow-up
Study population	Romanian adoptees (n = 155) three study groups by months of institutionalization before adoption <6 mos (n = 58) 6–24 mos (n = 59) 24–42 mos (n = 48) Control group (n = 52) Domestic adoption <5 mos	Romanian adoptees (n = 75) Study groups adopted at age: <4 mos (n = 29) >8 mos (n = 46) Control group (n = 46) Canadian-born, not adopted
Analysis compares	Each of three groups with controls and with each other Domestic UK adoption Romanian adoption <6 mos 6–24 mos 24–42 mos	Romanian adoptees Early adoptees: <4 mos of age at adoption RO: >8 mos of age at adoption Control: not adopted
Follow-up assessments	At age of 4 years if adopted at <24 mos of age At age of 6 years for all children	Time 1: median of 11 mos in adoptive/birth home Time 2: median of 39 mos in adoptive/birth home
Cognition	At adoption (Denver) 59% of study population with DQ <50 At age of 6 years (McCarthy GCI) Study population with GCI <80 2.3% for <6 mos 12.0% for 6–24 mos 32.6% for 24–42 mos 2% of control population with GCI <80 Cognitive deficits correlate with head circumference	Mean IQ 3 years after adoption (Stanford-Binet) <4 mos of age at adoption: no difference from control 8–24 mos of age at adoption: mean IQ = 90 (range: 65–127) >24 mos of age at adoption: mean IQ = 69 (range: 52–98)
Attachment	Percentage of children with disorganized attachment patterns Control group (3.8%) <6 mos (8.95%) 6–24 mos (24.5%) 24–42 mos (33.3%)	Percentage of children with insecure attachment: Nonadopted (42%) <4 mos at adoption (35%) >8 mos at adoption (63%)
Quasiautistic features	6% quasiautistic symptoms 6% mild symptoms of autism	At time 2: 41% of RO's continued stereotypical behaviors
Behavioral concerns	Severe inattention/overactivity symptoms Control group (9.6%) <6 mos (13.6%) 6–24 mos (32.1%) 24–42 mos (38.6%)	At time 2: 29% of RO's with externalizing behavior concerns

Abbreviations: Denver, Revised Denver Pre-Screening Developmental Questionnaire; DQ, generates developmental quotient; GCI, generates general cognitive index; McCarthy, McCarthy Scales of Children's Abilities; mos, months; RO, Romanian orphan.

Cognitive development

Delayed development of fine motor, gross motor, language, and social skills is widely reported for children immediately after international adoption (D. Johnson, MD, PhD, results for the Minnesota Adoption Project, personal communication, 2004) (see the article by Miller elsewhere in this issue) [6–9,15, 18,19]. In the ERA study, at the time of adoption, 59% of children demonstrated a development quotient less than 50 (suggesting severe developmental delays) as assessed with the Revised Denver Pre-Screening Developmental Questionnaire and McCarthy Scales of Children's Abilities at the time of adoption [11]. Limited information is available about the long-term epidemiology of significant and persistent developmental disorders in international adoptees, however.

One study in Denmark suggests an increased risk of "moderate" developmental difficulties with increased age at adoption. Nord and coworkers [16] describe a cohort of children adopted in 1992 and 1993 and evaluated via parent questionnaire in 1999 with a 92% parent response rate. According to parental response when the children were 7 to 10 years of age, 81% of children were assessed by their parents to be functioning "without any problems" at home and at school, 13% had lasting moderate difficulties (eg, learning difficulties, attention deficit, linguistic difficulties), and 6% had severe disturbances (eg, mental retardation, autism, cerebral palsy.) The older children were at the time of adoption, the greater was the proportion with moderate difficulties (10% for children less than 1 year of age at adoption versus 35% for children adopted after 3 years of age.) This increased risk of moderate difficulties is consistent with exposure to multiple developmental detractors before adoption, because many environmental factors have been linked to the long-term risk of modest (rather than severe) cognitive impairment [1].

The longitudinal Romanian adoption studies also suggest that although many children seem to develop typically after adoption, a substantial number of post-institutionalized children demonstrate significant cognitive difficulties [7–15]. The British and Canadian longitudinal studies of Romanian adoptees suggest a "dose-response" relation between the length of a child's institutionalization and a reduction in his or her cognitive abilities in preschool and early school years.

The ERA study in the United Kingdom found that although more than half of the children demonstrated severe developmental delays at the time of adoption, most of these children demonstrated cognition within the average range at follow-up. Investigators reported cognitive impairment at 6 years of age (defined as a McCarthy general cognitive index [GCI] <80) in 15.4% of the postinstitutionalized adoptees from Romania compared with similar impairment in only 2.0% of domestically adopted infants. There was a linear association in the ERA study between cognitive impairment and duration of institutionalization, with 2.3%, 12.0%, and 32.6% of children presenting with cognitive limitations after less than 6 months, 6 to 24 months, or 24 to 42 months of institutionalization before adoption, respectively. Although all children who resided in institutions did not demonstrate significant cognitive impairment, the children who had the greatest cognitive deficits over time were also those who spent the longest time in an institution and who had presented with the most severe subnutrition at the time of adoption. Cognitive deficits were also significantly correlated with smaller head circumference at the time of adoption and with head circumference at 6 years of age. Investigators considered the possible correlation of head circumference with malnutrition, but these factors were found to be independent predicators of cognitive outcomes in their analysis. The presence of cognitive deficits at 4 years of age was stable at follow-up 2 years later.

Similarly, rapid developmental catch-up after adoption but an increased risk of significant developmental delays after adoption was reported in the Canadian-Romanian adoption study. Ames [14] also found that the longer a child resided in an institution, the greater was the chance of cognitive difficulties as measured by performance on the Stanford-Binet test 3 years after adoption. Although the mean IQ of children adopted from Romania before 4 months of age did not differ significantly from that of the Canadian-born control group, the mean IQ was 90 (range: 65–127) for children with 8 to 24 months of institutional living and 69 (range: 52–98) for children spending more than 2 years in institutional care [14,15].

Language development

Most international adoptees are acquiring a second language in their adoptive country while losing their primary language from their native country. Language development for children acquiring their second language while losing their first language is described as qualitatively and quantitatively different from the tasks of acquiring a primary language or simultaneously developing language skills in more than one language. Glennen and Masters [19] described the development of English language skills in infants and toddlers adopted from Eastern Europe as occurring along a trajectory similar to but achieving typical developmental milestones slower than children with native language development in English. It is important to note that the children described in this study were relatively young at the time of adoption and language assessment (primarily infants and toddlers); therefore, they have not yet been followed into school age, when increased expectations for understanding complex language and executive functioning may emphasize a child's higher order language based deficits.

Older children have a more complex task than infants after international adoption into a family and culture that require a completely new language. They need a significantly higher level of language capacity to perform similar to same-aged peers when expressing their needs and for understanding what is being said to them in home, school, and social settings. Particularly for children with previous knowledge of their native language, assessment of a child's language abilities at the time of adoption is helpful in gauging the child's necessarily language support in educational and social settings. Children adopted internationally from institutions beyond infancy may present with a combination of challenges related to acquisition of their new primary language, including poor primary language development given limited conversational language exposure in institutions. Although acquisition of a second language may take years, children adopted from institutions should be considered to be at risk of language disorders given the relative paucity of language input in their preadoptive environments [19–22]. Especially for children adopted during preschool and school years, a child's functional language may be present well before a child understands much of the routine conversational language expected in home and school settings.

Pediatric providers should consider the following when assessing a child's language difficulties and school performance after international adoption:

- Is the child's hearing normal?
- What was the child's language proficiency before adoption?
- How long has the child been in his or her new language environment?
- What level of language is expected in home, social, and school environments for this child to be proficient?

Behavioral problems in context

In the most basic terms, a child's "behavior" may represent a learned adaptive or maladaptive behavior reinforced by a child's environment. Alternatively, the same behavior may be a manifestation of a child's neurologically based behavioral or psychiatric disorder. Several caveats are important when considering the prevalence of behavioral concerns in any population, but particularly with respect to international adoptees transitioning into their new home environments:

1. Identification of a "behavioral problem" is relative to the observer and the situation, because behaviors that may be concerning in one setting (eg, stealing food at an airport) may be adaptive in another setting (eg, stealing food in an orphanage).
2. Unlike direct evaluation or assessments of a child's skills, reports of a child's behaviors rely heavily on necessarily subjective parent, caretaker, or teacher questionnaires.
3. "Behavioral problems" may be the primary concern or may reflect an underlying difficulty (eg, cognitive impairments, specific learning difficulty, or mood concern).

One fundamental question that remains unanswered in the literature is whether the fact of a child's adoption alone increases his or her risk for behavioral concerns. Adopted children and adolescents (including those adopted domestically and internationally) are overrepresented among those receiving inpatient or outpatient mental health services, with at least a four- to five-fold relative risk reported for adoptees [23–25]. These studies do not uniformly control for the presence or absence of a variety of preadoptive factors, however, such as a child's genetic predisposition to behavioral and/or mental health disorders, prenatal substance abuse and/or exposure, preadoptive neglect, physical or sexual abuse, and time and/or type of dependent care.

Specific to adoptees, behaviors that may present as potentially problematic may in fact represent a typical response to an atypical stress and may be ameliorated or exacerbated by family and community responses to the child's situation. Pavao [26] has described behaviors that may be identified as problematic in certain settings for children (eg, daydreaming in class, speaking about issues of loss) which should instead be viewed as "normative stages" for an adoptive person along a normal emotional health trajectory. In addition, a family's response to an adoptive child over time may be influenced by unresolved trauma and/or loss related to infertility. Identity development may also involve factors beyond adoption that may be presenting as a child's behaviors, such as a child who is transracially adopted being identified as "different" within the family and community. Over time, the capacity of a child's family and local community and culture to support that child's healthy emotional development may affect the child's long-term emotional health and behaviors.

For internationally adopted children, a child's risk of behavioral concerns is influenced by that child's genetic predispositions and actual life experiences— not just the information reported to families before or at the time of their child's adoption. In general, information about a birth parent's history of behavior concerns or mental illness is often extremely limited, with scarce information provided about a child's birth mother and often nonexistent information about a child's birth father. Maternal substance use or mental illness may not be reported for a specific child; however, the absence of information should not imply that no concerns are present. In addition, as is true with all adoptees, extended family history may not be available at the time of adoption, and birth parents who are young at the time of a child's adoption may later develop mental health disorders that were not evident at the time of adoption.

Routine postadoptive behaviors

For internationally adopted children, it is crucial to differentiate a child's behaviors before adoption and immediately after adoption from those remaining over the long term. Children adopted from depriving institutions may present with behavioral symptoms suggestive of self-stimulation in the context of extreme deprivation. Gesell and Amatruda [27] described the spectrum and time course of behavioral concerns for children residing in institutions in 1941. More than six decades later, children adopted from institutions in 2005 continue to present with self-stimulatory behaviors, such as rocking, head banging, or shaking, and visual stimulation with hand wiggling or flapping. "Quasiautistic" behaviors were found in 12% of 111 children described at the time of adoption from Romania in the ERA study [7]. Self-injurious behaviors, such as biting or hitting oneself, may also be seen. Aggressive behaviors, such as hitting, kicking, or biting others, may have developed as a form of self-defense before adoption. In another article in this issue, Miller reviews other typical postadoptive behaviors for children after international adoption.

Typically, infants and toddlers demonstrate a significant reduction in the frequency and intensity of their self-stimulatory, self-injurious, and aggressive behaviors within weeks to months after international adoption. Some children continue to present with "autistic features," however, including decreased communication attempts, decreased social interactions (reduced nonverbal interactions and eye contact), and stereotypical behaviors. In the ERA study, 6% of children were reported to have persistent autistic features [7]. The prevalence of autistic behaviors after internationally adopted children have resided with their families for several years is not known, but our clinical experience suggests an increased prevalence of autistic behaviors after adoption in the setting of preadoptive deprivation.

Long-term behavioral concerns for international adoptees

Numerous investigators have reviewed behavioral concerns for children after international adoption, although most have presented results of convenience samples or specialized clinic populations. In contrast, Verhulst and coworkers [23–25] investigated behavioral problems for 10- to 15-year-olds as reported by their parents after international adoption to the Netherlands compared with same-aged peers in the Netherlands. One significant advantage of this study in contrast to many others describing international adoptees' behavioral concerns is that the study population reflects the demographics of the entire population of children internationally adopted at that time. In surveying parents of all international adoptees to the Netherlands who were born between January 1, 1972 and December 31, 1975, Verhulst and colleagues [23–25] compared the behaviors of 2148 children (reflecting 64.9% of children adopted in the Netherlands during this period; no statistically significant differences between demographics of responders and nonresponders) with those of 933 same-aged children from the general population as reported by their parents on the Achenbach Child Behavioral Checklist (ACBL), a standardized assessment measure. The children described in this study were adopted from a variety of countries reflective of international adoption practices worldwide in the 1970s and 1980s, with children born in Korea accounting for 32%, those born in Columbia accounting for 14.6%, those born in India accounting for 9.5%, those born in Indonesia accounting for 7.9%, those born in Bangladesh accounting for 6.7%, and those born in all other countries accounting for 20.3% of the sample population. Although children adopted worldwide since the 1970s and 1980s include more children from China and Eastern Europe than included in these studies, preadoptive conditions have not significantly improved and more children reside in orphanages with less individual attention from caretakers.

Verhulst and coworkers [23–25] reported that despite preadoptive experiences, most internationally adopted children had behavioral scores similar to those of nonadopted Dutch children. Approximately three times as many 12- to 15-year-old adopted girls scored in the clinically significant range on the Schizoid scale (including such items as "strange behavior," "stares blankly," "daydreams or gets lost in her thoughts," or "hears things that are not there"), however. Approximately four times as many 12- to 15-year-old adopted boys presented with delinquent behaviors (including such items as "lying and cheating," "steals inside or outside the home," "vandalism," "hangs around children who get into trouble," and "truancy"), and nearly three times as many 12- to 15-year-old adopted boys were reported to have "hyperactive" behaviors. Importantly, adopted children were rated as better than nonadopted children in sports and nonsports activities [23]. The authors also concluded that older age at placement increased a child's likelihood of being rated in a clinically significant range on a behavioral scale [24].

Several caveats are important when examining parent reports, which are the main source of children's behavioral concerns. First, it is crucial to consider confounding factors that may present as behavioral problems for children. For example, learning or attention problems may have contributed to some of the symptoms leading to elevated scores for adopted children with respect to behaviors noted in school or related to completing homework. In fact, 13.2% of the adopted children (versus 4.4% of the nonadopted children) described in the Netherlands study were attending special schools [23]. Second, parental expectations are naturally related to one's own experience with educational and professional success and may therefore influence one's ratings of their children. In the studies of Verhulst and colleagues [23–25], adopted children from lower socioeconomic adoptive homes were reported to have better academic performance, fewer school problems, and higher total competence scores than children from higher socioeconomic homes. The authors also caution readers with respect to generalizing their findings, given the variation in age and experiences at the time of adoption for international adoptees and the changing preadoptive conditions for international adoptees.

Both longitudinal studies of adoptees from Romania (see Table 1) suggest an increase in behavioral symptoms years after adoption. The ERA Study Team surveyed parents and teachers with the Revised Rutter Parent and Teacher Scales at 4 years (preschool version) and 6 years (school version) to identify behavioral concerns for children. By 6 years of age, length of institutionalization was positively linearly correlated with reports of inattention and/or overactivity (I/O) symptoms by parents and teachers but not with reports of conduct difficulties or emotional difficulties [28]. A child's risk of I/O symptoms as reported by parents and teachers increased with length of institutionalization (13.6%, 32.1%, and 38.6% of children had severe I/O symptoms when adopted from Romania at <6 months, 6–24 months, and 24–42 months, respectively, compared with 9.6% of children in the control group). Importantly, parent- or teacher-reported symptoms of "inattention" or "overactivity" may reflect cognitive, learning, and language concerns as well as primary difficulties regulating attention and activity. Investigators did find that the risk of I/O symptoms was increased with severe malnutrition or cognitive impairment but that a child's risk was not fully explained by correcting for a child's degree of malnutrition or cognitive deficits alone. Similarly, the Canadian-Romanian adoption study found that 29% of RO children (adopted from Romania after 8 months of age) continued to have externalizing behavioral concerns at time 2 (after 3 years with their adoptive families.) Although eating, sleeping, and stereotypical behaviors of concern had decreased between time 1 (less than 1 year after adoption) and time 2, 41% of children continued with some stereotypical behaviors, although their frequency had decreased for all children [14,29–31].

Attachment after international adoption

There has been great interest in understanding how early deprivation and institutional care affect children's abilities to form secure and stable attachments with caregivers and how these abilities may be improved after placement into a nurturing and attentive home environment. Bowlby [32] has defined attachment as a biologically rooted motivational system that matures during the first several years of life and motivates the young child to seek comfort, support, and nurturance from discriminated attachment figures. Selective attachment unfolds over the first year of life, and when all goes well, a child uses a preferred attachment figure as a "secure base" from which to venture out and explore and a safe haven to which to return in times of danger [32,33]. The fragmented and inadequate caregiving that exists within orphanages before international adoption can lead to frequent failed or missed opportunities for relationship connections, thus placing children at high risk of attachment disturbances after adoption. Although cases of internationally adopted children with severe reactive attachment disorders have garnered the most attention, it is important to consider the spectrum of relational difficulties that children who have sustained early deprivation and loss may experience.

Forming attachments

When a woman gives birth and becomes a parent, a period of enormous change, upheaval, and transition begins for the parents and the baby. Under optimal circumstances, parents enter into a state that Winnicott [34] terms *primary maternal preoccupation*, where parents become intensely identified and engrossed with their infant during the first few months of life. During this period of heightened sensitivity, seemingly minor everyday moments occur that expose the infant to new and important information about the world, including "everyday" interactions with the parent. When a parent picks up a crying infant in a timely way and settles the infant with nurturance and sensitive handling, the baby begins to develop positive and predictable expectations about the world and starts to understand something about his or her capacities to modify the environment and world. Armed with the confidence that these discoveries bring, the baby begins to explore, to reach and grab, and to use gesture and affect to get the attention of others. This baby, who is "wired" for interaction, becomes an increasingly active participant in the social dance with a caregiver. In addition, babies can start to tolerate small shifts and perturbations in their environment and stimuli [35].

At the same time, parents, of course, are not able to read all the baby's signals correctly all the time and could never be continuously available for interaction. These "mismatches," which result in small tolerable frustrations and disappointments for babies, begin the process of helping them to develop regulatory strategies that allow them to begin to manage a complicated world in an organized way without experiencing overwhelming shame, despair, and disorganization. Winnicott [36] refers to the "ordinary devoted mother" as one who is able to adapt to the parenting role and provide a protective cocoon around her infant that buffers the child from undue stress and filters the amount of environmental stimulation and challenges to which the infant is exposed. Winnicott [34,36] and Weitzman and coworkers [35] have emphasized that parents do not need to be of superhuman talent or heroes; they simply need to do a "good enough" job in meeting their child's basic human, emotional, and developmental needs for things to go reasonably well.

So, in what seems like routine everyday moments lay elegance and complexity, because these moments ultimately result in infants successfully developing secure attachment relationships, an internal felt sense of safety and trust, and an emerging sense of the self.

Zeanah and colleagues [37–39] describe the first year and a half of life as comprising four phases that reflect increasing relationship discrimination coupled with a child's increasing capacity for exploration and discovery. The period from birth to 2 months is called Orientation/Limited Discrimination. During this period, although infants can distinguish the sounds and smells of the caregiver, they do not discriminate in relationships. From 2 to 7 months of age, infants are in a period of Discrimination/Limited Preference. Babies may show greater comfort with a preferred caregiver but typically remain social with everyone, and preferences are not strongly expressed. A significant shift occurs between 7 and 12 months, when infants enter the period of Hierarchy of Preferred Caregivers. At this point, infants have developed strong preferences for caregivers and are acutely sensitive to their absence or to the approach of others. Hence, this is the period when stranger awareness or separation protest begins to emerge. Between 12 and 20 months, toddlers enter into the fourth phase, Secure Base, where they use the attachment figure as a "home base" from which to venture out and explore, knowing that they can return to the safety and security of the caregiver when distressed or frightened.

Early studies of attachment in orphanages

For the thousands of children reared in orphanages, nonnurturing homes, or multiple foster homes or orphanages, exposure to the good enough care of the ordinary devoted mother described by Winnicott [36] is often denied. Some of the earliest work on the effects of institutional care on children's development and attachment came not from orphanages in the developing world but from orphanages in America and Britain. These studies were some of the first to describe the effect of deprivation on children's social-emotional and overall development by studying children who "participated" in an extraordinarily unfortunate but natural experiment that happened when children were reared in orphanages. These studies were critical in establishing the link between attachment disturbances and the lack of opportunity in the first years of life to develop selective attachments as a result of neglectful, overwhelmed, inattentive, or even abusive caregiving. They also contributed to shaping current definitions of attachment disorders.

Provence and Lipton [4] studied 75 institutionalized children in New Haven, Connecticut. Children's physical needs were adequately met, but they experienced limited emotional nurturance and interactions. It was believed that if the children formed close relationships with caregivers, this might interfere with their ability to form a relationship with future adoptive parents. In this study, it was noted that differences in behavior could be noted as early as 2 months of age, when these infants showed less vocalization. The institutionalized children displayed intense visual interest in adults; however, the children did not pass through the four phases described previously but instead remained in a period of limited discrimination. These children showed greater recognition and preference for familiar objects than for familiar people, which stands in contrast to typical development. By 1 year of age, children showed little initiation of social interactions and, overall, had constricted and limited affect. During times of distress, there was little evidence that they activated an attachment system, and they rarely sought out help or nurturance from a caregiver. Even after placement, these children continued to display persistent problems in their relationships with others and in self-regulation. Many of the children displayed indiscriminate sociability, with relationships remaining superficial.

Tizard and Hodges [40] followed a group of 65 children reared in residential nurseries in Britain for their first 2 to 4 years of life and reported findings similar to those of Provence and Lipton [4]. These were considered "high-quality" institutions, where basic needs were adequately met, staff-to-child ratios were good, and play materials were present. Caregivers in this setting were also discouraged from developing close personal relationships, and children were exposed to an average of 24 different caregivers by the age of 2 years and to an average of 50 by the age of 4 years. Between the ages of 2 and 4 years, children were adopted, returned to their biologic parents, or remained in institutional care. This is a landmark study in that it is the only longitudinal study of institutionalized children that has followed children for 16 years and thus described the effects of early deprivation on children's development after many years.

- At the age of 4.5 years, most children showed preferences for particular caregivers. Caregivers of institutionalized children, however, noted that they showed "shallow affections," and most were reported "not to care deeply about anyone." Despite the superficial quality of their relationships, institutional children were also noted to follow caregivers around more than noninstitutionalized children and were the only children in the sample who were described as "clinging." Institutional children were also described as attention seeking, clingy, and indiscriminately friendly with strangers. In contrast, all but four of the adopted children were thought by their adoptive mothers to be attached.
- At the age of 8 years, few children remained in institutional care. Of the children who had been in institutional care at the age of 4.5 years, some had been adopted, some were placed in foster homes, and some were returned to their biologic parents. Most adoptive parents and those of a comparison group of never-institutionalized children reported that their child was closely attached to them, but only 54% of mothers of returned children and 43% of foster mothers felt this way. The indiscriminate sociability and attention seeking seen in institutional and placed children at the age of 4 years had greatly diminished by the age of 8 years but was still significantly more likely to be present in this group than in never-institutionalized children.
- At the age of 16 years, problems with peer relationships seemed to replace the indiscriminate sociability seen earlier. These teenagers were reported to be more adult oriented, less likely to have a best friend, and less able to use good judgment in selecting friends.

These early studies of institutionalized children showed that deficits in forming relationships with others could be seen in early infancy and that the effects of early deprivation could still be seen many years after adoption. Of note, most children who had not developed selective attachments in the first year of life displayed a range of behaviors that might seem incongruent, such as the coexistence of indiscriminate sociability and clinginess.

Defining attachment disturbances

Attachment has been classified based on patterns of infant behaviors and has most typically been assessed using the Ainsworth Strange Situation procedure on 12- to 18-month-old infants [41,42]. The procedure introduces a series of increasing stressors to the child (introduction of a stranger into the room and separation from the caregiver), and behavior during the reunion of the child and the caregiver is assessed. Classification of attachment is determined by noting the child's ability to use the caregiver to regulate emotion and how well the child is able to reorganize and resume exploratory play. Based on observations of specific behavioral interactions, children are determined to be securely or insecurely attached. Insecure attachment is further divided into anxious-avoidant, anxious-resistant, and disorganized/disoriented. Although these patterns have been linked to later social-emotional competency, self-reliance, empathy, and flexibility, they do not represent attachment disorders that require treatment and are commonly seen in typically developing children.

Attachment disorders have been classified in the *Diagnostic and Statistical Manual of Mental Disorders*, fourth edition (DSM-IV) as having two clinical patterns. The first type, emotionally withdrawn, describes children who are excessively inhibited and hypervigilant and display ambivalent responses to caregivers. The second type, disinhibited, is characterized by indiscriminate sociability and some failure to show selective attachments. Zeanah and colleagues [37–39] have expanded on this classification by delineating three categories of disorders: disorders of nonattachment, secure base distortions, and disrupted attachment disorder. Because most of the literature examining institutionalized and postinstitutionalized children's attachment has described attachment disorders according to the DSM-IV, these expanded classifications are not further discussed here.

Recent studies of attachment

Two longitudinal studies (see Table 1) and several smaller studies have examined attachment in postinstitutionalized Romanian adoptees, extending the findings of earlier studies by using laboratory assessments and standardized measures to assess attachment. It is important to note that these studies primarily assessed children who were reared in the harshest and most neglectful Romanian orphanages. Although children being adopted today may not come from such poor-quality institutions, and thus some of the findings may not fully generalize, the general principles regarding the development of secure attachment relationships and the effects of early deprivation and loss remain salient.

Quality of attachment

The Canadian-Romanian study assessed differences in attachment security among three groups of children: those adopted into Canada after at least 8 months in a Romanian orphanage and two comparison groups of children, Canadian-born nonadopted children and a group of Romanian-born children adopted before the age of 4 months [29,30,43]. All three groups of children were assessed at two time points: at a median of 11 months and 39 months of living in the adoptive home. The later placed children scored significantly lower in parents' security of attachment ratings than the other two groups at the first assessment; however, by the second assessment, parent ratings of attachment security were no longer different between the groups.

Attachment patterns, as assessed by a laboratory evaluation similar to the Strange Situation, however, revealed that 63% of late adoptees displayed insecure attachment patterns as compared with 42% of nonadopted children. These findings were similar to attachment patterns seen in children at the age of 4 years in the other longitudinal study, the ERA study, where only 33% of children with 6 to 24 months of institutional care were rated as securely attached compared with 55% of adoptees who were adopted into England before 6 months of age. A study of Romanian adoptees in Toronto also replicated these findings [44].

The English-Romanian Study assessed attachment in children at the age of 4 and 6 years in two ways. First, at the age of 4 and 6 years, the presence of three disinhibited behaviors was measured: (1) indication that the child lacked differentiation between adults, (2) indication that the child would readily go off with a stranger, and (3) indication that the child showed a definite lack of checking back with the parent in new and anxiety-provoking situations. One inhibited behavior, which was later dropped from the analyses, was also measured. These behaviors correspond to DSM-IV classifications of reactive attachment disorders. Second, at the age of 4 years, a separation-reunion procedure similar to the Strange Situation was conducted in the child's home. Children were classified as secure, insecure-avoidant, insecure-dependent, insecure-disorganized, or insecure-other. This last category was reserved for the children who did not fit into any particular classification named previously.

This study found a linear relation at the ages of 4 and 6 years between the duration of deprivation and the frequency of attachment disorder behavior, but there was substantial variability in the duration of deprivation among those exhibiting moderate to high levels of attachment disorder behaviors. This means that it was not only the children with the longest period of deprivation who displayed the highest levels of attachment disorder behaviors. In fact, 38% of children with a significant length of early deprivation displayed no attachment disorder behaviors at all. For the group of children with more than 6 months of institutional care, however, the rates of severe attachment disorder behaviors were substantially higher when compared with Romanian and UK children adopted before 6 months of age, with approximately 30% of the children adopted between 24 and 42 months of age exhibiting severe behaviors. These behaviors were stable between 4 and 6 years, with more than half of the sample showing no change in ratings of attachment security over time.

The findings of this study are confusing, however, because this study also found large numbers of early adoptees with mild or even severe attachment disturbances, which is contrary to what one would expect. This suggests that the ability of these measures to detect true attachment disturbance may be limited because of inaccuracy in parent report or the measures themselves and may overestimate attachment disturbances.

The Canadian-Romanian Study and the ERA study found that children with prolonged institutional care had significantly more atypical insecure attachment classifications and disorganized attachment strategies than the other groups but did not have increases in more typical forms of insecurity (eg, insecure-avoidant, insecure-dependent).

To summarize, both longitudinal studies of children adopted from Romania suggest that the length of a child's deprivation is negatively associated with security of attachment and attachment disorder behaviors. Although laboratory assessments of these patterns do not seem to change significantly over time, parents' assessments of attachment security did significantly improve over time. There was variability in which children had the most severe attachment behaviors, which raises questions regarding the key features of institutional care that contribute to developing severe attachment disturbance beyond the length of deprivation. Finally, the children with the most institutional care had more atypical and disorganized attachment patterns, suggesting that one must look beyond whether adoptees are simply securely or insecurely attached and consider the type of insecure attachment strategy. Future studies are needed to determine if there is a unique attachment typology seen specifically in postinstitution-alized children.

Indiscriminate sociability

Early studies [4,45] described a pattern of behavior among children who have experienced institutional care that included approaching strangers without caution. O'Connor and coworkers [10–13] have pointed out that although this behavior is referred to as indiscriminate sociability or indiscriminate friendliness, it is often neither social nor friendly. Contact is often superficial, and there is a scripted quality to the interactions, which lack reciprocity. Over time, one begins to notice that these approaches toward strangers do not seem to be driven by an interest in social connectedness and more often are internally driven or have the goal of meeting a child's desire for something.

There has been significant debate about how indiscriminate sociability relates to attachment disorders. In one of the described subtypes of attachment disorders (disinhibited subtype), there is the assumption that in the presence of this behavior, the child has no preferred or discriminated attachment figure. In children with a history of institutional care, however, indiscriminate sociability has been seen in children with secure attachment patterns in more than one study.

In the Canadian-Romanian study, indiscriminate sociability was determined with two of the questions thought to measure more extreme indiscriminate behaviors (whether children wandered without distress and whether children would be willing to go home with a stranger) by asking parents about behaviors children showed when encountering new adults. Late adoptees displayed significantly more indiscriminate sociability than the other two groups. Initially, only 6% of parents identified indiscriminate sociability as a concern, and there was no relation between indiscriminate sociability and parent ratings of attachment security. On follow-up at a median of 39 months in the adoptive home, there was no decrease in indiscriminate sociability for late adoptees, but this behavior did diminish in early adoptees, suggesting that the indiscriminate sociability in older adoptees was a more enduring behavior. Seventy-one percent of parents of late adoptees now reported that their child was "overly friendly."

Overall, there was no relation between indiscriminate sociability and security of attachment, although if parents responded positively to the two "extreme" questions, there was a higher likelihood of being insecurely attached. These findings led the Chisholm [29] to conclude that indiscriminate sociability was not always necessarily indicative of an attachment disorder, except possibly when more extreme indiscriminate behaviors were present.

In the ERA study, many of the children rated as insecure-other and all the children who had severe attachment disorder behaviors displayed indiscriminate sociability. These same children seemed to have difficulty in regulating arousal and excitement. Similar to the study by Chisholm [29], this study also found the coexistence of secure attachment patterns and indiscriminate sociability in some children. These authors concluded that the way attachment is measured in children without selective attachment may be flawed; therefore, children may falsely seem to be securely attached when they are not.

Zeanah and colleagues [33,38,46] examined a group of institutionalized Romanian children to characterize the relation between indiscriminate sociability and the presence of a preferred attachment figure. Children aged 11 to 68 months who were living in an orphanage in Bucharest, Romania on a standard unit where children are cared for by multiple caregivers were compared with children living on a "pilot" unit that aimed to provide a more consistent caregiving environment by reducing the number of caregivers. Twice as many children on the standard unit displayed indiscriminate sociability compared with the children on the pilot unit. Similar to the other studies, many children displayed indiscriminate sociability and a preferred caregiver. Zeanah and coworkers [33,39] raised the possibility that although indiscriminate sociability is a clinically significant entity, it may represent something other than a disorder of attachment. They suggested that this might represent a disorder of impulsivity or a disturbance in the regulation of attachment.

These studies examining indiscriminate sociability suggest that this behavior is highly prevalent among children who have experienced institutional care for more than the first 6 months of life and may have been an adaptive behavior in an orphanage. It is often an enduring behavior that remains long after the child has settled into the adoptive home. Parents initially may not identify this as a problem and may even find it endearing, but this assessment may change over time. It is challenging for pediatricians to know how to counsel families whose children display indiscriminate sociability. On one hand, it is clearly not synonymous with an attachment disorder, which may reassure parents; however, conversely, the child who wanders off or would go home with a stranger is highly vulnerable, and, potentially, these children may not show good judgment when choosing friends or when approaching adults. Pediatricians should routinely inquire about and observe for the more extreme indiscriminately sociable behaviors.

Relation between attachment and parenting

There has been interest in understanding how children's security of attachment relates to their relationships with a parent. One can imagine how children who are disinhibited in their interactions or display atypical strategies for obtaining proximity, comfort, and security from a parent, even if they have identified the parent as a preferred attachment figure, might influence how parents respond to them, interpret their signals and cues, and maintain engagement and reciprocity in their interactions.

The Canadian-Romanian Study examined parent stress. Parents in all three groups (early Romanian adoptees, late Romanian adoptees, and nonadopted comparison group) demonstrated a similar commitment to the parenting role. In the follow-up study of this cohort, there was a significant relation between insecure attachment and increased parenting stress. These children had lower cognitive scores and more behavior problems, and parents were reported to be in a lower socioeconomic group. Parents of children with indiscriminate sociability also had significantly increased parent stress. When evaluating and caring for children with suspected attachment disturbances and indiscriminate sociability, it is critical to consider the impact of raising this type of child on the parent. Pediatric providers need to remember to ask parents how they are managing stress in these situations and to provide support and intervention when necessary.

Parenting

When one considers parenting the adopted child, one must first consider the similarities and differences that exist for the adoptive parent. What do adoptive parents hold in common with the parents of biologic children? To name a few traits, they share similar concerns for the child's well-being, they have hopes and dreams for the child's future, and they want to give and receive love. One must consider, too, that there are ways in which adoptive and biologic parents diverge.

Many adoptive families begin adoption with their own potentially unresolved histories of grief and loss as related to failed pregnancies, loss of fertility, and loss of the imagined family or child [47]. In addition, adoptive parents often are unable to talk with others about the complexity of their feelings as they bring their new child into their home. This includes acknowledging their own and their child's losses, possible feelings of rejection and hurt, concern for their child's future, and the challenges of parenting a child who comes into a family beyond infancy.

The early upheaval experienced by a new mother who just gave birth is often responded to with support and understanding. Adoptive families of the older infant or child often report that society often expects them to fall in love with their child immediately and vice versa. When they experience a range of feelings that one would expect during such a period of upheaval, adoptive parents report that their extended family, friends, and members of the society at large often have difficulty in acknowledging their difficult feelings; they often insist on reminding adoptive parents who voice anxiety or ambivalence that they chose to adopt and that they have finally gotten their long-awaited child. In other words, they asked for this, so how can they complain?

As many of the articles in this issue have shown, many children enter adoptive families with difficulties in the areas of development, behavior, and attachment. These increased needs may potentially exacerbate or significantly tax parents who may be feeling vulnerable, scared, or alone.

Studies of internationally adopted children have shown different features of the child as mediators of parenting stress. For example, in the Canadian-Romanian study, it was found that parenting stress was most significantly related to child behavior problems and the number of children adopted and was negatively correlated with attachment security, family income, and maternal age. The presence of developmental delays and medical problems and the number of siblings were not related to parenting stress [14,48,49]. Behavior problems of significance included increased distractibility and decreased concentration. Similar findings of the relation between parent stress and behavior problems have been shown in studies of parenting in special needs adoptions [50]. In those studies, medical conditions, mental retardation, and sensory impairment did not significantly relate to the quality of the parent-child relationship and developmental delays and learning disability were only moderately associated with impaired parent-child relationships. Behavior problems, however, were strongly associated with difficulties in the parent-child relationship.

Parents may have been less prepared for the behavior problems, and this may contribute to why they are more stressful. Studies have revealed that when parents were asked about all the things that they were concerned about in their child shortly after adoption, 55% reported potential medical problems and 49% reported developmental delay; however, only 18% indicated that behavior problems were a concern [48,49].

These findings contrast with the studies of parenting from the ERA Study, where it was determined that cognitive delays were the primary mediator of impaired parent-child relationships [12,13,50,51]. Prior studies have suggested that delayed children are often less affectively responsive in social interactions and that parents of delayed children may show decreased positive affect toward the child [52,53].

In the ERA study, there were improvements in the parent-child relationship noted over time, and these improvements were primarily mediated by catch-up in cognitive development. The children who were the most delayed on arrival and demonstrated the greatest developmental catch-up constituted the group with the greatest gains in the quality of parent-child relationships.

Working with children and families after international adoption

Overall, almost all adoptive parents express satisfaction with adoption, and this does not diminish over time [51], suggesting that adoptive parents take pleasure in their child's accomplishments and successes. The group of adopted children who experienced sustained early deprivation, separation, and loss before adoption are a heterogeneous group of children who are generally at higher risk for developmental delay, behavior problems, and attachment disturbances, however. Although there is certain to be improvement in a child's development over time after placement in a nurturing and loving home, some of the vulnerabilities conferred from early adversity may be lasting in subtle or not so subtle ways and can have a profound effect on children, parents, and siblings. Although adoptive parents would presumably fit Winnicott's definition of the good enough parent [34,36] as much as nonadoptive parents, unfortunately, this may not be enough in this complex setting. In fact, there are data to suggest that adoptive parents think that parenting a child who experienced early deprivation is more involved parenting [54]. Unfortunately, interventions are scarce that can help parents to develop the skills that may be required to become "good enough and then some" parents to this group of children [35].

Implications for primary care providers

Primary care providers working with internationally adopted children and their families need to be aware of the potential vulnerabilities of adoptive families so as to support them more fully by listening to, recognizing, understanding, and empathizing with their child's and family's needs. Internationally adopted children, especially those with a history of institutional living before adoption, are at greater risk for a range of developmental, behavioral, and attachment concerns, which affect families in a number of ways. As a result, development, behavior, attachment, parent stress, and parent-child interactions need to be monitored routinely and systematically during primary care visits so that appropriate services for children and families can be provided if needed. This is especially true in the first years after adoption when there is significant transition for the parents and the children.

Children adopted internationally and their families are a heterogeneous group. Pediatricians must be thoughtful to individualize the care of adoptive children and not make assumptions shortly after adoption that the family has instantly reconfigured as a consolidated family unit. It is critical to avoid using "standard" parenting advice that may not apply to children who have experienced loss, deprivation, separation, and instability in their early lives. By listening to families, carefully evaluating children, and monitoring progress over time, pediatricians can avoid the pitfall of oversimplifying and underestimating the complexity and challenges that these families face. Instead, pediatric primary care providers can play a key role in maximizing the potential of an internationally adopted child and his or her family.

References

[1] Pennington B. The development of psychopathology: nature and nurture. New York: Guilford Press; 2002.

[2] Gunnar M, Bruce J, Grotevant H. International adoption of institutionally reared children: research and policy. Dev Psychopathol 2000;12:677–93.

[3] Spitz R. Hospitalism: an inquiry into the genesis of psychiatric conditions in early childhood. In: Eissler RS, editor. Psychoanalytic study of the child. New Haven, CT: Yale University Press; 1945.

[4] Provence S, Lipton RC. Infants in institutions. New York: International Universities Press; 1962.

[5] Dennis W. Children of the crèche. New York: Appleton-Century-Crofts; 1973.

[6] Rutter M. Maternal deprivation. In: Bornstein MH, editor. Handbook of parenting, vol. 4. Applied and practical parenting. Mahwah, NJ: Erlbaum; 1995. p. 3–31.

[7] Rutter M, Andersen-Wood L, Beckett C, et al. Quasi-autistic patterns following severe early global privation. J Child Psychol Psychiatry 1999;40:537–49.

[8] Rutter M, O'Connor T, Thomas G. Are there biological programming effects for psychological development? Findings from a study of Romanian adoptees. Dev Psychol 2004;40(1): 81–94.

[9] Rutter M, Kreppner J, O'Connor TG for the English and Romanian Adoptees Study Team. Specificity and heterogeneity in children's responses to profound institutional privation. Br J Psychiatry 2001;179:97–103.

[10] O'Connor TG, Rutter M for the English and Romanian Adoptees Study Team. Attachment disorder behavior following early severe deprivation: extension and longitudinal follow-up. J Am Acad Child Adolesc Psychiatry 2000;39:703–12.

[11] O'Connor TG, Rutter M, Beckett C, et al for the English and Romanian Adoptees Study Team. The effects of global severe privation on cognitive competence: extension and longitudinal follow-up. Child Dev 2000;71:376–90.

[12] O'Connor TG, Bredenkamp D, Michael R, The English and Romanian Adoptees Study Team. Attachment disturbances and disorders in children exposed to early severe deprivation. Infant Ment Health J 1999;20:10–29.

[13] O'Connor TG, Marvin R, Rutter M, et al for the English and Romanian Adoptees Study Team. Child-parent attachment following early institutional deprivation. Dev Psychopathol 2003;15: 19–38.

[14] Ames E. The development of Romanian orphanage children adopted to Canada (final report to the National Welfare Grants Program: Human Resources Development Canada). Burnaby, BC: Simon Fraser University; 1997.

[15] LeMare L. Follow-up on the Romanian Adoptee study. Presented at the Joint Council on International Children's Services, Washington DC, April 10, 2002.

[16] Nord L, et al. Survey made by Smabornscentret in Arhus and Adoption Center Arhus, Denmark concerning children placed in adoption with Danish families through AC Denmark in 1992 and1993. Nordic Research Conference, 35 Years with Intercountry Adoptions. Goteborg: Nordic Research Council; 2001. p. 13–5.

[17] Cederblad M. Adoption—but at what cost? Swedish government report. 2003. Available at http://www.nia.se/english/utredneng.pdf. Accessed July 15, 2005.

[18] Johnson DE, Dole K. International adoptions: implications for early intervention. Infants Young Child 1999;11(4):34–45.

[19] Glennen S, Masters M. Typical and atypical language development in infants and toddlers adopted from Eastern Europe. Am J Speech Lang Pathol 2002;11(4):417–33.

[20] Gindis B. Language-related issues for international adoptees and adoptive families. In: Tepper T, Hannon L, Sanstrom D, editors. International adoption: challenges and opportunities. Meadowlands, PA: Parent Network for the Post-Institutionalized Child; 2000. p. 89–97.

[21] Federici R. Help for the hopeless child: a guide for families (with special discussion for assessing and treating the post-institutionalized child. 2nd edition. Alexandria, VA: Ronald S. Federici and Associates; 2003.

[22] Schecter JD. Observations on adopted children. Arch Gen Psychiatry 1960;3:45–56.

[23] Verhulst FC, Althaus M, Versluis-den Bieman H. Problem behavior in international adoptees: I. An epidemiological study. J Am Acad Child Adolesc Psychiatry 1990;29:94–103.

[24] Verhulst FC, Althaus M, Versluis-den Bieman H. Problem behavior in international adoptees: II. Age at placement. J Am Acad Child Adolesc Psychiatry 1990;29:104–11.

[25] Verhulst FC, Versluis-den Bieman H, van der Ende J, et al. Problem behavior in international adoptees: III. Diagnosis of child psychiatric disorders. J Am Acad Child Adolesc Psychiatry 1990;29:420–8.

[26] Pavao J. The family of adoption. Boston: Beacon Press; 1998.

[27] Gesell A, Amatruda C. Developmental diagnosis: normal and abnormal neuropsychologic development in infancy and early childhood. In: Knobloch H, Pasamanick B, editors. Developmental diagnosis. 3rd edition. Hagerstow, MD: Harper and Row; 1941. p. 1–506.

[28] Kreppner M, O'Connor TG, Rutter M for the English and Romanian Adoptees Study Team. Can inattention/overactivity be an institutional deprivation syndrome? J Abnorm Child Psychol 2001; 29(6):513–8.

[29] Chisholm K. A three year follow-up of attachment and indiscriminate friendliness in children adopted from Romanian orphanages. Child Development 1998;69:1092–106.

[30] Chisholm K, Carter M, Ames E, et al. Attachment security and indiscriminately friendly behavior in children adopted from Romanian orphanages. Dev Psychopathol 1995;7:283–94.

[31] Fisher L, Ames E, Chisholm K, et al. Problems reported by parents of Romanian orphans adopted to British Columbia. Int J Behav Dev 1997;20:67–82.

[32] Bowlby J. Attachment and loss, vol. 1. Attachment. New York: Basic Books; 1982.

[33] Zeanah C. Disturbances of attachment in young children adopted from institutions. J Dev Behav Pediatr 2000;21:230–6.

[34] Winnicott DW. Primary maternal preoccupation. In: Winnicott DW, editor. Collected papers: through pediatrics to psycho-analysis. New York: Basic Books; 1956.

[35] Weitzman CC, Senturias Y, Trivedi P, et al. Nonverbal social communication of international adoptees. Presented at the 2004 Pediatric Academic Society Annual Meeting. San Francisco, May, 2004.

[36] Winnicott DW. The ordinary devoted mother. In: Winnicott C, Shepherd R, Davis M, editors. Babies and their mothers. Reading, MA: Addison-Wesley Publishing Company; 1987. p. 3–14.

[37] Zeanah C. Before it's too late: assessment and treatment of attachment disorders. Presented at the Annual Meeting of the Society for Developmental-Behavioral Pediatrics, Pittsburgh, PA, September 18–22, 2003.

[38] Zeanah C, Smyke A, Dumitrescu A. Attachment disturbances in young children. II: indiscriminate behavior and institutional care. J Am Acad Child Adolesc Psychiatry 2002;41:983–9.

[39] Zeanah C, Boris N. Disturbances and disorders of attachment in early childhood. In: Zeanah CH, editor. Handbook of infant mental health. New York: Guilford Press; 2000. p. 353–68.

[40] Tizard B, Hodges J. The effect of early institutional rearing on the development of eight year old children. J Child Psychol Psychiatry 1978;19:99–118.

[41] Carlson E, Sampson M, Sroufe LA. Implications of attachment theory and research for developmental-behavioral pediatrics. J Dev Behav Pediatr 2003;24:364–79.

[42] Ainsworth MDS, Blehar MC, Waters E, et al. Patterns of attachment: a psychological study of the strange situation. Hillsdale, NJ: Erlbaum; 1978.

[43] Floyd FJ, Philippe KA. Parental interactions with children with and without mental retardation: behavior management, coerciveness, and positive exchange. Am J Ment Retard 1993;97: 673–84.

[44] Marcovitch S, Goldberg S, Gold A, et al. Determinants of behavioral problems in Romanian children adopted in Ontario. Int J Behav Dev 1997;20:17–31.

[45] Tizard B, Ress J. The effect of early institutional rearing on the behavior problems and affectional relationships of four-year-old children. J Child Psychol Psychiatry 1974;16:61–73.

[46] Smyke A, Dumitrescu A, Zeanah C. Attachment disturbances in young children. I: the continuum of caretaking casualty. J Am Acad Child Adolesc Psychiatry 2002;41:972–82.

[47] Waterman B. Mourning the loss builds the bond: primal communication between foster, adoptive and stepmother and child. J Loss Trauma 2001;6:277–300.

[48] Mainemer H, Gilman L, Ames E. Parenting stress in families adopting children from Romanian orphanages. J Fam Issues 1998;19:164–80.

[49] Mainemer H, Gilman L. The experiences of Canadian parents adopting children from Romanian orphanages [abstract]. Canadian Psychology 1992;33:503.

[50] Rosenthal J, Groze V, Aquilar G. Adoption outcomes for children with handicaps. Child Welfare 1991;70(6):623–36.

[51] Groothues C, Beckett C, O'Connor TG. Successful outcomes: a follow-up study of children adopted from Romania into the UK. Adoption Quarterly 2001;5:5–22.

[52] Murray A, Hornbaker AV. Maternal directive and facilitative interaction styles: associations with language and cognitive development of low risk and high risk toddlers. Dev Psychopathol 1997;9:507–16.

[53] Croft C, O'Connor TG, Keaveney L, et al for the English and Romanian Adoption Study Team. Longitudinal change in parenting associated with developmental delay and catch-up. J Child Psychol Psychiatry 2001;42:649–59.

[54] Rochford C. The experience of families who parent an adopted Romanian child. Dissertation Abstracts International Section A: Humanities and Social Sciences 1996;57:2[A].

PEDIATRIC CLINICS
OF NORTH AMERICA

ELSEVIER
SAUNDERS

Pediatr Clin N Am 52 (2005) 1421–1444

Strategies for Addressing Long-Term Issues After Institutionalization

Lisa Nalven, MD, MA, FAAP[a,b,]*

[a]*Developmental Pediatrics–Adoption Screening and Evaluation Program, Valley Center for Child Development, 505 Goffle Road, Ridgewood, NJ 07450, USA*
[b]*Department of Pediatrics, Columbia University College of Physicians and Surgeons, New York, NY, USA*

Any child can exhibit developmental and/or behavioral difficulties; however, a child who has been adopted internationally after institutional (ie, orphanage) care is at increased risk. Because of their prior histories and experiences, these children can present with a complex profile of developmental and behavioral issues that requires a comprehensive approach to evaluation and intervention. This article reviews typical developmental and behavioral concerns seen in post-institutionalized children, discusses considerations pertinent to evaluating this population of children, provides examples of the developmental and/or behavioral profiles of children who exhibit long-term issues, and discusses the strategies and resources available to provide appropriate evaluations and therapeutic interventions for these children.

Background

There are many factors that influence a child's development and behavior. In the general population, 15% to 20% of all children exhibit some type of developmental or behavioral concern that may require intervention. These difficulties are generally attributable to underlying differences in brain development related to a child's genetics, prenatal insults, and postnatal environmental factors. Most children have milder difficulties, such as problems with attention, language, or reading. Only a small percentage have more significant difficulties, such as mental retardation

---

* Valley Center for Child Development, 505 Goffle Road, Ridgewood, NJ 07450.
E-mail address: nalvli@valleyhealth.com

doi:10.1016/j.pcl.2005.06.010   *pediatric.theclinics.com*

(1%–2%) or cerebral palsy (<1%). Children can have specific medical histories that increase the risk of developmental and/or behavioral problems, such as micro-cephaly, premature birth, low birth weight, prenatal alcohol exposure, genetic disorders, or chronic medical conditions. In addition, specific factors like malnutrition, abuse, and neglect can all have long-lasting deleterious effects on children's long-term development and behavior. Children who are raised in environments of "privation" (eg, orphanages, neglect by primary caregivers) are at increased risk for a variety of developmental and behavioral challenges. Human brains have increased susceptibility to these factors during early child-hood, which can impact "critical periods" in specific areas of brain development.

Current reports in the literature suggest that 50% to 90% of children in-ternationally adopted from a variety of countries primarily using orphanage care (eg, Russia, Romania, China) exhibit developmental delays at the time of their initial evaluation and that a significant proportion of these children are delayed in multiple areas (eg, language, cognition, and motor skills) [1–5]. Follow-up of these children described that some children exhibited typical development, par-ticularly those who were adopted at less than 6 months of age, whereas children who were in orphanages longer, had medical problems, or demonstrated more significant growth delays at adoption exhibited a greater degree of developmental delay and behavioral difficulties. Children typically make rapid gains shortly after joining their adoptive families. There are some children who are extremely resilient, and after their initial adjustment, they "catch up" entirely, without any obvious evidence of being influenced by their early experiences. Most children continue to make progress (but at a slower rate) through school years and may have mild difficulties that persist. There are some children who continue to experience more significant developmental and/or behavioral difficulties and require a great deal of ongoing supportive services [1,4,6–11]. The variability in progress for children is a function of the underlying cause(s) of their difficulties and the strategies and resources used to improve on a child's deficits.

Developmental evaluation of the postinstitutionalized child

Considerations in developmental evaluation

Initial and follow-up developmental evaluations are time-consuming. A 15- to 30-minute routine pediatric visit from which a clinician develops a *gestalt* de-velopmental assessment has been demonstrated not to be sufficient for identifying developmental concerns and formulating an appropriate diagnosis. Studies have shown that general pediatricians generally do not make accurate appraisals of a child's intelligence (IQ) when compared with formal psychometric testing and tend to underidentify the presence and degree of cognitive impairment [12,13]. Deficits in residency training, limitations of the general pediatric office setting, limited time for visits, individual factors, and biases all contribute to the chal-lenges of making developmental diagnoses in the primary care setting [14].

Language barriers also have an impact on the clinician's and parent's ability to assess a child's development after international adoption. Children's language is often used as an indicator or proxy for intelligence. Given that most clinicians and parents do not speak the child's native language, accurate assessment of the child's skills is difficult if not impossible. For the older child who speaks another language and has not yet mastered English, casual observation without formal testing is not an accurate assessment of a child's abilities. In addition, most young children adopted from orphanages are delayed in their primary language because of lack of stimulation and opportunity to engage in language. Therefore, language is not a reliable indicator of a child's overall intelligence, general problem-solving ability, or long-term developmental potential.

Children may present with a range of developmental and/or behavioral challenges. There are children whose delays or behavioral issues are significant, and therefore quite apparent on observation in the general pediatric office setting, such as children presenting with autism or severe developmental delays. For children with more subtle or complex difficulties, however, the extent of impairment often is not clear and may only be evident to the pediatrician because of a parent's expressed concerns. Both groups of children require specialized evaluations and interventions, which are often beyond the scope of general pediatric practice.

Complexity of diagnostic considerations and interventions

The multifactorial nature of a postinstitutionalized child's developmental and/or behavioral challenges requires that all possible causes be identified and addressed. What seem to be similar difficulties in learning and behavior may have many different underlying causes (Box 1). Postinstitutionalized children are exposed to a variety of pre- and postnatal factors that have an impact on brain wiring and function. A clear understanding of a given child's profile of brain functioning is essential to understanding why he or she is having difficulty in learning or is exhibiting certain behaviors. Appropriate treatment requires accurately identifying the underlying causes and additional factors that may impede or support a child's progress. This usually requires multidisciplinary evaluations and interventions as well as long-term monitoring of a child's progress.

Case 1

Sonya was adopted from the Ukraine at 18 months of age. She presented with global delay, failure to thrive, and microcephaly. Sonya received early intervention services and made dramatic gains in her development. Although initially demonstrating catch-up with respect to her physical growth, she was of short stature and had persistent microcephaly and mildly dysmorphic features. As a result of persistent difficulties, she was evaluated by a developmental pediatrician and a child development team. Medical evaluation, including genetic testing and assessment of dysmorphology, did not identify a specific cause for Sonya's difficulties.

Box 1. Observed behaviors and possible diagnoses

Behaviors exhibited

> Difficulty in communicating needs
> Poor school performance
> Poor eye contact
> Poor or inappropriate social interaction
> Noncompliant/defiant behavior
> Inattentive/hyperactive
> Aggression
> Atypical behaviors (eg, self-stimulatory)

Diagnoses to be considered

> Prenatal brain injury
> Trauma (physical, emotional)
> Neurologic disorder
> Learning disabilities
> Emotional difficulties
> Learned behaviors

At 3 years of age, Sonya transitioned into a specialized language-based pre-school program, where she continued to receive speech and language and occupational therapies. In her classroom, she became social with peers and acquired age-appropriate preacademic skills, and significant behavioral issues were not observed. At home, she continued to demonstrate issues around "control" and remained hypervigilant when with her family in routine community settings. Sonya intermittently attended play therapy, and her parents were offered support for addressing behavioral issues. In contrast to Sonya' controlling style, her parents had a quiet soft demeanor and needed help in responding to her behavior.

Comprehensive testing was performed through Sonya's local school system before her transition to kindergarten, demonstrating her intelligence to be within the "normal" range. Language skills were generally in the normal range as well, although she had relative weaknesses with tasks requiring the use of more abstract concepts. Her hypervigilance and guarded manner continued outside home and school environments. Based on this assessment and on her previous success with a specialized preschool program, Sonya entered a mainstream classroom without additional support. Early in the school year, Sonya began to regress: toileting accidents, disorganized drawings, social withdrawal, and concerns for attention deficit/hyperactivity disorder (ADHD) were expressed by the teacher. Sonya seemed to be overwhelmed by the demands of the busy classroom and could not demonstrate the skills she had previously mastered. Her comfort level and strengths as exhibited in a small, structured, supportive classroom disappeared in a less structured and more demanding environment. Without environmental support, Sonya's anxiety became overwhelming and severely compromised her ability to function in her classroom.

A recommendation was made for Sonya to transition to a smaller classroom for children with learning disabilities so as to receive support for her academic subjects, with opportunities to join the mainstream class for activities, such as art, gym, and music. Her private therapist was recontacted to work with Sonya and her family and to consult with the school regarding her emotional needs, because these issues overshadowed the gains she had made with regard to academic skills. Sonya, although making significant gains, had persistent difficulties with more complex language functions, nonverbal memories, and emotional dysregulation that interfered with her ability to function without any support.

Genetic influences, prenatal insults, and postnatal trauma all may have been involved in the development of this child's neural circuitry, which has been permanently altered and requires long-term intervention, even with "normal intelligence." As increasing demands were placed on Sonya, they exceeded her capacity to respond by using her cognitive abilities and to regulate her emotions, resulting in what was perceived to be a behavioral problem. Interventions were required to support the weaknesses in her cognitive profile and to assist her with processing and managing her inner emotional life.

Initial evaluation

Children adopted from institutional settings are considered at "high risk" for developmental and behavioral difficulties, and most warrant a systematic evaluation documenting their profile of strengths and weaknesses to guide appropriate interventions. Ideally, postarrival developmental evaluations should be performed by professionals who are experienced in child development, familiar with the effects of institutional living, and knowledgeable about the specific risk factors pertinent to a particular child's profile. Because of the range of potential issues for postinstitutionalized children, a multidisciplinary approach is recommended, which may include some or all of the following for a given child: a general pediatrician, developmental pediatrician, child neurologist, pediatric psychologist/neuropsychologist, occupational therapist, physical therapist, speech/language therapist, nutritionist, and early childhood educator.

Within a few weeks after a child joins his or her adoptive family, a detailed baseline evaluation that reviews available history and includes physical and developmental evaluations should be performed. The initial evaluation should document the age level at which a child is functioning in various domains of development (eg, cognitive, fine motor, gross motor, expressive/receptive language, socioemotional, self-help) and determine if the delays observed are consistent with what is known about postinstitutionalized children or attributable to other factors. Standardized instruments in conjunction with functional observations help to provide a complete picture of a child's profile of strengths and weaknesses and the direction for intervention. A baseline physical and neuro-motor evaluation is also important to identify findings that are consistent with orphanage care (low muscle tone, pattern of growth failure and delays) versus those that point to other factors (increased muscle tone, focal neurologic findings, dysmorphic features) and may require additional medical evaluation by appropriate specialists, such as a developmental pediatrician, pediatric neurologist, or geneticist. Baseline assessments should help to determine whether interventions are required immediately or can be deferred while the child is adjusting to his or her new home and being monitored. Parents should be provided with guidance to support their child's development and transition into family life (see the articles by Miller and Schulte and Springer elsewhere in this issue).

Follow-up assessment

During an initial adjustment period after international adoption, a child must become accustomed to living in a family, hearing a new language, and learning about an entirely new environment and way of living. With infants and toddlers, many families settle into a comfortable routine within a month of being together. Older children typically take longer to adjust, because years of prior experiences need to be incorporated into their new life and expectations for normal functioning in home, school, and social settings are greater. Families often benefit from working with qualified professionals to develop strategies that foster bonding and skill development during the initial adjustment period or shortly thereafter. Professional guidance is particularly important if a child is demonstrating continued developmental delays or having difficulty in adjusting to family living or if new difficulties emerge over time.

Children with developmental delays or challenging behaviors require ongoing monitoring to determine if they are making appropriate progress. Ongoing developmental evaluation, initially every 3 to 4 months, is important to determine whether a child is making expected progress and would benefit from skilled developmental and/or behavioral interventions. For a child with an early pattern of milder delays and behaviors consistent with institutionalization, guidance and monitoring without immediately initiating therapeutic services may be sufficient. Comparing the number of months a child is with his or her family with the number of months gained in skills is often a good measure of progress. To catch up, a child must demonstrate greater than 1 month of developmental progress for each month that he or she is with his or her family. The rate of learning and behavioral adjustment shortly after arrival and through the first 6 months can provide some insight into how "intact" a child's neurocognitive profile may be in the long term.

If a child's history or initial physical examination identifies known risk factors (eg, prematurity, prenatal alcohol exposure, seizures, significant malnutrition or failure to thrive, abuse), ongoing evaluation and specific interventions are indicated. Even if a child demonstrates early developmental catch-up, difficulties with higher order cognitive skills as well as with behavioral and emotional regulation may not be evident until school age. Thus, for children who do not exhibit significant difficulties early on, parents may later identify increasing concerns as the children grow older and demands increase. Providers should have a low threshold for referring any child with a history of institutionalization and associated risk factors who later presents with any type of developmental or behavioral difficulty for comprehensive evaluations. Guided by a child's neuro-developmental profile, ongoing involvement of pediatric specialists, such as a developmental pediatrician, neurologist, or psychiatrist, may assist in integrating the results of multidisciplinary evaluations, making recommendations for specific interventions, performing additional medical evaluations, or prescribing medication.

Case 2

Lilly is a 15-month-old child adopted from a Chinese orphanage at 11 months of age. On joining her family, she was "developmentally delayed." At her initial primary care visit, immunizations were given, but further medical testing and developmental assessments were not performed. Four months after arrival, she was brought to a developmental pediatrician because little developmental progress was observed. Per parent report, Lilly had a rudimentary combat crawl that primarily relied on her arms, would not weight bear on her legs, manipulated toys in her hands but did not expand her exploration, vocalized a /k/ sound and "ah," and had difficulty taking pureed foods from a spoon. Since joining her family, Lilly had demonstrated improved head control, an emerging ability to balance when placed in a sitting position, turning to her English name, and recognizing family members. The results of her physical examination were remarkable for poor muscle strength and tone, but there were no focal findings.

Occupational, physical, speech and language, and feeding therapies were recommended for Lilly, and her parents were given written handouts with activities to support Lilly's skill development. Routine medical testing for children adopted internationally was ordered, including an audiologic evaluation (see the article by Schulte and Springer elsewhere in this issue). A follow-up appointment in several months was scheduled to review Lilly's progress with intervention and to determine if additional medical testing for evaluation of the developmental delay was indicated. Four months after arrival, Lilly had not made adequate gains in her skills and was not demonstrating catch-up in her development. Although the available history did not document any additional risk factors beyond orphanage care, Lilly's learning profile is not progressing as expected and increases the concern for ongoing issues.

Accessing developmental and behavioral evaluations and services

Within the American educational and health care systems, developmental and/ or behavioral evaluations for children can be accessed through private and public resources. Private resources include hospitals with child development centers, pediatric therapy and rehabilitation centers, and community practices. The specific provider or the services for a "developmental or behavioral" issue may not be reimbursed by health insurance. In some cases, an initial evaluation is covered but not any of the recommended therapies (eg, speech, occupational, and physical therapies) recommended as a result of the evaluation. Behavioral and mental health resources for children are often difficult to access, and health care plans often have designated providers who may not have expertise in working with this specific population. Because developmental and/or behavioral difficulties often require ongoing treatment, the cost of private services without insurance coverage can be staggering and not a viable option for many families. Given the relatively modest cost of developmental and behavioral evaluations relative to the cost of providing ongoing developmental and/or behavioral therapeutic interventions, private resources (eg, developmental pediatrician, child psychiatrist, educational psychologist, speech/language therapist) can be used to confirm a family's concerns. The results of these evaluations and resulting recommendations can then be presented to the community- and school-based developmental and educational programs to guide the services that a child can receive through the public sector at no cost to the family. Families may choose to use private resources or therapies to augment the services their children are receiving through public programs.

Publicly funded resources for children with developmental issues are mandated through state and federal laws, and therefore can be requested by a parent without a referral from a physician, insurance provider, or other professional provider. The Education for All Handicapped Act (PL94-142) and the Individual with Disabilities Act (IDEA, PL99-457, reauthorized in 2004) guarantee evaluation and services for eligible children from birth to the age of 21 years. Although based in federal law, services and funding are administered at the state level, leading to some variability across the country based on the process and services provided in particular communities. Some services may be contracted to private providers. Pediatricians should be familiar with their local guidelines for accessing public resources and help parents to become advocates for their child's needs through early intervention and school programs.

Early intervention

Early intervention typically provides evaluation and therapy for children from birth to 3 years of age. To initiate the process, parents or other providers contact the state-designated agency to request an evaluation. Typically, a telephone call to the appropriate agency is all that is required to initiate the process, with later completion of written consent. There are specific time lines required for agency response, evaluation, and implementation of services, and parents may discontinue their involvement with the program at any time. A multidisciplinary evaluation should be conducted to establish a child's developmental skills in each domain of functioning. Speech and language, occupational, and physical therapists; early childhood specialists; educators; and social workers may all be involved in the assessment process. In some states, baseline medical evaluations by a developmental pediatrician, neurologist, orthopedist, audiologist, or other specialist may be included (Box 2). To qualify for therapeutic services, some state guidelines require 33% delay in one domain of development or 25% delay in two or more domains. If a child qualifies for services, an individualized family service plan (IFSP) is written, which outlines the goals and objectives of the services and the types of interventions that are to be provided. Services may include various therapies, case management, and parent support. Children who do not qualify for services but are thought to be at risk for developmental issues may be enrolled in a "tracking" program with periodic assessment of their development. If a parent disagrees with the evaluation outcome, there are procedures to appeal denial of services.

At the state level, the services received and the cost to the family vary based on local regulations and resources. In some cases, only evaluation is provided and families bear the burden of identifying and paying for the cost of intervention services. In other states, there are limited to extensive services provided at no cost to families or using a sliding scale model based on family income. Home-based versus center-based provision of services also varies by state. Once in the program, periodic re-evaluation should be performed, usually every 6 months or sooner if needed. If it is thought that a child continues to need services after 3 years of age, help with transitioning to an appropriate preschool program should be provided and initiated at least 90 days before the child's third birthday.

Special education

From the age of 3 years (preschool) until the age of 21 years, the public school district is responsible for the evaluation and provision of services for children with developmental challenges under legislation for special education services. Evaluation by a child's school district can be initiated by the school or parent but

---

Box 2. Evaluations for early intervention and special education services

- Developmental/intelligence (IQ) testing
- Achievement/learning assessment
- Occupational therapy (fine motor, graphomotor, visual-motor, visual perceptual, self-help)
- Physical therapy (gross motor)
- Speech/language therapy
- Social/emotional
- Medical (may involve developmental pediatrician, pediatric neurologist, or child psychiatrist)

requires that parents provide a written request and consent for the process to be initiated. A child may be receiving services through early intervention or privately, receiving no services and attending public or private school, or not in school when the request for evaluation is made. As with early intervention, there are specific time lines and procedures for the evaluation process, meeting with parents, and making a decision as to whether or not to provide special education services for a child. Intake and testing should occur according to state-specified guidelines and procedures. A multidisciplinary evaluation of areas of concern is performed, which may involve some of or all the domains listed in Box 2.

Formal testing and an assessment of a child's ability to function at an age- or grade-appropriate level determine his or her eligibility for special education services. For example, a child may not be deemed eligible for special educational services because he or she may have areas of weakness that do not meet criteria for a disability requiring services, or he or she may exhibit difficulties that do not occur at school or do not affect his or her academic progress. If there is a disagreement between parents and the school district's recommendations, there are guidelines for appeals, due process, and second opinions.

According to federal guidelines, children must meet criteria for a category of disability in order to receive special education services (Box 3). Variations of the classification guidelines may occur from state to state. The specific category does not necessarily determine the type of services a child receives, because children with a similar diagnostic classification may have a range of challenges, but rather determines that a child is eligible for services. At the preschool level, children are often classified under a general heading of developmentally delayed, because the final diagnosis is not often clear at a young age.

If a child is determined to be eligible for services, an individualized education plan (IEP) is written, which outlines the child's difficulties, goals and objec-

---

Box 3. Special education categories

- Vision impaired
- Hearing impaired
- Traumatic brain injury
- Autistic
- Learning disabled
- Emotionally disturbed
- Multiply disabled
- Communication impaired
- Mental retardation
- Orthopedic impairment
- Other health impaired (medical issues that interfere with school performance, including ADHD)
- Preschool handicapped

tives to address those difficulties, and specific interventions to be provided (eg, specific therapies, instruction, teaching and classroom modifications, equipment, transportation, summer programming). A child's classroom placements should be in the "least restrictive environment" that meets the child's learning needs. Interventions may include classroom or work modification; an in-class aide; and specialized instruction and/or therapies in the classroom or in a separate classroom, self-contained classroom, or specialized school. For some children, a mainstream classroom with interventions that target a specific weakness is sufficient. Other children, because of more significant impairments, may require a school that specializes in meeting their physical, learning, behavioral, or emotional needs.

A child's IEP must be reviewed and updated each year to ensure that the child continues to receive appropriate services. This includes a summary of the child's "present level of performance." A complete re-evaluation is required every 3 years (or earlier if indicated) and on transition to different stages of programming (eg, transition to kindergarten or middle school) to review a child's diagnoses and necessary interventions.

If a child has areas of weakness that do not meet criteria for special education services, there are several other options for a child to receive academic support. Basic skill or supplemental instruction can be provided to give additional support in academic areas, such as reading or mathematics, but the intensity of the intervention and strategies used may differ greatly from those provided under special education. For physical or mental disabilities that affect academic functioning but do not meet criteria for special education services, the Rehabilitation Act of 1973 (PL93-112) may be helpful. Section 504 of the Rehabilitation Act comes under the American Disabilities Act (not special education law) and applies to institutions that receive federal funds, such as public schools. The focus of this law is to prevent discrimination against individuals with disabilities who require modifications so that a disabling condition does not interfere with access to or performing one's job. Typically, this law has been directed toward physical disabilities (eg, ramps for wheel chairs), but it has also has been applied in the school setting to include children with ADHD, a medical condition that interferes with a child's school performance. Under this law, a 504 Plan can be written to provide modifications that support a child's success in school (eg, preferential seating, untimed tests). Unlike special education interventions, 504 Plan modifications do not come with federal funding support and different guidelines and procedures apply.

Parents may also turn to private resources for support. This option may be useful to augment services that are being provided at school but is not a substitute for services that a child may need during the school day. For many children, an hour of tutoring or therapy after school does little to support them during the 6-hour school day, where they are constantly being challenged. The classroom setting requires specific neurocognitive skills of children to demonstrate their academic and social competence. For children with significant deficits, replacement instruction and in-class accommodations are necessary.

Private resources are also appropriate if a child has areas of weakness that do not meet criteria for school support but would benefit from remediation. Although not qualifying for public services, children with the milder deficits can benefit from thoughtful intervention and can demonstrate gains that have a positive impact on their ability to function. In these cases, after-school tutoring, occupational therapy, speech therapy, or other interventions may helpful. Children who exhibit a mild or focused weakness may be able to carry over skills acquired in a private therapy session into the classroom setting (Fig. 1).

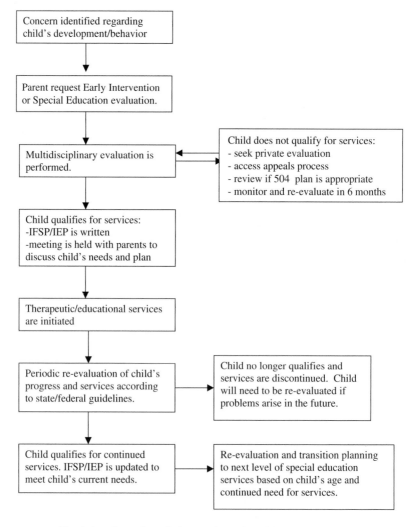

Fig. 1. A pathway for early intervention and special education services.

Therapists

Therapists who work with children are trained in a variety of disciplines, and their involvement is determined by a child's specific needs. These professionals may work directly with a child to address skill mastery (eg, occupational or speech therapist) or to address emotional issues (eg, child psychiatrist, psychologist, social worker). For some children, physical nurturing, emotional reassurance, and consistency may suffice, whereas for others, more directed therapy may be necessary for a child to work through and process prior experiences. As children become more verbal and function at more abstract and higher cognitive levels, "play therapy" may evolve into a more talk-oriented cognitive therapy model. Some children may benefit from using medication to help manage their behavioral and/or emotional difficulties, allowing them to be more available to benefit from other modes of therapeutic intervention.

In addition to working directly with a child, therapists should provide parents with specific tools and strategies for supporting their child, for responding to difficult situations, and for structuring their family's household and activities to meet their child's needs. Parents may not come to their role with skills that match their child's specific issues, but this does not mean that they are poor parents. Parent training can make them "experts" in meeting their child's needs. This applies whether working on fine motor skills, language, behavior, or emotional issues.

When identifying a therapist of any type, parents and referring providers should ask about the therapist's prior experience in working with children adopted from institutions abroad, primary age group of his or her clients, diagnoses with which he or she is familiar, theoretic framework, and type of interventions offered through his or her practice. Contacting local adoptive parent groups who have resource lists or agencies that work with the state foster care system can provide recommendations of professionals with appropriate expertise. Parents should be wary of professionals who offer "cure" and unique interventions that are not generally endorsed by professional peers (see the article by Costello on complementary and alternative therapies elsewhere in this issue).

Community resources

Supportive services for families are important for children with a range of developmental, behavioral, or emotional challenges. Some families may need to learn a limited set of skills to meet their child's needs. Others may need to learn to advocate for their child to receive appropriate educational and mental health and/or disability services and resources. Some families may need tangible day-to-day support. State agencies (eg, Department of Developmental Disabilities, Department of Mental Retardation) and private organizations (eg, Young Men's Christian Association [YMCA], Young Women's Christian Association [YWCA]) may offer recreational activities, transportation, and in-home support services as well as respite resources. Making families aware of these resources can help them to support their child's development while allowing them to attend to other children at home, be able to participate in the community, and preserve the well-being of their family. In some cases, a child's emotional and behavioral needs exceed a family's ability to manage the situation appropriately while the child remains in their home. In some cases, the safety of the child or of family members is at risk and an out-of-home therapeutic living arrangement may be required. If this becomes a consideration, families require knowledge of public and private agencies and funding mechanisms as well as family emotional support.

Key considerations pertinent in evaluation of international adoptees

Evaluation of language development

When evaluating a child adopted from an orphanage abroad, it is critical to consider a child's preadoptive history, including exposure to a learning environment, and the limitations of a cognitive or learning assessment obtained before a child becomes fluent in his or her new language. One specific challenge, particularly when assessing preschool- or school-aged international adoptees, is determining a child's language competence. Professionals who are not familiar with children with this type of history often attribute a child's difficulties solely to the fact that he or she simply has not yet learned English; thus, problems are thought to be attributable to English as a second language (ESL) issues. In fact, many of the children we see in the infant to toddler stage have not mastered their primary language (eg, Russian, Chinese) at an age-appropriate level (eg, a 2-year-old who only babbles) at the time of their adoption. Older children may speak their native language but still exhibit language delays and/or disorders because of living in a language-poor environment or neurologic issues. If a child demonstrates difficulties and/or delays in his or her primary language, this represents a language "disorder" and affects a child's ability to learn English. For children who are truly language delayed, remediation is essential and requires formal speech and language therapy. In contrast, a child whose primary language is age appropriate should be able to learn English without significant difficulty; an ESL approach would be appropriate with explanation to the school that unlike other typical ESL children, international adoptees are losing their primary language while learning a second. Importantly, when assessing a child's development within several months of adoption and planning for appropriate intervention, it is important to assess a child's language and other abilities in his or her native language.

Young children are often learning English words in their first weeks with their families. Once immersed in English, children lose their native language at a quicker rate than they acquire English. As a result, there is a window of opportunity for assessment that is lost if formal evaluation is deferred. By law, early intervention programs and school districts must evaluate a child in his or her native language to determine if any type of delay is present. Although not ideal, for infants and toddlers who have limited language (although receptive skills may be better developed than expressive skills), delay can be documented based on the child's history provided by the agency and/or orphanage or on a limited sound and word repertoire at initial evaluation even if testing in the child's native language is not performed. Children aged 3 years and older typically have developed some language proficiency and should have testing in their native language within a month after arrival to obtain the most accurate assessment of their language abilities. This can be difficult to achieve in an appropriate time frame through public resources, and parents may choose to seek private resources to obtain an assessment before the child loses her or his highest level of language mastery in the native language.

Limitations of catch-up and acculturation

Although internationally adopted children typically have a period of adjustment, growth and developmental catch-up, and acculturation, this process does not go on indefinitely. Rutter [6] studied young children adopted from Romania who were re-evaluated at 4 and 6 years of age. Difficulties that were present at the 4-year evaluation persisted at 6 years, and the gains that were documented at 4 years were maintained at 6 years. Thus, it is not acceptable to continue to attribute learning and behavioral difficulties to second language issues or to an ongoing need to adjust, leading to the conclusion that a child just needs more time to catch up. The impact of malnutrition, stress, trauma, and deprivation on early brain wiring may have significant implications for higher order cognitive functions, which may be evident at the time of adoption or may not become apparent until grade school, when demands increase. Moreover, deficits in brain function attributable to prematurity or fetal alcohol exposure do not fade or disappear over time.

Differential diagnosis of a child's difficulties

Similar behaviors may stem from many different causes, including but not limited to prenatal brain injury, prenatal substance exposure, trauma (physical or emotional), neurologic disorders, learning disabilities, emotional difficulties, or learned behaviors. Although a child adopted from an orphanage may have issues similar to those of a child who has not experienced privation, postinstitutionalized children are at increased risk and may have multiple factors that contribute to developmental, learning, behavioral, or emotional difficulties. Language delay could be representative of ESL, an isolated language disorder, a sign of mental retardation, selective mutism, hearing impairment, or a combination of factors. Learned behaviors that may have been adaptive in the orphanage setting may be a poor match for family and school functioning. A comprehensive evaluation of a child is necessary to identify potential causes and comorbidities of a child's difficulties and to design appropriate interventions.

Cognitive impairment and learning disabilities

A child's early delays in skill acquisition and learning may persist over time; in such a case, the diagnosis should eventually be reformulated and better described as meeting criteria for mental retardation or a specific learning disability. Children with less severe learning issues may first present with behavioral or emotional difficulties because they do not understand the material expected of them in the classroom setting. Learning disabilities and mild mental retardation cannot be diagnosed if a proper assessment is not performed.

Interventions for learning difficulties include educational remediation and necessary accommodations throughout the school years. Although a child with a learning disability may initially demonstrate significant gains with intervention, there are some areas that may always remain weak. For example, children with early language delays are known to be at increased risk for later language-based learning issues, such as difficulty in reading (ie, dyslexia.) With appropriate intervention, children with dyslexia can become accurate readers. Although these children learn to read at grade level, they continue to be slower readers into adulthood. As a result, an intervention that starts as remediation in grade school with specialized reading instruction becomes a need for accommodations, such as extra time for reading and taking tests, through high school [15].

The school experience requires that children engage in all subjects independent of ability or interest. For children with more significant cognitive-adaptive impairment, appropriate educational interventions to teach academic and life skills are necessary to support optimal current and future functioning. For children with milder learning difficulties, school may always be difficult. Nevertheless, they can be successful in life if they receive appropriate support and parents have appropriate expectations. In the end, individuals self-select their future academic or vocational pursuits based on their individual aptitudes.

Attention deficit/hyperactivity disorder

As with many preschool and school-aged children, parents often wonder if their internationally adopted child has ADHD. ADHD is said to affect 4% to 10% of the school population [16]. Although internationally adopted children may present with the core symptoms of inattention and/or distractibility, impulsivity, or hyperactivity associated with a diagnosis of ADHD [17], their preadoptive experiences may have contributed to their symptoms and require consideration of a comprehensive differential diagnosis of their "ADHD symptoms" (Box 4). A thorough evaluation to rule in or to exclude other causes for a child's observed behaviors and common comorbidities is essential. If the primary diagnosis is not ADHD but perhaps depression resulting in inattention, the appropriate intervention for a child is vastly different. Children who have cognitive impairment or learning issues are less likely to attend because of poor comprehension of the material presented, not necessarily because of a primary difficulty with attention, and they may act out because of frustration rather than poor impulse control.

Box 4. Differential diagnosis of attention deficit/hyperactivity disorder symptoms

- Adjustment reaction
- Age-appropriate behavior in an active child
- Language delay
- Learning disability
- Cognitive impairment (mental retardation)
- Anxiety (including PTSD)
- Depression
- Autistic spectrum disorder (including pervasive developmental disorders)

Moreover, it is estimated that 40% to 60% of children with ADHD also have learning difficulties or other comorbid conditions, such as anxiety or depression [16]. In these cases, stimulant medications are not the sole treatment recommended. Intervention needs to be multimodal to address all the impairments that negatively affect a child's functioning in home and school settings.

Case 3

Alexander is a 10-year-old adopted from Russia at 2 years of age. Alexander was first evaluated at the age of 6 years because of concerns about possible ADHD. At the initial evaluation, physical examination revealed that Alexander had facial features and growth characteristics consistent with fetal alcohol syndrome (FAS), which had not been previously diagnosed. Alexander was attached to his parents but was indiscriminately friendly in social settings. His parents had explicitly taught him to use formal greetings and shake hands, but he needed a reminder not to hug the examiner.

Formal psychoeducational evaluation demonstrated Alexander's intelligence to be in the average range, but he had relative weaknesses with visual spatial and visual perceptual skills as well as difficulties with social comprehension, organization, inattention, and impulsivity. Medication was initiated to address the symptoms of inattention and impulsivity. Behavioral management strategies and information about FAS were discussed with Alexander's parents. Based on the psychoeducational testing, recommendations were made for a special education classification with educational interventions.

Alexander attended a parochial school, and although state and federal guidelines require special education services be provided, these services were not as extensive as those available in a public school. Because the school provided close supervision that would address social and safety concerns, Alexander remained at the parochial school through the third grade. At that time, the academic support he required could no longer be provided in his private school setting, and he transitioned to a public school program. Increased academic support was provided with Alexander attending a resource room for some academic subjects, but modifications for his mainstream classroom were not implemented. The school and teacher continued to view Alexander as a child with normal intelligence, ADHD symptoms, and learning weaknesses and did not have an understanding of the larger neurocognitive issues seen in children with FAS.

During his most recent school year in the fifth grade, Alexander remained pleasant and outgoing, but a more complete neurocognitive profile of a child with FAS became more evident. Alexander increasingly demonstrated poor judgment and did not learn from his prior experiences at an age when children are expected to begin to exhibit more independence and require less adult supervision. Alexander has "borrowed" his mother's cell phone and has walked out of the house and taken a ride with someone he recognized from church rather than waiting for his father to drive him to school. His teacher supervised him packing up his backpack at the end of the school day, but Alexander would put work back in his locker if he did not like the assignment or thought that it was already completed. He continued to be smaller than his peers, was frequently teased, and tended to "hang out" with the children who were most likely to get into trouble. His teacher thinks that because he is in the fifth grade, he should be more "responsible" and not need additional support or supervision from parents or teachers.

Alexander's parents continued to advocate for ongoing academic and behavioral support at school, including appropriate modification of his work assignments, support for organizational skills, and improved supervision. They limited Alexander's social activities to those at their church with adult supervision. Alexander's parents were directed to information to help mitigate the "secondary morbidities" (eg, school failure, trouble with the law, substance abuse) seen in children with FAS, which are a result of the neurologic dysfunction caused by alcohol exposure during fetal brain development [18]. Despite normal intelligence, Alexander is going to require lifelong support.

FAS and other alcohol-related disabilities are the result of alcohol's direct injury to the developing fetus, which can produce characteristic facial dysmorphology, impair physical growth, and compromise central nervous system (CNS) development and function (see the article on prenatal substance exposure by Davies and Bledsoe elsewhere in this issue). Comprehensive evaluation revealed that Alexander's inattentive and impulsive behaviors, which were thought to represent ADHD symptoms, had much broader implications for diagnosis, and interventions were recommended.

Reactive attachment disorder

In contrast to ADHD, which is thought to be relatively common in the general pediatric population, reactive attachment disorder (RAD) is quite rare. Children with RAD present with "markedly disturbed and developmentally inappropriate social relatedness" and have a history of "grossly pathologic care" [17]. Pathologic care can include abuse, neglect, or the lack of a stable primary caregiver and is nearly universal for children adopted from an orphanage. Typical bonding and attachment challenges are expected as a child becomes part of his or her family; however, not all children who experience pathologic care develop RAD symptoms. Professionals and parents are often quick to raise this diagnostic consideration with an adopted child, even if a child has been adopted as a young infant or may have been in a nurturing environment since infancy.

Ultimately, consideration of a diagnosis of RAD in the context of planning further assessment of a child's difficulties is recommended for children who do not seem to have formed a special relationship with family members and who do not exhibit the ability to empathize with others, feel remorse, or control their impulses. According to the *Diagnostic and Statistical Manual of Mental Disorders*, fourth edition (DSM-IV) classification, children may present with an "inhibited" subtype (avoidant, hypervigilant, and withdrawn) or "disinhibited" subtype (indiscriminately friendly with strangers) of RAD. Any diagnosis of an attachment disorder requires a careful evaluation of a child's pre- and post-adoptive history, current levels of function across domains, and past and current behaviors as well as a review of medical issues. Although a child may manifest outward behaviors suggesting the possible diagnosis of RAD, the underlying issue may not be the child's inability to form selective attachments but another developmental or behavioral disorder (Box 5) [17].

Case 4

Jeff was adopted from Moldova at 10 months of age. He was malnourished and "very active" at the time of his adoption. His growth and development were reported to catch up quickly, but his kindergarten teacher reported that he could not remain in the class without the support of a one-to-one aide. Jeff's parents were concerned about his activity level, oppositional behavior, and obsessions. Jeff's first consultation was at an ADHD clinic. Parents and teachers completed questionnaires, but Jeff was not interviewed or evaluated. A diagnosis

---

Box 5. Differential diagnosis of reactive attachment disorder symptoms

- Adjustment reaction
- Depression
- Learning disability
- Cognitive impairment (mental retardation)
- Parent-child relational problem
- Autistic spectrum disorder (including pervasive developmental disorders)
- ADHD
- Oppositional/defiant disorder

of the combined type of ADHD was made, and medications were started with limited benefit.

A second consultation was performed at an "attachment center." Parents completed questionnaires and were interviewed. Jeff was not interviewed or evaluated, and a diagnosis of RAD was made. The family began work with a therapist. At 6 years of age, Jeff was seen at a child development clinic. Comprehensive evaluation revealed multiple tics (vocal and motor), obsessive and compulsive features, a verbal IQ much higher than the nonverbal IQ, deficits in executive functioning, neurologic "soft signs," and visual impairments.

A discussion was held with Jeff's parents and his teacher about the cognitive, emotional, and social implications of the neurobehavioral profile. Educational interventions were provided, as were eye glasses, social skills training, and medication for the obsessive features. Weaknesses in a child's cognitive profile can affect his social competency with family and friends. Without a full understanding of Jeff's profile, appropriate interventions had not been implemented. Understanding of a child's neurocognitive profile is important in understanding the child's behavioral and emotional response to situations. If a child has difficulties with abstract language or has features of a nonverbal learning disability, understanding facial expressions and emotions can be difficult and may make a child seem unattached [19].

Treatment for RAD, as opposed to a learning disability, focuses on helping the child develop trusting and secure relationships with individuals who are significant in his or her life. Treatments are multimodal and are based on a child's developmental age, with the goal of facilitating the parent-child relationship. Providing parents with appropriate support and strategies for working with their child is critical.

Posttraumatic stress disorder

Posttraumatic stress disorder (PTSD) is precipitated by a traumatic event or series of events that result in a real or perceived threat to an individual's or another's safety and manifests as feelings of intense fear, helplessness, or horror, and thus overwhelming anxiety, for the affected person. Children with symptoms of PTSD may present with disorganized or agitated behavior, sleep disturbances, flashbacks, hypervigilance, poor concentration, irritability, avoidance, and withdrawal in certain situations that arouse memories of previously traumatic events [17]. Alternate criteria for PTSD, which expand on DSM-IV criteria, have been suggested for the preschool-aged group, which adjust manifestations for their developmental level (eg, regression in previously attained skills like toileting or language, changes in play behaviors, extreme temper tantrums). Reconceptualization of the manifestations of PTSD suggests that this disorder is more prevalent in the pediatric population than previously reported, particularly for children in high-risk populations [20].

Adoptive parents often are not aware of the details of a child's prior living situation and experiences; therefore, they may not be aware of prior trauma and the risk for PTSD and may misinterpret a child's behavior. More obvious symptoms of PTSD may not be evident until a child experiences an event that triggers a memory or is able to act on or verbalize his or her past experiences and emotions. A child may have seemed "fine" at a young age; however, as the child reprocesses his or her experiences at different developmental ages and the demands of functioning in a family and in the community become more complex, symptoms may become more apparent (eg, although being successfully toilet trained at home and in public places, a child refuses to use the white-tiled institutional-appearing bathroom at school and has extreme tantrums to avoid entering the bathroom). PTSD should be considered in children who are being evaluated for ADHD, RAD, or other difficulties, such as anxiety, developmental regression, or oppositional behaviors.

Case 5

Suzanna is an 8-year-old child adopted at 6 years of age from Russia. She had been orphaned at 5 years of age after she witnessed her mother being murdered by a boyfriend. Suzanna was cared for by an uncle for 1 year, and little information was available about her life experiences during this period. After adoption, Suzanna had been enrolled in the first grade with ESL support and began to learn English rapidly. Because of the circumstances of Suzanna's life, her mother initiated a relationship with a therapist experienced in adoption, but progress was reported to be slow. Suzanna and her mother came for developmental and be-havioral evaluation in the third grade because of significant behavioral issues at home and in school. At home, she was exhibiting extremes of behavior: calm and wanting to be held, humorous and playful, unable to fall asleep, oppositional behaviors, and screaming fits. Her mother reported that she was not doing well in school and had not made friends. Suzanna was disruptive in class, repeatedly getting out of her seat and not following the teacher's instructions. Her erratic behavior resulted in her dismissal from the after-school child care program. The school district had refused to perform any evaluations because her performance was not "significantly" below grade level, and they thought that her difficulties were attributable to ESL and, possibly, ADHD symptoms.

During her first visit to the office, Suzanna arrived in a fancy holiday dress and party shoes. Her mother indicated that she was not willing to fight with her daughter over clothing. Suzanna was pleasant, somewhat coy, and resistant but complied with the examiner's requests. On observation, her English was fluent for casual conversation. At the second visit, Suzanna arrived in black pants and shirt that had a leopard-spotted trim and a headband with ears. She crawled around the waiting area, climbed on furniture, acted like a cat, and refused to comply with any requests. She appeared disorganized and fearful.

Psychoeducational testing performed at a separate evaluation revealed average intelligence with weakness in more complex language skills, including social comprehension, as well as some difficulty with reading fluency. Based on Suzanna's history, current behavior, and cognitive profile, her behavior was thought to be most consistent with PTSD with some dissociative features. She did not present with symptoms of ADHD or with significant language impairment beyond that expected of a child with 2 years of English language exposure. Recommendations were made for academic support and for collaboration between Suzanna's therapist and her school providers so that they could understand the cause of her behaviors and develop an IEP that would appropriately address her needs. A trial of medication to address anxiety and hyperarousal was initiated, with a modest reduction in symptoms. The school district did not follow through on recommendations; thus, difficulties persisted in this environment. Suzanna's mother engaged an advocate and pursued due process to have her daughter enrolled in an approved private school, at the district's expense, to meet her daughter's academic and emotional needs.

PTSD must be considered in the differential diagnosis of children who have a history of residing in institutions. Although a child's history may not explicitly describe traumatizing events, they may have occurred. Moreover, it is the child's perception of events (eg, life in the orphanage) that influences the development of symptoms. Interventions that are specifically directed at helping a child feel safe and process past experiences are essential, and medication management may be necessary. Parents need to understand their child's prior experiences and continue to develop strategies to help the child feel safe.

Summary

Children adopted from institutional settings or other situations in which neglect or abuse is prevalent are at increased risk for presenting with developmental and/or behavioral and emotional challenges. Experienced evaluators and therapists are essential to provide families with a thorough understanding of their child's history and current neurocognitive status and to direct interventions to address developmental and/or behavioral symptoms. As a result of the complexity of a child's difficulties, evaluations and interventions are often multidisciplinary. Interventions should be directed toward supporting the child and the family. Parents need accurate information about their child's strengths and weaknesses and recommendations about available resources so as to develop an appropriate intervention plan supporting their child.

Many children do well, and although there remain issues associated with the process of adoption that are always part of their lives, they may not require ongoing specialized interventions. There are children who have mild but ongoing issues that are manageable with limited interventions. There is also a group of children who have more significant issues that persist or becoming increasingly problematic. Short- and long-term management of a child's issues requires careful diagnostic evaluation and periodic re-evaluation. If the child's deficits and difficulties are not correctly delineated, the appropriate mode of intervention cannot be initiated and progress remains elusive. Children may require short-term interventions during their initial adjustment and catch-up periods or may require long-term interventions to address underlying neurodevelopmental differences that persist. When a child exhibits persistent global delays that are determined to represent mental retardation or cerebral palsy, lifelong accommodations and support are required. What about the child who has symptoms of a learning disability, attachment difficulties, anxiety, PTSD, or ADHD? These disorders may improve over time but often do not resolve completely. With appropriate intervention, these neurocognitive deficits can be mediated into more functional outcomes. Pediatricians are who are aware of the complex long-term issues that can affect a postinstitutionalized child are in a unique position to support and work with a child and his or her family to achieve the best possible long-term outcome (see Appendix).

Appendix: Resources

National Information Center for Children and Youth with Disabilities
www.nichcy.org
800-695-0285
Council for Exceptional Children
www.cec.sped.org
800-CEC-SPED
Learning Disabilities Association of America
www.ldanatl.org
412-341-1515
National Center for Learning Disabilities
www.ncld.org
888-575-7373
Children with Attention Deficit Disorder
www.chadd.org
800-233-4050

References

[1] Ames EW, Chishom K, Fisher L, et al. The development of Romanian children adopted to Canada: final report. Burnaby (BC): National Welfare Grants Program, Human Resources Development Canada; 1997.
[2] Miller LC, Kiernan MT, Mathers MI, et al. Developmental and nutritional status of internationally adopted children. Arch Pediatr Adolesc Med 1995;149:40–4.
[3] Miller LC, Hendrie NW. Health of children adopted from China. Pediatrics 2000;105(6):e76.
[4] Benoit TC, Jocelyn LJ, Moddermann DM, et al. Romanian adoption: the Manitoba experience. Arch Pediatr Adolesc Med 1996;150:1278–82.
[5] Johnson DE, Miller LC, Iverson S, et al. The health of children adopted from Romania. JAMA 1992;268:3446–51.
[6] Rutter M for the English and Romanian Adoptees Study Team. Developmental catch-up and deficit, following adoption after severe global early privation. J Child Psychol Psychiatry 1998;39(4):465–76.

[7] Rutter M, Anderson-Wood L, Beckett C, et al. Quasi-autistic patterns following severe early global privation. J Child Psychol Psychiatry 1999;40(4):537–49.

[8] O'Conner TG, Rutter M, Beckett C, et al for the English and Romanian Adoptees Study Team. The effects of global severe privation on cognitive competence: extension and longitudinal follow-up. Child Dev 2000;71(2):376–90.

[9] Verhulst FC, Althaus M, Versluis-den Bieman HJM. Problem behavior in international adoptees: II. Age at placement. J Am Acad Child Adolesc Psychiatry 1990;29(1):104–11.

[10] Verhulst FC, Althaus M, Versluis-den Bieman HJM. Problem behavior in international adoptees: III. Diagnosis of child psychiatric disorders. J Am Acad Child Adolesc Psychiatry 1990;29(3): 420–8.

[11] Verhulst FC, Althaus M, Versluis-den Bieman HJM. Damaging backgrounds: later adjustment of international adoptees. J Am Acad Child Adolesc Psychiatry 1992;3(3):518–24.

[12] Korsch B, Cobb K, Ashe B. Pediatricians' appraisal of patients' intelligence. Pediatrics 1961; 27:990–1003.

[13] Bierman JM, Connor A, Vaage M, et al. Pediatricians' assessment of the intelligence of two-year-olds and their mental test scores. Pediatrics 1964;34:680–90.

[14] Glascoe FP, Dworkin PH. Obstacles to effective developmental surveillance: errors in clinical reasoning. J Dev Behav Pediatr 1993;14:344–9.

[15] Shaywitz SE, Shaywitz BA. Dyslexia (specific reading disability). Pediatr Rev 2003;24(5): 147–52.

[16] American Academy of Pediatrics. Clinical practice guideline: diagnosis and evaluation of the child with attention deficit/hyperactivity disorder. Pediatrics 2000;105(5):1158–70.

[17] American Psychiatric Association. Diagnostic and statistical manual of mental disorders. 4th edition. Washington, DC: American Psychiatric Association; 1994.

[18] Streissguth A. Primary and secondary disabilities. In: Streissguth A, editor. Fetal alcohol syndrome: a guide for families and communities. Baltimore, MD: Paul H Brookes Publishing Company; 1998. p. 95–119.

[19] Albers L, Nalven L. Behavioral concerns in international adoptees. Presented at the Medical Institute, Joint Council of International Children's Services, Washington, DC, April 10, 2002.

[20] Sheering MS, Zeanah CH, Myers L, et al. New findings on alternative criteria for PTSD in preschool children. J Am Acad Child Adolesc Psychiatry 2003;42(5):561–70.

PEDIATRIC CLINICS
OF NORTH AMERICA

Pediatr Clin N Am 52 (2005) 1445–1461

ELSEVIER
SAUNDERS

Education and Internationally Adopted Children: Working Collaboratively With Schools

Kathryn N. Dole, MS, OTR/L[a,b,*]

[a]International Adoption Clinic, Fairview–University Medical Center, University of Minnesota,
MMC 211, 420 Delaware Street SE, Minneapolis, MN 55455, USA
[b]Department of Special Education, Minneapolis Public Schools, 2225 E. Lake Street,
Minneapolis, MN 55407, USA

Physicians, nurse practitioners, and other health care workers often are called on to assist families as they make decisions about a range of issues related to their internationally adopted child's schooling. Families have questions about when to start their child in school, what type of school is best, how to access special education, what speech and language issues should be of concern, and how to deal with behavioral problems. Physicians and health care workers often are not prepared to address these concerns with families, and they may find themselves in the difficult position of being asked to make recommendations about educational issues with which they are not familiar. In many cases, the health care professional's only current contact with schools is in relation to the education and life experiences of their own children, which, in all likelihood, are vastly different from those of an internationally adopted child. To give parents accurate and informed information regarding their child's education, physicians and health care workers need to familiarize themselves with federal and state regulations affecting schools, what services children are entitled to, and what the limitations of school services are as well as what local educational resources are available and how to access them.

Helping families to work collaboratively with their child's school may be the first and most important step in securing a strong educational environment

* International Adoption Clinic, University of Minnesota, MMC 211, 420 Delaware Street SE,
Minneapolis, MN 55455.
  E-mail address: dolex001@umn.edu

0031-3955/05/$ – see front matter © 2005 Elsevier Inc. All rights reserved.
doi:10.1016/j.pcl.2005.06.007   *pediatric.theclinics.com*

for the internationally adopted child. Families often seek the assistance of medical personnel when they are having difficulty with the school or when the school is not providing what the family thinks is needed for their child. Medical personnel are often asked for school advice, although this may not be an area in which they have familiarity or understanding. As a result, they may give families inaccurate or incomplete information. For example, in a medical setting, a child with gait problems who is able to ambulate may receive physical therapy (PT) for improving the quality of his or her gait, whereas in the educational system, this child would receive PT only if he or she were unable to move safely between classes.

At the same time, medical personnel can assist educators who often are not aware of or familiar with the medical and environmental factors that can affect an internationally adopted child's ability to learn and succeed in school. The medical professional can be an excellent resource to assist school staff in understanding the health care needs of the adopted child. Children who have the benefit of medical and educational staff working together with their families have the best chance of maximizing their learning potential.

Educational considerations

Educational programs vary from state to state and from city to city; thus, becoming familiar with local programs is essential when assisting families seeking help in this area. Services also vary depending on the age of the child. Early intervention programs for infants and toddlers, which are often provided in special education, have different eligibility criteria than special education programs for high school students. Understanding programming and the process involved in obtaining access to these programs helps to ensure that children receive appropriate services and prevents undue frustration for families if their child happens not to qualify for certain school programs. It also prepares them to seek other resources outside the education realm if needs exist that the school may not be able to provide or may not be responsible for providing.

Parents adopting older children may or may not be familiar with their school system, and they frequently have not contacted the school before deciding to adopt. Families adopting infants or toddlers often do not consider educational issues or resources before adoption because they may not consider them as immediate needs. Parents adopting special needs or older children should be encouraged to communicate with their local school district as soon as they know that their child may need school services. This is appropriate even before the family accepts a referral from their adoption agency, because the family benefits from having information about the resources that are available for their child. Many children join their families during the school year, and if they are of school age, planning ahead for their transition into the school makes this as comfortable and successful as possible.

Assisting parents in understanding that the school's responsibility is to educate their child rather than to meet all their child's medical needs can help the family to understand why the child may not be eligible for what parents think should be provided. At the same time, parents should have access to information regarding what their child is entitled to through the public education system. For example, families adopting children with physical limitations, such as cerebral palsy, want to know if their child is eligible for special education. If not, do they need to get therapy through the medical field, or do they need both sets of services? In many cases, families assume that the school is going to meet most of their child's needs, but this is often not the case.

Medical and educational issues for internationally adopted children

Children who are adopted internationally have unique medical and educational needs. Many factors unique to his or her experience can negatively influence a child's development. These factors include prenatal care, genetic background, malnutrition, sensory deprivation, neglect, physical and sexual abuse, prenatal alcohol exposure, and multiple placements before adoption, just to name a few. These children frequently arrive with little or no birth information and no background information about the birth family. This lack of information adds to the challenge of determining which issues may influence a child's long-term developmental outcome and educational needs. Fortunately, there is a great deal of information related to the most common medical diagnoses and health concerns facing these children [1]. Although many conditions are easily treated and present no long-term effects on development or learning, others can have significant ramifications for a child's motor, cognitive, or emotional and/or behavioral development, which, in turn, can greatly influence the child's academic progress and overall school success. Therefore, these children benefit from receiving a comprehensive evaluation when they arrive in the United States.

Obtaining a comprehensive medical and developmental evaluation is one of the most important recommendations that the physician can give parents of newly adopted children. Numerous clinics specializing in the evaluation of international adoptees have been created throughout the country (a partial clinic listing is available at the University of Minnesota's International Adoption Clinic web site: http://www.umniac.org). These specialty clinics can provide primary care providers and families with insight into the factors that may influence their child's development and can assist in providing information and strategies to aid the child who is showing the effects of early deprivation or institutionalization.

International adoption specialty clinics have the experience and expertise to assist families in identifying and prioritizing internationally adopted children's issues. For example, at the University of Minnesota, a child who exhibits developmental delay as well as medical and nutritional problems has the medical and nutritional issues addressed immediately, even before being referred to an early intervention program. This is because as the medical and nutritional problems resolve and the child has the benefit of the care and nurturing of his or her new family, the developmental concerns may also resolve and intervention may not be needed.

Current research indicates that the older the child is at the time of adoption, the greater is the chance that the negative effects of institutionalization may affect his or her development [2]. In many cases, internationally adopted children demonstrate inconsistent skills and behaviors (eg, speech skills may be delayed, although motor skills are within normal limits). Parents frequently report that these children have immature socially inappropriate behaviors that interfere with school success, making friends, and developing healthy attachments.

No two children who are adopted internationally are exactly alike. A 6-month-old full-term child with normal growth adopted from South Korea who has only ever lived in foster care may have quite different educational issues than a 24-month-old born prematurely and placed in an institution who currently is showing poor growth and a small head size. An 8-year-old who has been in an institution his entire life, has limited speech in his native language, and has suffered from malnutrition and suboptimal care has different needs than an 8-year-old who lived with his biologic family for 6 years before being removed from that situation because of neglect and is currently suffering from severe anxiety.

Educational factors

All children are entitled to a public education, and children with disabilities are entitled to a free appropriate public education (FAPE). Although federal laws regulate education to some degree, state laws and states' interpretation of federal law can result in programs that vary from state to state. For example, in some states, early intervention programs are regulated under the department of education, whereas in others, they are located under the department of health. This can influence how funding is distributed and how programs prioritize needs as well as who provides direct services to children. As a result, the same early intervention PT a child receives that is provided under a medical or health model in one state may be provided under an educational model in another state. Although the training and professional requirements of the physical therapist are the same in both states, the manner in which he or she provides and implements these services may be different. This can be confusing to families and health care providers. Adding to this confusion is at what point the orders are to be written to address the child's needs. In a hospital or outpatient clinic, the physician or nurse practitioner can write orders for rehabilitation services and the therapy is started as soon as the order is received. In the school setting, however, the school's team of evaluators may determine whether the child receives the services rather than an outside physician. In that case, it is only after the school team determines that the child needs the services that the physician order can be requested.

Parents also should consider having their child evaluated outside the school system. If the need is immediate or short term, it may be better to access medically based therapy, which is usually much faster to implement. Also, although evaluations done outside the school system may be used to help families when they are requesting school services, it is important to understand that the school must do its own assessment to determine eligibility; the school is not required to use any outside evaluations in making this determination.

Types of schools

There are primarily two groups of schools available for children: public (including charter schools) and nonpublic (including private schools and home schools). Each type of school has benefits and limitations, and parents must make school decisions based on their child's needs. Parents also must be prepared to try several different programs before finding the right school for their child and be willing to continually monitor their child's progress, modifying programming as needed.

Regular public schools

Regular public schools are the option chosen by most parents; they are open to all children, and schools must follow federal and state education laws and regulations. Funding is often problematic, because public schools face increasing financial challenges associated with rising costs, increasing needs of children, and fiscal resource restriction. Costs of programs like special education have placed a burden on schools, because the government has increased mandates but has not provided adequate funding. Currently, special education funding is at approximately 15%, a small fraction of the actual cost of providing these services [3].

The No Child Left Behind (NCLB) legislation passed in 2002 has placed increased accountability on public schools for ensuring positive outcomes for students. Although the intent of the legislation is to improve educational outcomes for children, it has placed increased expectations on schools to meet those outcomes, which are considered by many to be unrealistic, especially for special education students and English language learners (ELLs).

Regular public schools provide a vast array of programs for children. Those who are adopted quite young and who have no developmental delays or medical problems generally enter the school system just like their peers, and they frequently progress through the system without any academic difficulty related to their adoption.

They participate in preschool screenings for vision and hearing as well as for early learning or readiness skills that schools have identified as necessary for success in kindergarten.

Charter schools

Charter schools are public schools that develop a "charter" with a local authority, frequently a state department of education or local school board. They generally are able to function without adhering to many of the regulations required of regular public schools, but they must detail their mission and organizational plan before they are permitted to open. They are frequently small schools and are allowed more autonomy, because it is believed that they are accountable to the granting authority to produce positive educational results. Charter schools are often developed around a similar population of students or families who want more control over their children's education, but they are expected to be open to all students. Because they are funded with public funds, charter schools are tuition-free, but they do not receive the same dollar amount per student as regular public schools because they are not required to provide the same range of services or to comply with NCLB legislation. When selecting a charter school, parents should evaluate the stability of the program, including the length of time the school has been open.

Private schools

Private schools are considered nonpublic schools, and as such, they have significant freedom in determining education curriculum and programming. Religious organizations or other groups that focus on specific educational goals and objectives may develop private schools. Families pay tuition, and additional funding is generally private, although some states allow families to use public vouchers toward tuition for their children attending private schools. Although they are not required to meet most state testing and graduation standards, private schools often focus on small class size, uphold high educational expectations, and frequently have academic entrance requirements. They also offer families more choice and control over their child's education. Internationally adopted children may benefit from the small class size and individualized programming but may not meet the entrance requirements of some private schools, or they may have behavioral issues that are not accepted in a private school setting.

Home schools

Home schooling is a type of nonpublic education provided in a family's home and generally taught by a parent. Communities may have home school cooperatives (groups of families who are home schooling their children collectively), or families may choose to educate their children independently. Although home schooling is legal in all states, regulations vary by state. Children may be home schooled full time or part time while also attending a more traditional public or private school. It is estimated that approximately 2% of children in the United States are home schooled. Families choose to home school for a variety of reasons, but it is especially popular with white middle-class families who have strong religious convictions [4].

At the University of Minnesota's International Adoption Clinic, anecdotal reports from parents of older internationally adopted children who have chosen to home school indicate that this has been a positive choice for them. This educational setting seems to be most effective if the parents have home schooled other children and are comfortable with this method of education. Many older postinstitutionalized children are immature and delayed in academics. Home schooling provides an environment that is small and individualized as well as a safe and secure situation while the child is transitioning to his or her new family. It allows for a highly structured day, which is also often helpful for a newly adopted child. Home schooling does not offer the social experiences that other types of schools do, so parents need to find other ways to incorporate social activities into their child's days.

Children who attend nonpublic schools are entitled to participate in public school activities and to take advantage of certain educational resources. Nonpublic school students who qualify for special education services can receive these services at their community school, but the public school is not required to provide the services within the nonpublic setting. Families who have their children in nonpublic schools may not be aware of the public education resources available to their children, and it may be beneficial for parents to discuss these possibilities with their local public school staff.

Public school programs that may benefit internationally adopted children

The most common public school programs used by internationally adopted children are early intervention services, Title I, ELL programs, 504 plans, and special education. Additionally, children can benefit from many educational resources that are not part of special education, including friendship groups, sports activities, and other extracurricular activities.

English language learners

Learning English is one of the most important aspects of development that internationally adopted children and their families should understand. School districts, faced with increasingly diverse populations speaking many different languages and dialects, are challenged to meet the needs of children whose native language is not English. Large urban school districts can have as many as 100 different languages, and even small communities are faced with children who are not native English speakers. Children who are identified as ELL or as limited English proficient (LEP) often participate in programs like English as a second language (ESL) or English for speakers of other languages (ESOL). The amount of service varies and is based on student need, which is determined by whether the student (1) first learned a language other than English, (2) comes from a home where the language usually spoken is not English, or (3) usually speaks a language other than English and scores significantly below the average score for students the same age on a nationally normed English reading or English language arts achievement test [5].

For internationally adopted children, the language issue can be complicated by additional factors, including the age of the child at adoption and whether or not the child was functioning at age level in his or her native language at the time of adoption. It is also important to know, whenever possible, if the child was with the birth family or in foster care for any length of time, because this is often the time when the child would have had the most exposure to one-on-one communication.

In addition, other development or medical problems can interfere with the child's acquisition of English. Frequent ear infections, common among children raised in institutions, can have a negative impact on hearing, which can result in decreased language and can also affect articulation.

Young children who have been institutionalized at an early age often have suffered from stressful environments of neglect, severe malnutrition, and possible abuse, which can have an impact on learning. They have often been in situations that do not foster one-on-one communication. In observation of two groups of children in a Chinese orphanage, children in one group who lived in foster homes on the orphanage grounds were compared with children living in the orphanage itself, and it was noted that the children in the foster homes had better social skills and more communication skills. It was thought that this finding was directly related to their environment and the opportunity to speak with caring adults about their daily activities on a regular basis (Pi-nian Chang, PhD, personal communication, 2003).

Children who are adopted from other countries vary from other non–English-speaking children in that they generally join English-speaking families and do not have extended family members who continue to communicate with them in their native language. As such, they are not bilingual, and English becomes their primary language. As a result, they often acquire English faster than children who live in non–English-speaking homes. Children who are adopted when they are younger than 18 months of age and have no other significant delays often learn English quickly, frequently communicating at or close to age level within 12 to 18 months [6]. Children adopted later take longer to catch up. Children adopted after the age of 24 months should have a speech and language screening to determine whether significant delays are present and whether a formal evaluation is needed. Most children adopted when they are older than 3 years of age should have a speech and language evaluation within the first year after arrival with their new families. If obvious disabilities exist or the family is concerned about delays in speech, they should consider having a speech and language evaluation completed as soon as possible.

Many school districts provide ELL services to children and often prefer to wait a least a year before evaluating a child for special education. This is not appropriate if the child has an identified disability known to affect learning, such as fetal alcohol syndrome. A child can receive ELL services in addition to special education. Families may be hesitant to ask for a special education evaluation or for their child to be labeled with a disability, but if the child has language issues and developmental delays, special evaluation should be a considered, because ELL services alone do not address learning or cognitive delays.

Title I

Title I was originally started in 1965 as part of the Elementary and Secondary Education Act (ESEA) and currently is included as part of the NCLB program. This federally funded program was designed to help children gain academic achievement as part of the "War on Poverty." Title I services are provided based on whether 40% or more of a school building's students fall below the poverty line [7] rather than on individual student eligibility, and schools receiving Title I funds can use them to serve all students in their building. Title I funds are used primarily to focus on increasing reading and mathematic skills. Internationally adopted children may participate in Title I programs with other children in their schools, but if the school does not meet the threshold, the adoptee would not have access to these additional academic programs.

504 Plans

The 504 plans are provided for regular education students who do not qualify for special education but need some support in their educational program to be successful in school. For example, a child who is doing well academically but needs access to a word processor because of poor motor coordination as the result of a brachial plexus injury could be provided, through a 504 plan, with access to a computer so that the disability does not prevent the child from making academic gains. The 504 plans are not meant to be used to obtain services that require the child to be eligible for special education.

Early intervention

Many states and communities have programs for children, such as Head Start and early childhood family education (ECFE), to help with enhancing development for young children. These programs may be educational in nature but are often not part of special education programs. Early intervention programs for young children are designed to help infants and toddlers who are at risk for significant developmental delays. Services can begin as early as birth based on the needs of the child.

Early intervention programs can also be provided as part of special education services in schools and are called early childhood special education (ECSE) services. These services are provided to children who are delayed in their development and at risk for continued delays because of a disability. Infants and toddlers must meet eligibility requirements and are frequently determined eligible under the developmental disability category. Referral methods and evaluation are discussed in the section on special education.

Special education

Special education services are based on legislation originally passed in 1975. The Education of All Handicapped Children Act (EAHCA), PL 94–142, required that an Individual Education Plan (IEP) be developed before any child with a disability could receive special education and related services. This law was amended in 1990 when the Individuals with Disabilities Act (IDEA) passed. The IDEA provides guidelines for determination of special education eligibility and for how services are provided to eligible children with disabilities [8]. The most recent reauthorization of this legislation was the Individuals with Disabilities Improvement Act of 2004 (IDEIA).

It is estimated that more that 45% of internationally adopted children have received some type of special education. (Dana Johnson, MD, PhD, personal communication, 2003). The type and duration of services vary depending on the age and needs of the child. It is important to understand the process of how a child qualifies for special education services, again remembering that there is variation from state to state on how special education laws are implemented. Families are entitled to due process protection under IDEA. They have rights to conciliation if they do not agree with the services provided, because conflicts often occur around misunderstandings between what the family wants and what the school is able to provide. Also, families can contact local advocacy groups for information about their rights and how to work with their school if they need additional support or information about services.

Referral for special education

Special education law requires that a child be evaluated for special education and that the child be determined eligible for services based on eligibility criteria that have been established by federal law and interpreted by the specific state's department of education. A child must qualify for special education before services like PT or occupational therapy (OT) can be provided.

Although the basic process is the same for children of all ages, there are a number of differences for young infants and toddlers. The process begins with a referral or request for a special education evaluation for the child. Parents may request this evaluation, and it is recommended that the parent give the school district a written request, because the district must then respond within a reasonable time, generally within 10 days of the request.

For some early intervention programs, a screening may be done before a formal evaluation to determine whether the child is likely to qualify for special education before proceeding with a more extensive assessment. Even if the child passes the screening, the parents can still request a complete assessment. For older school-aged children, the district must provide prereferral interventions to see if the child's education improves before proceeding to a formal evaluation. This ensures that children are not placed in special education unnecessarily. The parents can, in some circumstances, request that the evaluation be completed immediately without prereferral interventions. This is most common in situations in which the child has a diagnosis known to be associated with a disability, such as Down syndrome or fetal alcohol syndrome.

Evaluation

When the special education evaluation process begins, the parents and school personnel meet as a team to determine what areas are to be evaluated and who is responsible for the various portions of the evaluation. Parents are considered part of the team and are encouraged to participate in this process. It is important for parents to be specific about what they think are the needs of their child and to share relevant information that can help the school to complete an evaluation that is as comprehensive as possible. Adoptive parents often do not have access to the same information about their child that birth parents usually have, such as accurate birth dates and genetic background. This lack of information can create a stressful situation for parents. In other cases, parents may prefer not to share all the details of their child's early life experiences. Health care professionals can assist parents in determining whether certain medical or historical information should remain private and whether withholding that information would or would not negatively affect the thoroughness of an assessment.

All tests and areas to be assessed must be written in an evaluation plan that is presented to the parents for their signature before the process can be initiated. Tests are to be racially and culturally nondiscriminatory and, unless unfeasible, are to be administered in the child's native language [9]. Because the school district may want to delay the evaluation to give the child time to transition to his or her new environment or because representatives of the school district believe that they cannot determine whether a delay is related to culture, race, or language rather than to a disability, determining the best time to complete a school-based assessment can be difficult, and health care providers can assist families with this question. If it seems that the child is not going to qualify for school-based services, it may be more helpful to obtain services outside the school district rather than to pursue special education.

The age of the child, length of time in institutions, type of care given before adoption, history of malnutrition, and other health-related issues should all be considered when determining the appropriate time to initiate an evaluation. Each child's situation is unique and must be looked at individually.

The areas most often assessed for special education include intellectual functioning; academic performance; communication; motor and/or physical development; sensory development; health and medical status; emotional, social, and behavioral development; functional skills; and transition areas. The district has 30 school days to report back to the parents with a completed evaluation, the results of which determine whether or not the child is eligible for special education.

Eligibility criteria vary depending on the disability category; however, in general, the child must be -1.5 to -2.0 SDs below the mean on standardized tools in addition to meeting other criteria, including any diagnoses or factors affecting the child's performance. Because the standardized tools most frequently used are not normed on institutionalized children, the use of these tests may not be valid. Also, because language is an issue, especially for older children, families report that they are often told their child cannot be evaluated for special education until she or he has been here for 1 year or more, reasoning that the child needs to have participation in an ESL program for that long before he or she can be tested. This is not true. A child who does not speak English can be evaluated using tools that are not language based or, in certain cases involving older children, through the use of an interpreter. It is important that the child be considered for an evaluation if he or she has a known disability or if delays seem to be greater than expected. Although results of evaluations done less than a year after arrival should always be viewed with caution, they are used as a starting point for the child's education. Most studies show that internationally adopted children continue to make gains in IQ scores over time [2].

Children can qualify for special education in the following disabilities categories, and others may be included if they are state approved:

- Autism spectrum disorder (ASD)
- Blind and/or visual impairment (B/VI)
- Deaf-hard of hearing (DHH)
- Deaf-blind (DB)
- Developmental cognitive disability (DCD)
- Developmental delay (DD, formerly ECSE)
- Emotional and/or behavior disorder (EBD)
- Other health impaired (OHI)
- Physical impairment (PI)
- Severely multiply impaired (SMI)
- Specific learning disorder (SLD)
- Speech and language impairment (S/LI)
- Traumatic brain injury (TBI)

Each disability area has separate eligibility criteria. Once a child has been determined to be eligible for special education, the team then determines where the child has needs and who is going to work with the child to meet those needs. This type of comprehensive evaluation is repeated every 3 years.

Individual education plan or individual family service plan

Once the evaluation has been completed and the child has been determined eligible, an individual family service plan (IFSP) for infants and young children or an IEP for older children is developed. This is often also the period when families request OT, PT, and speech therapy. It is important to understand that speech therapy is a related service but has eligibility criteria that a child must meet to receive services. Speech therapy is also a service that can be provided alone (ie, the child can receive speech therapy through the school district if he or she meets the eligibility criteria for speech impairment, even if he or she does not meet criteria in any other area).

It is different for OT and PT. They are also considered related services (along with audiology, psychologic services, recreation, counseling, school health services, and social work services), but OT and PT do not have eligibility criteria. They can be provided only if they relate to other educational goals and if the student needs these services to be successful in the school environment. For example, if the child has fine motor needs, the team decides who is going to provide this service. It could be the teacher or OT, determined by who can best meet the child's need. Many children have suffered from sensory deprivation in institutions, and families often request OT to assist with this.

The IEP includes the child's present level of performance in each area, the identified needs, and the appropriate goals and objectives to address those needs. The IEP also includes the location where services are to be provided, along with the amount of time and frequency of the services.

Implementation of the individual education plan

IEPs and IFSPs are developed and then reviewed on an annual basis. These are also reviewed during the school year to monitor progress and can be modified with parent input as needed. The team, which includes the parents, educational personnel, and others involved in the child's care, determines the goals and objectives for the child's plan. Again, it is important to remember that these are educational goals or goals to support the child's educational program. Services are provided in the least restrictive environment (LRE), which, for older children, is usually the school. Younger children can receive services in a daycare or preschool setting. The LRE is especially important to consider with young postinstitutionalized children, because it is often beneficial for a young child to participate in a setting with children exhibiting typical behavior. This allows the child to model appropriate behavior while receiving services from special education professionals.

Considerations for internationally adopted children

When making decisions about school needs and placement for adopted children, keep the following issues in mind.

Age at adoption

Parents of young children have some time to make decisions, but parents adopting school-aged children need to make decisions about placement quickly.

Families and schools often want the child to be placed with same-age peers, but this may not be the most appropriate setting, especially if the child has significant cognitive, social, emotional, and language delays. It may be helpful to wait a few weeks before enrolling the student to get a better feel for where the child is most likely to be successful. Whenever possible, it is best to minimize classroom change so that the child does not have to adjust to new routines and people.

Length of time with adoptive family

Children often show major progress in development even after a short time with their new family. Allowing time for this transition is helpful in determining the child's long-term needs. The rate of change or catch-up may decrease over time; thus, the longer the child is with the family, the better is the chance that schools and families can obtain an accurate picture of the child's strengths and needs.

Previous environment

The number and type of preadoption living situations play an important part in how the child functions in her or his new home and school. Postinstitutionalized children benefit from consistency and routine in their days at home and at school. They require structure and clear boundaries with behavior management that includes natural consequences.

Speech

Children often are perceived as understanding more English than they do. It is often difficult for children to understand and follow directions in the classroom; thus, the teacher may think that the child has an attention problem when, in fact, it is a language delay. Children often acquire social or conversational English quickly, but language that is needed to be successful in the academic setting is slower to develop. This fact should be taken into account when determining grade placement.

Use of interpreters

Infants and toddlers usually do not benefit from the use of interpreters. Children less than 5 years of age may initially benefit from having an interpreter, but if they are spoken to only in English, they generally no longer use their native language after 6 to 8 months. They may seem confused and upset when spoken to in their native language, perhaps because they think or worry that they are going to be returned to their native country. Children older than 5 years of age, especially if old enough to be working on academics in school, benefit from having some things interpreted for them for a period after arrival.

One possibility would be for a family to use an interpreter on a weekly basis to review classroom information with the older child. Interpretive services can be helpful for as long as 1 year, depending on the child's age and language skill, but generally are used for a much shorter time. Parents also often report that the child quickly refuses to use his or her native language and wants to use only English. If interpreters are used, it is important that information be translated accurately; thus, care should be taken in the selection of interpreters working with internationally adopted children.

Anxiety and hypervigilance

Many internationally adopted children suffer from anxiety, which can greatly interfere with the ability to learn. If a child is anxious and worried about what is going to happen, he or she cannot focus on learning. Providing counseling or emotional support is important; children respond to structure and a warm loving environment but may need more professional intervention and patience from the professionals working with the child.

Behavior and social emotional issues

Attention problems, temper tantrums, attachment issues, limited play skills, and poor interactive skills can be among the most difficult problems that internationally adopted children face. They often need to be taught how to behave in social situations and how to respond to others around them. Many parents say that their child is immature and that this is one of the most challenging areas to deal with. Teachers report that children often have difficulty in making friends and relating to their peers.

Suggestions for families seeking educational programming

- Obtain a comprehensive medical and developmental evaluation, including emotional and social development.
- Identify medical and educational factors that may interfere with the child's ability to be successful in the school setting.
- Prioritize medical and developmental issues. For example, it is important to have a child's hearing assessed before a speech and language evaluation is done.
- Learn about the local school district. Most school districts post information on the Web, and information from federal and state education departments is also available on-line.
- Use international adoption web sites that give specific information about any disabilities or issues that affect the child.
- Visit the school, and make an appointment to speak with the administrators and teachers who are going to interact with the child. Request a teacher who is open to working with a child who may be challenging to deal with.

- Collaborate, collaborate, and collaborate.
- Become familiar with education-related laws.
- Remember that the school's job is to educate children rather than to solve or resolve all the issues that affect the child's school success.
- It is often difficult to sort out what may be causing a particular problem for a child. Knowing what behaviors are typical or atypical, postinstitutionalized behavior or behavior related to a disability can be challenging for schools and parents.
- Visit the school regularly, and offer to share information that may help the school to understand the child better.
- Remember that the child is one of many in the classroom.

Summary

Health care workers play an important role in helping international adoptees adjust to their new families and in maximizing their success in the educational environment. Schools are different than medical settings, and health care workers who dispense advice to families are of greatest assistance if they work closely with their local education department to understand fully how children can best be served in schools.

Acknowledgments

The author thanks the clinic staff of the International Adoption Clinic at the University of Minnesota, including Drs. Dana Johnson, Angela Sidler, Stacene Maroushek, Pi-nian Chang, and Maria Kroupina, and Sandra Iverson as well as Mary Chesney, Mary Jo Spencer, and Susan Jacobson for their clinical observations and knowledge of internationally adopted children and their families.

References

[1] Johnson DE. Medical and developmental sequelae of early childhood institutionalization in international adoptees from Romania and the Russian Federation. In: Nelson C, editor. The effects of early adversity on neurobehavioral development. Mahwah, NJ: Lawrence Erlbaum Associates; 2000. p. 113–62.
[2] Ames E. The development of Romanian orphanage children adopted to Canada. 1st edition. Burnaby, British Columbia: Simon Fraser University; 1997.
[3] Parrish T, Harr J, Wolman J, et al. State special education finance systems, 1999–2000. Center for Special Education Finance. Palo Alto (CA): American Institutes for Research; 2004.
[4] McLoughlin CS, Chambers H. Home schooling: a guide for parents. Bethesda (MD): National Association of School Psychologists; 2004.
[5] Hallberg G, Harrison C, Lamker D, et al. A special education cross-cultural resource guide for

educators who work with English language learners. Minneapolis (MN): Minneapolis Public Schools; 2003.

[6] Glennon S. Typical and atypical language development in infants and toddlers adopted from Eastern Europe. Am J Speech Lang Pathol 2002;11:417–33.

[7] Braden JP, Schroeder JL. High-stakes testing and No Child Left Behind: information and strategies for educators. Bethesda (MD): National Association of School Psychologists; 2004.

[8] US Department of Education. 22nd annual report to Congress on the implementation of the Individuals with Disabilities Education Act (IDEA). Washington, DC: US Government Printing Office; 2000.

[9] US Congress. Individuals with Disabilities Education Act amendments of 1997. Washington, DC: US Government Printing Office; 1997.

ELSEVIER
SAUNDERS

PEDIATRIC CLINICS
OF NORTH AMERICA

Pediatr Clin N Am 52 (2005) 1463–1478

Complementary and Alternative Therapies: Considerations for Families After International Adoption

Eileen Costello, MD

Southern Jamaica Plain Health Center, 640 Centre Street, Jamaica Plain, MA 02130, USA

Parents of children with atypical development often seek help from their primary care pediatrician. The incidence of developmental and/or behavioral challenges and atypical development is increased in adopted children. As the number of children adopted internationally increases, requests for advice from a knowledgeable and trusted clinician about specific therapeutic options also increase. As a result, primary care pediatric providers should be informed about the risks and benefits of potential therapies for families. The more traditional therapies, based on the biopsychosocial model of health, are covered elsewhere in this issue. Here, the less traditional yet extremely popular complementary and alternative therapies that many families pursue with or without the knowledge of their child's primary care provider are addressed. Not every possible complementary or alternative intervention is discussed; rather, the focus is on the most commonly used approaches advocated for children with developmental challenges as well as on other techniques that have generated huge interest despite potential danger or expense.

The increased use of complementary and alternative medicine (CAM) among the US population is well documented [1]. Rates of using CAM in children range from 20% to 40%; in many cases, the pediatrician is unaware of the use of these therapies in his or her patients [2,3]. The severity of an illness and parental use of CAM are strong factors determining its use in children [4]. Families of children with neurodevelopmental disorders, such as attention deficit disorder (ADD) and attention deficit hyperactivity disorder (ADHD), report frequent use of complementary treatments [4].

E-mail address: quirkykids@aol.com

Studies by Levy and colleagues [5,6] at The Children's Hospital of Philadelphia suggest that 30% of children in their autism program were using alternative treatments and 9% were using potentially harmful treatments. The statement of the American Academy of Pediatrics (AAP) on counseling families regarding the use of CAM cites data suggesting that up to 50% of children with autism are using some form of complementary medicine (National Council for Reliable Health Information; available at: www.ncaf.org).

Children may present with a range of developmental concerns after international adoption, with diagnoses often including a range of autistic spectrum disorders (ASDs; eg, autism, pervasive developmental disorders, Asperger disorder.) Up to 16% of children adopted from extremely depriving environments, such as orphanages in Romania, presented with autistic or "quasiautistic" symptoms [7].

Likely targets for intervention with respect to international adoptees may include symptoms of disorders of attachment, sensory defensiveness, repetitive behaviors, impaired language development (as distinct from speech development), disorders of learning and attention, organizational difficulty, executive dysfunction, processing disorders, and social impairments. New parents of adopted children, especially those for whom this is a first child, may present with concerns in any of these areas. As a result, therapies used in this population that are considered complementary or alternative, although in common use for children with a range of developmental concerns, include sensory integration treatment (SIT), pragmatic language therapy, dietary manipulation, chelation for toxic metals, antifungal therapy for presumed overgrowth of yeast, auditory integration training (AIT), avoidance of childhood immunizations, administration of secretin, and attachment therapies.

Definitions: complementary and alternative medicine

What constitutes an alternative or complementary therapy? What should we keep in mind when evaluating such a therapy? In general, an alternative therapy is one outside the domain of typical medical practice that is offered in place of or as a substitute for conventional therapies. Complementary therapies are used to complement more "mainstream" therapies. In the case of therapies directed at children with developmental disabilities, however, there is a blurring of the line between conventional and complementary and alternative therapies. For example, little credible evidence exists to support approaches outside intensive educational and/or behavioral programs and certain pharmacologic agents.

Many families avail themselves of some combination of traditional and nontraditional therapies. Parents of children with developmental disabilities are often frustrated by their child's slow progress with conventional therapies and have their own ideas about causes of their child's disabilities. Decisions about subsequent therapies for their child are often based on these beliefs. There has been an explosion of Internet web sites devoted to controversial treatments for children with developmental disabilities, and pediatricians must be informed about some of their claims. In addition, parents of internationally adopted children are quick to perceive that most pediatric providers have little or no experience with children from institutional settings and may seek counsel from other providers claiming to have expertise in this area. Thus, pediatricians must inform parents that no one knows all the answers for this group of children and that it is not in the child's best interest to abandon the more traditional educational and medical approaches when there are not immediate results.

Complementary and alternative therapies for developmental disorders are, by definition, unproven by long-term experience or scientific studies. These therapies have been characterized in a number of different ways. The AAP uses Nickel's model for defining a treatment as "controversial," based on the following characteristics [8]:

- Treatments based on an overly simplified scientific theory (eg, casein-free and gluten-free diet, chelation of heavy metals)
- Therapies claimed to be effective for more than one condition (eg, craniosacral therapy for ADHD, learning disabilities, ASDs, and developmental delay)
- Claims that children respond dramatically and that some are cured, particularly if treated early
- Use of case reports or anecdotal data rather than carefully designed studies to support claims for treatment
- Failure to identify specific treatment objectives or target behaviors
- Treatments stated to have unremarkable or no adverse effects, leading proponents to deny the need to conduct controlled studies

Another description of complementary and alternative therapies by Hyman and Levy divides nontraditional approaches into four categories as follows [9]:

1. Unproven biologic treatments that are commonly used but have no basis in theory (eg, medical therapies like high-dose vitamins or antifungal agents)
2. Unproven benign biologic treatments that have some basis in theory (eg, dietary manipulation, including the gluten-free and casein-free diet)
3. Unproven and potentially harmful biologic treatments (eg, chelation of presumed toxins, avoidance of childhood immunizations or antibiotics)
4. Nonbiologic treatments (eg, auditory integration therapy, craniosacral therapy)

Considering therapeutic risks and benefits

Several considerations are important when counseling parents regarding these interventions. First, all health care providers have a responsibility to ensure that a therapy does no harm to a child. Parents are often under the impression that an alternative therapy is less likely to be harmful than one in the mainstream or one recommended by their pediatrician. As a result, it is a pediatric provider's responsibility to be informed about the potential hazards of an intervention. Second, parents need to be informed about what type of therapists practice a given intervention and what credentials they should have. Third, any intervention should be specifically targeted toward a particular symptom that is impeding the child's forward progress. Fourth, all families faced with such decisions need to consider issues of time, money, and the "schlepp factor," including the needs of other children in the family and the logistics of who is going to get a child to these appointments. Finally, the number of potential interventions is extensive and continuously growing, such that any one child may receive or benefit from several interventions simultaneously.

Assessment of a child's response to a given therapy is critical. Parents would do well to consider what is a reasonable goal for their child within the next year and to reassess in a year's time whether a given therapy is having the desired impact. In a field with so few hard data, each family does its own data collection and creates its own therapeutic program. The pediatrician can play an important role in helping parents to assess progress from an intervention.

In the sections that follow, each of the more commonly used alternative or complementary therapies is introduced, along with the behavior or difficulty it is intended to address. In some cases, additional training is required or expected of the therapist, and that training or certification is described as well. The theory underlying each therapy is explained. It is important to keep in mind that there is little scientific basis for most of these therapies and that appreciating them sometimes requires a "leap of faith" for providers trained in evidence-based thinking. Families of children with development disabilities are much less likely to be skeptical, and the desire to participate in a therapy purported to help may overwhelm any instinct to question the theory or the therapy. Most parents of affected children are willing try anything that makes a certain amount of sense to them and that they believe is unlikely to be harmful.

Specific therapies

Pragmatic language therapy

Virtually all children with developmental differences have some degree of language impairment. It is important to distinguish the inevitable transition that all internationally adopted children undergo to some degree while acquiring their new primary language from the language impairment of the developmentally delayed child. This is especially challenging when neither the parent nor the pediatric provider understands the child's primary language.

Impaired language functioning, as opposed to impaired speech, impedes a child's ability to learn; to process spoken or written language; and to get along in the social environment of his school, community, or family. Whether or not there are any language-processing issues, the internationally adopted child is likely to suffer language impairments because of the requirement to transition from a first language to a second language virtually overnight. For the older adopted child, the task of learning a new second language occurs while losing the first language. Although basic proficiency in a new language takes, on average, 1 to 3 years, cognitive academic linguistic proficiency can take 5 to 9 years to achieve (Hope Dickinson, PhD, personal communication, 2005). Participating in school and learning at grade level require that a child has acquired language proficiency in a new language or that specific accommodations are provided. This lag in acquisition of adequate language functioning can create a great disadvantage in an academic setting and puts the child at risk for under-diagnosis as well as overdiagnosis of a primary learning or attentional disorder.

The nonverbal aspects of communication are particularly difficult for a child transitioning to an entirely new culture, where unspoken rules of communication are even more foreign. This challenge in understanding the interpersonal components of communication is exactly what pragmatic language therapy purports to address. Children are grouped according to age and language abilities and given concrete coaching to improve their ability to read nonverbal cues, including facial expressions, tone of voice, and the body language of the speaker. They are helped to understand the give and take of conversation, such as turn taking, starting and ending a conversation, and the relevance of one's partner in conversation. For example, a child would speak differently to his school principal than he would speak to a teammate at baseball practice. Children are taught to assess the level of interest of the listener and how to demonstrate that they themselves are interested in a given topic of conversation. Cooperative games with a common goal, where children are required to work together, are often used when working with younger children. Observing a television program or videotape without the sound helps children to interpret the important nonverbal aspects of communication.

Pragmatic language groups are usually conducted by speech and language pathologists with special training. In some areas, psychologists or social workers are organizing "friendship groups" or "social skills groups" with the same goals in mind. Although there are few data to support this type of therapy, there are wait lists at most centers that offer them and "pragmatics" has moved into the mainstream of therapeutic options for many children perceived to have challenges with interpersonal interactions. Many schools are incorporating pragmatics into their speech and language programs [10]. Pragmatic language therapy is increasing in use throughout the country for children with disorders of language and communication. Although many children with atypical development, especially those characterized as quasiautistic after international adoption, are extremely verbal, few are skilled at using their language for effective interpersonal communication, and fewer still are able to see another person's point of view. In addition, some children with a history of significant trauma or institutionalization may have learned survival skills ("street smarts") and are astute at reading social cues. In fact, these children are sometimes indiscriminately charming or friendly to strangers but may not appreciate the nuances of routine conversations. This combination can create safety concerns for young children.

Little risk of harm is associated with pragmatic language therapy, and it is typically provided by professionals with specific training in speech and language therapy. Many intensive educational programs have incorporated these treatments into children's daily schedules, and children may have specific individualized educational plan (IEP) goals and objectives linked to pragmatic language therapy goals. Insurance coverage for this therapy is variable and often depends on the qualifications of the specialists providing the service and the diagnostic and billing codes used for these services.

Sensory integration treatment

SIT is rapidly becoming the most familiar of the complementary therapies directed at atypically developing children. Many children with autistic features and other developmental disorders have difficulty in processing sensory information. There is evidence that previously institutionalized children have higher rates of difficulty with sensory processing as well [11]. SIT is based on the theory that a child's ability to integrate sensory information—especially touch, body position, and body movement—and to respond appropriately lays the groundwork for "appropriate occupational behavior, including self-care and self-management, play, and academic skills" [11]. Cognition as well as physical, social, and emotional development depend on these abilities [11]. Children with dysfunction of sensory integration can be expected to have difficulties at home, at school, and in the greater community.

Difficulty in processing sensory stimuli in infancy may present as a case of colic that does not go away, with an arching, screaming, hard-to-console, and hard-to-feed infant who seems uncomfortable in his own skin. In its most severe form, sensory "defensiveness" can interfere with a child's ability to eat, to tolerate physical contact or the typical noise level in a home or classroom, or to enjoy usual childhood activities like swimming or swinging or going to a movie. More often, a child becomes irritable or uncomfortable in response to a seemingly mild sensory stimulus, such as the tags on the back of his shirt, the seams in his socks, or the waistband on his pants [12]. This irritability can be difficult for caretakers to interpret, particularly in a preverbal child or a child who is not yet verbal in English. Parents are often desperate for help and advice and many turn to SIT, often at the recommendation of an early intervention program.

A SIT program varies according to the presenting complaint. A "sensory diet" is developed for an individual child and could involve prescribed periods of "brushing" of the skin with a stiff surgical brush to decrease tactile sensitivity, using a soft oral brush to gradually address oral defensiveness or food aversions, or swinging on a large swing with close supervision to help a child with proprioception or a sense of gravity. "Gravitational insecurity," the inability to tolerate having one's feet off the ground, is a frequent characteristic of children with purported sensory integration difficulties. A great deal of literature has been devoted to this topic, yet there is little evidence-based literature to support it. Third-party payers have been slow to cover the expense. Many early intervention and school systems routinely incorporation sensory integration approaches in their treatment plans, however. With respect to efficacy, we cannot be certain whether the intense attention itself, the particular type of therapy, or simply the passage of time is responsible for a child's improvement.

Sensory integration evaluation and treatment should be conducted by an occupational or physical therapist with certification in SIT. With a certified therapist, there is at least some consistency in approach, enabling a more meaningful assessment of progress or response to treatment. A typical program lasts from 6 months to several years, with frequent assessments throughout the treatment. Like pragmatic language therapy, little risk of harm is associated with SIT and children enjoy it. Nevertheless, consideration should be given to the cost to families with respect to the time, money, and potentially missed opportunities to pursue other activities that may be displaced by pursuing SIT. For example, children who have been diagnosed with an ASD should not receive SIT in place of educational and behavioral interventions that are known to be beneficial. Rather, SIT can be included in a program based primarily on the behavioral and educational interventions.

Chelation therapy

Geographic clusters of developmentally delayed children and the high rates of developmental disorders in adopted children from particular countries lead many parents to question their child's possible exposure to environmental toxins. Concerned parents sometimes seek evaluation of this question and therapeutic inventions directed at a presumed toxin. Increased lead levels are far more likely to occur in the internationally adopted child, but lead poisoning is receiving less attention than other metals by alternative practitioners. Although numerous epidemiologic studies have provided no evidence for a link between environmental toxin exposure and autism, mercury remains the heavy metal most frequently linked in some circles with the development of the ASDs. This connection is based on the known association with high tissue levels of mercury and subsequent damage to the developing brain.

The most common method for determining a child's mercury exposure is hair analysis in nonstandardized laboratories, supported by the (false) belief that the level of mercury in the hair correlates with tissue levels and can direct toward a helpful diagnosis or treatment. Acceptable versus toxic ranges of specific heavy metals and minerals in human hair have not been determined. In addition, there is no standardization of the testing process among commercial laboratories that conduct hair analysis [13]. Nevertheless, based on the results of hair sample analysis, chelation treatments with agents like succimer, dimercaprol, D-penicillamine, and N-acetylcysteine have been recommended for children with elevated levels of mercury to promote excretion of the offending agent.

Although chelation agents enhance elimination of mercury from the body, three important facts must be kept in mind with respect to their purported use in children presenting with developmental disorders: (1) data from the Centers for Disease Control and Prevention and the Institute of Medicine do not support a relation between mercury exposure from vaccines and autism, (2) no evidence exists to suggest improved developmental outcomes for children who have undergone chelation therapy, and (3) chelating agents themselves are potentially toxic to the liver and may cause allergic reactions [14]. The American Institute of Nutrition/American Society for Clinical Nutrition and the American Medical Association [15] have made strong statements opposing hair analysis as a determinant of any type of therapy.

Gluten-free and casein-free diet

Dietary manipulation is a common alternative therapy used by parents for their children with developmental and attention difficulties. Fifty-four percent of families referred for evaluation for ADHD indicated using complementary and alternative therapies to help their child, and 16% indicated using dietary changes to manage symptoms [4]. Thirty-eight percent of pediatricians participating in a 1997 quality improvement program reported patients using alternative therapies for ADHD, and the most common was dietary manipulation [16]. With dietary interventions, parents may feel increased control over their child's treatment and may believe that a more natural intervention is less likely to be harmful than other options, such as the use of prescription medications.

A popular diet proposed for a child with an ASD diagnosis is a diet free of dairy and wheat proteins, referred to as the glutein-free and casein-free diet. Although the gluten-free diet is a well-documented and lifesaving treatment for children with celiac disease or gluten-sensitive enteropathy, its use for children with autistic features has no supporting scientific evidence.

The theory underlying this dietary intervention is that certain children have increased gut permeability to peptides from glutein and casein and that the selective absorption of these opioid-like peptides is related to the onset of autistic symptomatology [17]. It has been suggested that elimination of these peptides from the diet can improve the long-term outcomes of children with autistic symptoms. A *Cochrane Review* in January 2004 found only one randomized controlled clinical trial of this topic, and the sample size was too small to draw any conclusions. Anecdotes from parents claiming huge success, and even cure, after using this diet with their children are available on many web sites (eg, https:www.cfgfdiet.com), however. Desperate parents may seek advice concerning how to implement this diet with their children. Avoidance of dairy and wheat in childhood is no small task, requiring extreme vigilance on the part of caretakers. Physicians involved with families choosing this route are advised to monitor growth and nutrition carefully, to evaluate the child on a more frequent basis, and to help families assess whether there is a response. Further nutritional consultation may be indicated to ensure that children are making appropriate weight and height gains and receiving adequate vitamins and minerals in their diet. The effort involved in maintaining such a restrictive diet, especially once a child is mostly away from home at school, is huge. Helping parents to assess whether or not there is a benefit is an important role for the pediatric provider.

Avoidance of childhood immunizations

In addition to avoiding certain nutrients in the diet, there is a growing movement to avoid routine childhood immunizations out of fear that there is an association between them and autistic symptomatology. Most pediatricians have encountered this in practice, and a great deal of attention has been paid to it in the pediatric literature. Fears about immunizations take many forms, including the following:

- The measles, mumps, and rubella (MMR) vaccine is responsible for increasing rates of autism diagnoses because it contains live measles virus [18].
- The mercury-based preservative thimerosal is poisoning children.
- Combined immunizations or multiple immunizations at the same time tax an immature immune system and create immune mediators that cause damage to a developing brain.
- MMR vaccine causes deficiency in vitamin A, which, in turn, causes autism.

A growing body of evidence disputes all these theories. Importantly, thimerosal was removed from diphtheria-tetanus (DPT), haemophims influenza type B (HIB), and hepatitis B vaccines in 1998, yet the trend toward increased diagnosis of ASDs has continued. Despite the accumulation of evidence to the contrary, Internet web sites have promoted these theories to families, taking advantage of the fear, anxiety, and confusion that most parents feel when parenting an already vulnerable child [19,20]. Parents often ask, "If my child is impaired now, will further vaccination make him worse?" Pediatricians must be informed about the relative benefits of childhood immunizations and be equipped to discuss them with parents [21]. It may be important to educate parents about the diseases the immunizations were developed to prevent. Younger parents may have no memory of or experience with childhood illnesses, such as measles or mumps, which themselves can have serious developmental consequences and are best avoided by prevention.

Antibiotics and antifungals

Antibiotics have been targeted as a cause and treatment for autistic symptoms. Antibiotics have been implicated in changing the gut flora of autistic children, which, in turn, may be treated with a more powerful antibiotic. Overwhelming yeast infection attributable to previous antibiotic treatment has been promoted as the cause of many medical and developmental syndromes, including autism [22]. Treatments aimed at ridding the body of harmful yeast include the use of probiotics and potentially dangerous doses of antifungal agents, such as nystatin or fluconazole. None of these treatments have been systematically studied [23]. Given the potential dangers, parents are best advised against seeking this type of treatment for their children.

Auditory integration training

Parents of children with learning, attention, or developmental disabilities may be told that their child is suffering from central auditory processing disorder (CAPD.) Proponents of CAPD suggest that children with this diagnosis have normal hearing but that information heard is not efficiently processed at the cerebral level, which makes learning new information especially challenging. Differentiating symptoms of CAPD from those related to disorders, such as ADHD, or specific language-based learning disorders is not clear in the literature or easy in clinical practice. This may be a case of the blind men and the elephant. A given disability can be seen in many different ways depending on the lens of the examiner.

Central auditory processing evaluations are conducted by audiologists with special training, require special equipment, and can cost up to $2000. This expense is not generally covered by third-party payers. The popular and expensive treatment recommended for children diagnosed with CAPD is AIT. It is in wide enough use around the United States that the AAP has created a policy statement describing its ineffectiveness [24]. AIT consists of half-hour sessions once or twice daily over a 10-day period. During each session, the child wears headphones to listen to music that has been modified by a computer according to his or her particular auditory sensitivities. Some types of AIT programs recommended repeating the 20 sessions again within a year's time.

There is a small body of literature discussing the outcomes of AIT programs, but no controlled studies support these assertions. AIT proponents claim that children who have been treated with AIT have improved expressive language and auditory comprehension, improved attention, and decreased irritability [25]. One published report documented no difference in improvements in behavior and verbal and performance IQ between children treated with AIT and those listening to unmodified music on their own, however [26]. Another author concluded that "no individual child was identified as benefiting clinically or educationally from the treatment" [27]. In addition, there is concern about the safety of these treatments based on potentially unsafe sound levels produced by the equipment. Given the resources of time and money required for this therapy as well as the lack of demonstrated efficacy, pediatric providers would do well to advise families against this therapy.

Craniosacral therapy

Because of the importance of avoiding unproven or potentially harmful therapies, a discussion of craniosacral therapy is in order. Craniosacral therapy may be performed by a number of professionals, including osteopaths, massage therapists, dentists, and physical therapists. It is routinely recommended to improve central nervous system functioning in general and autism, infantile colic, learning disabilities, and ADD in particular.

The theory underlying craniosacral therapy is that human brain pulsations can be detected by fingertips over the cranium, that restriction of movement of the cranial sutures interferes with the flow of cerebrospinal fluid, and that this is related to a number of disease states. Through gentle manipulation of the cranium, diagnoses can be made and improvements in neurologic function can begin. Information promoting this therapy is readily available on web sites (eg, www.upledgerinstitute.com).

Current literature does not support the use of craniosacral therapy. In 1999, a Canadian group reviewed the available literature discussing craniosacral therapy and concluded that evidence was insufficient to recommend it to patients or to third-party payers [28]. In 2002, two faculty members at the New England College of Osteopathic Medicine came to the same conclusion and recommended that this form of treatment be removed from their college curriculum [29]. This information is slow to make its way to families in need of help, however. Despite lack of evidence supporting the effectiveness of this therapy, craniosacral therapy may be recommended or offered by early intervention programs.

Secretin

Secretin is an intestinal polypeptide that has been promoted as a potential treatment for autistic behavior. A 1998 television program reported an article that described significant improvement in the behavior of three autistic children who received secretin as part of their preparation for a gastrointestinal procedure. Specifically, the authors reported improved eye contact, alertness, and expressive language [30]. Demand for secretin became so intense after this report that a national shortage of the substance ensued.

Since 1998, a number of studies have failed to demonstrate efficacy of a single or multiple doses of secretin on the behavior of autistic children. A double-blind, placebo-controlled, crossover study of secretin in 2003 reported two significant findings. Single-dose secretin was not effective in changing behavior or communication in ASD children when compared with placebo [31]. Furthermore, to determine if parents might note subtle changes not demonstrated by more standardized measures, parents were questioned regarding their ability to distinguish when their child received secretin rather than a placebo, and vice versa. Families were unable to determine reliably which treatment their child was receiving, and the authors concluded that there is no clinical evidence to support secretin treatment [32].

Attachment therapy

Children who join their families after international adoption, particularly those adopted from institutions or beyond infancy, have an increased risk of difficulties with developing healthy attachment relationships. The importance of and challenges to healthy attachment after international adoption are described elsewhere in this issue (see the article by Weitzman and Albers). Importantly, children presenting with attachment challenges commonly have impairments in many other areas of their functioning, including cognitive, language, or emotional challenges (including posttraumatic stress disorder), which must be assessed and remediated in conjunction with supporting a healthy attachment between the parent and child.

As with any recommended treatment, appropriate assessment and diagnosis regarding a child's possible attachment difficulties and comorbidities are important. The manifestations of attachment difficulties in children beyond infancy and the range of typical attachment trajectories for children and their parents after international adoption are not well described in the literature, however. In addition, appropriate diagnosis of an "attachment disorder" must take into account a child's knowledge of expected social interactions, language skills, and possible comorbidities. Finally, knowledgeable professionals who can support families with their child's important transition, including attachment within the family, are hard to find.

Given the theoretic risk and challenges in understanding and addressing attachment difficulties for this population of children, adoptive parents face a great deal of uncertainty with respect to the "best approach" to fostering healthy attachment relationships with their child. Adoptive parents commonly hear about their child's risk of "attachment problems" before adoption; however, frequently, they do not know about the range of typical postadoption attachment behaviors for children or strategies for promoting healthy attachment or other factors that may confound a child's ability to develop healthy attachment relationships. Families may seek support through their primary care providers, community therapists, parent groups, or on-line when they are concerned about their child's challenging behaviors or indiscriminate friendliness. Individuals may consult Internet resources and can complete a questionnaire that may characterize their child with symptoms of an attachment disorder solely based on questionnaires completed on-line.

"Attachment therapy" may mean many different things to parents and providers. For example, Theraplay, is described as an attachment-based play therapy through which therapists and parents engage children in play with the goal to decrease negative behaviors. In contrast, "holding therapy" involves a therapist or parent physically restraining a child to allow him or her to feel safe and to tolerate "affective intensity" during the therapy session. To others, attachment therapy may be part of a more global approach, including psychotherapy, with parents to support them in addressing their child's challenging behaviors and providing psychoeducation regarding their child's current level of functioning and the impact of earlier trauma and institutionalization on their child's emotional health.

The cost of these interventions may range from $75 to $150 per hour to several thousand dollars per week for an intensive residential treatment program. There is no empiric evidence supporting the efficacy of any of these treatment approaches [33]. Many anecdotal reports of these therapies' successes are available to families via written testimonies, on-line data, and in-person conversations, however. As a result, families continue to seek a range of attachment therapies to address their children's difficulties.

Unfortunately, several deaths of children after international adoption have been attributed to attachment therapies. The American Academy of Child and Adolescent Psychiatry and the American Psychiatric Association have issued statements opposing coercive therapies for children with suspected attachment disorders [34,35]. A recent practice parameter outlines specific strategies for working with children with suspected attachment difficulties and outlines the challenges in diagnosing children beyond infancy with attachment difficulties [33].

Pediatric providers working with families of a child at risk for or diagnosed with an attachment disorder can support families by appreciating the impact of possible attachment concerns while discussing with families the importance of addressing potential comorbidities, including learning and emotional difficulties. Providers must discuss with families what strategies are being used with a given child's attachment therapy. Coercive therapies such as holding therapy or "rebirthing therapy" are clearly contraindicated [33]. In addition, families and those they work with to address their children's development of healthy relationships must balance the cost of unproven therapies with the potential risks to children.

Community activities

A number of families turn to activities in their home communities that have the potential to be therapeutic for their children's social development. Scouting, martial arts, theater groups, and team sports, for example, have the advantage of contact with typically developing children while promoting a sense of community at the same time. Because many children with atypical development have particular interests or skills, programs incorporating the interests or skills have great potential to help with socializing and self-esteem. Robotics or mathematic clubs and music or choral groups are wonderful places for all kinds of kids. There are increasing numbers of programs designed to address the motor and social issues common to the child with atypical development. These programs generally take place in a gymnasium or similar large space, where small groups of children work with a counselor toward a common goal, which can only be reached through a cooperative effort that requires communication. A brief session at the end of the game enables children to talk about their experience and their feelings about working together. Many parents provide powerful anecdotes supporting the success of these activities [36]. Community activities are more likely to be affordable and convenient and may allow parents to observe their child's participation and progress. In addition, community-based activities are more likely to allow participation of the whole family, increase interaction with more typically developing children, and are not perceived as "therapy" by the child.

Summary

Children who are internationally adopted are at increased risk of developmental and behavioral concerns, including attention disorders, learning disorders, and ASDs. In attempting to promote their child's optimal development and well-being, parents of internationally adopted children are faced with the additional stress of having many unanswered and unanswerable questions about their child's early origins. As a result, internationally adopted children and their parents need the support and counsel of their pediatrician as they grow and develop into adulthood.

A combination of traditional, complementary, and alternative therapies is the rule rather than the exception for most children with developmental challenges. The training of today's pediatricians is unlikely to have included the study of alternative and complementary treatments, although most American medical schools are currently offering such courses in their curriculum. The next generation of providers should be better equipped to address questions regarding these therapies in practice.

Counseling families regarding the use of interventions outside mainstream recommendations requires pediatric care providers to walk a fine line between being open to new ideas and providing realistic expectations for families. To best serve the children in our care, we must be as informed as possible, maintain an open mind to parental concerns, and, perhaps most importantly, warn against potentially dangerous interventions while maintaining a supportive and compassionate stance.

Given the paucity of scientific evidence-based data to support the various therapies that parents of children with developmental disabilities ask about, pediatricians can learn most about them from the families themselves. Inquiring about what program a family has designed to help their child can inform the practicing pediatrician about the range of therapies available in the community. Families with internationally adopted children may be more likely to engage in questionable therapies because of the unique stress of sudden parenthood of a child with a developmental challenge. Pediatric providers are entitled to explain their own comfort level with options that parents may choose, particularly with regard to avoidance of immunizations or any avoidance of or use of a medication that could be of potential harm to a child. The ability to discuss these topics openly provides the best possible partnership between providers and parents for the optimal care of the child.

References

[1] Eisenberg D, Davis R, Ettner S, et al. Trends in alternative medicine use in the United States. 1990–1997. JAMA 1998;280:1569–75.

[2] Ottolini MC, Hamburger EK, Loprieto JO, et al. Complementary and alternative medicine use among children in the Washington DC area. Ambul Pediatr 2001;1(20):122–5.

[3] Sawni-Sikand A, Schubiner H, Thomas RL. Use of complementary/alternative therapies among children in primary care pediatrics. Ambul Pediatr 2002;2(2):99–103.

[4] Chan E, Rappaport L, Kemper K. Complementary and alternative therapies in childhood attention and hyperactivity problems. J Dev Behav Pediatr 2003;24(1):4–8.

[5] Levy S, Hyman S. Use of complementary and alternative treatments for children with autistic spectrum disorders is increasing. Pediatr Ann 2003;32:10.

[6] Levy S, Mandell D, Merhar S, et al. Use of complementary and alternative medicine among children recently diagnosed with autistic spectrum disorder. J Dev Behav Pediatr 2003; 24:6.

[7] Rutter M, Andersen-Wood L, Beckett C, et al. Quasi-autistic patterns following severe early global privation. J Child Psychol Psychiatry 1999;40:537–49.

[8] Nickel RE. Controversial therapies for young children with developmental disabilities. Infants Young Child 1996;8:29–40.

[9] Hyman SL, Levy SE. Autistic spectrum disorders: when traditional medicine is not enough. Contemp Pediatr 2000;17:101–6.

[10] Prizant B, Schuler A, Wetherby A, et al. Enhancing language and communication development: language approaches. In: Cohen D, Volkmar F, editors. Handbook of autism and pervasive developmental disorders. 2nd edition. Hoboken, NJ: Wiley; 1997. p. 572–602.

[11] Cermak SA, Danhauer LA. Sensory processing in the post-institutionalized child. Am J Occup Ther 1997;51:500–7.

[12] Kranowitz CS. The out-of sync child: recognizing and coping with sensory integration dysfunction. New York: Perigee; 1998.

[13] Seidel S, Kreutzer R, Smith D, et al. Assessment of commercial laboratories performing hair mineral analysis. JAMA 2001;285:1.

[14] American Academy of Pediatrics, Committee on Children with Disabilities. Technical report. The pediatrician's role in the diagnosis and management of autistic spectrum disorder in children. Pediatrics 2001;107:5.

[15] American Medical Association. Hair analysis: a potential for medical abuse. American Medical Association: Policy #H-175.995 (Sub. Res. 67, 1–84; reaffirmed by CLRPD Red 3, 1–94).

[16] American Academy of Pediatrics. Monitoring children with attention deficit hyperactivity disorder. Ambulatory Care Quality Improvement Program. Elk Grove Village, IL: American Academy of Pediatrics; 1997.

[17] Seroussi K. Unraveling the mystery of autism and pervasive developmental disorder: a mother's story of research and recovery. New York: Broadway; 2002.

[18] Wakefield AJ, Murch SH, Anthony A, et al. Ileal-nodular hyperplasia, non-specific colitis, and pervasive developmental disorders in children. Lancet 1998;351:9103.

[19] Stratton K, Gable A, McCormick M, editors. Thimerosal-containing vaccines and neuro-developmental disorders. Institute of Medicine, Immunization Safety Review Committee. Washington, DC: National Academies Press; 2001.

[20] Stratton K, Gable A, McComick M, editors. Immunization safety review: thimerosal-containing vaccines and neurodevelopmental disorders. Washington, DC: Institute of Medicine, National Academies Press; 2000.

[21] American Academy of PediatricsCommittee on Children with Disabilities. Counseling families who chose complementary and alternative medicine for their child with chronic illness or disability. Pediatrics 2001;107(3):598–601.

[22] Finegold SM, Molitoris D, Song Y. Gastrointestinal microflora studies in late-onset autism. Clin Infect Dis 2002;34(Suppl 1):56–516.

[23] Levy S, Hyman S. Use of complementary and alternative treatments for children with autistic spectrum disorders is increasing. Pediatr Ann 2003;32:10.

[24] American Academy of Pediatrics, Committee on Children with Disabilities. Policy statement on auditory integration training and facilitated communication for autism. Pediatrics 1998;102(2): 431–3.

[25] Bellis TJ. When the brain can't hear: unraveling the mystery of auditory processing disorder. New York: Pocket Books; 2002.

[26] Bettison S. Long term effects of auditory training on children with autism. J Autism Dev Disord 1996;26:361–7.

[27] Mudford OC, Cross BA, Breen S, et al. Auditory integration training for children with autism: no behavioral benefits detected. Am J Ment Retard 2000;105:2.

[28] Kazanjian A, et al. A systematic review and appraisal of the scientific evidence on craniosacral therapy. British Columbia Office of Health and Technology Assessment. 1999.

[29] Hartman SE, Norton JM. Interexaminer reliability and cranial osteopathy. Scientific Review of Alternative Medicine 2002;6:1.

[30] Horvarh K, Stefenatois G, Sokolski KN, et al. Improved social and language skills after secretin administration in patients with autistic spectrum disorders. J Assoc Acad Minor Phys 1998;1:9–15.

[31] Levy SE, Souders MC, Wray J, et al. Children with autistic spectrum disorders. I: comparison of placebo and single dose of human synthetic secretin. Arch Dis Child 2003;88:731–6.

[32] Coplan J, Souder MC, Mulberg AE, et al. Children with autistic spectrum disorders. II: parents are unable to distinguish secretin from placebo under double-blind conditions. Arch Dis Child 2003;88:737–9.

[33] American Academy of Child and Adolescent Psychiatry. Practice parameter for the assessment and treatment of children and adolescents diagnosed with reactive attachment disorder of infancy and early childhood. Washington, DC: American Academy of Child and Adolescent Psychiatry; 2005.

[34] American Academy of Child and Adolescent Psychiatry. Position statement: coercive interventions for reactive attachment disorder. Washington, DC: American Academy of Child and Adolescent Psychiatry; 2003.

[35] American Psychiatric Association. Position statement: reactive attachment disorder. Washington, DC: American Psychiatric Association; 2002.

[36] Klass P, Costello E. Quirky kids: understanding and helping your child who doesn't fit in-when to worry and when not to worry. New York: Ballantine Books; 2003.

ELSEVIER
SAUNDERS

PEDIATRIC CLINICS
OF NORTH AMERICA

Pediatr Clin N Am 52 (2005) 1479–1494

Special Topics in International Adoption

Jerri Ann Jenista, MD

Department of Pediatrics and Emergency Medicine, St. Joseph Mercy Hospital, PO Box 996, Ann Arbor, MI 48106, USA

As international adoption has become more "mainstream," the issues recently addressed in domestic adoption have become more important in adoptions involving children originating in other countries. Certain groups of prospective adoptive parents, such as gay or lesbian couples, single parents, and parents with disabilities, have begun to apply to adopt in ever increasing numbers. Children who may have been considered unadoptable in the past are now routinely being offered to prospective adoptive parents. The numbers and ages of the children placed and the spacing between adoptions have come under scrutiny. The rates of adoption dissolutions and disruptions are being examined carefully by the receiving and sending countries.

Research on the difficulties in these special circumstances and the outcome for the children involved is in the most preliminary stages. Currently, many of the kinds of situations described here are considered "experimental programs." The laws and policies of the sending countries explicitly prohibit some, and some are issues for the parents and professionals caring for children after adoption. This article attempts to summarize what information is already known and outlines areas in which research is desperately needed.

Adoptive parents: same-sex couples

Probably the most contentious issue in domestic adoption today concerning adoptive parents is whether or not gay or lesbian households are the appropriate placement for any child [1]. Some states prohibit gay or lesbian persons from foster care or adoption programs run by governmental agencies. Some explicitly

E-mail address: jaenista@aol.com

prohibit adoptions by such individuals, although the same persons may provide foster care. Although no state has laws specifically permitting adoption by both of the unrelated partners of the same sex, some individual courts do allow such proceedings [2]. Recently, a few states have passed laws allowing "second-parent" adoption by the partner of a person who already has an adopted or biologic child. A summary of the current laws and "same-sex–friendly" states and jurisdictions is available (www.lambdalegal.org). Authoritative and non-judgmental articles on gay and lesbian adoption with references to many re-sources for parents and professionals are widely available [1,3–5]. It is difficult to collect any statistics on the numbers of children adopted by gay or lesbian persons as it is likely, in many situations, that one of the partners adopts as a single person, without any mention of sexual preference.

The outcome for children raised by same-sex parents is a topic of great in-terest. Studies, however, are hampered by numerous issues [6,7]. Many couples raise children for whom one of the partners is the biologic parent; the child may have been conceived during a previous heterosexual relationship, through arti-ficial insemination, or through an informal relationship set up explicitly to pro-duce a child. Some of these children may continue to have relationships with the biologic parent of the other sex, perhaps mitigating some of the proposed "damage" that might be inflicted by growing up with homosexual parents. Most studies, however, tend to show that children raised in such households have more similarities than differences compared with children raised in households headed by heterosexual couples or single parents [1,7–12].

Few studies of children adopted by same-sex partners exist. Most of these studies have examined small groups of parents and children, provide only short-term outcomes, and are probably not truly representative, because the parents studied tend to be volunteers or members of activist or support groups. It seems that such families may be a valuable resource for the many children waiting for permanent families, however, and there are moves among some private adoption agencies to consider same-sex couples as a viable alternative resource for these "waiting children" [13,14].

There are some additional issues for such families, for example, whether to "come out" publicly about the composition of the household and to deal with the combined stigmatization of being adopted and being raised by same-sex parents [12,15,16]. There may be significant anxiety shared by the adoptive partners about custody issues, legal ability to consent to medical or educational interventions, health insurance, and disability and death benefits in a situation in which one partner is the legal parent and the other has no formal relationship with the child [17] Because of these issues and their impact on the children involved, the American Academy of Pediatrics has issued a statement supporting "co-parent" or second-parent adoption [17] to ensure that the child has the full legal benefits offered through each of the parents. This controversial statement has been vilified as encouraging or approving of families headed by same-sex cou-ples; however, careful reading of the document indicates that the policy is in-tended to ensure the best interests of the children already living in such households. The concept behind the policy statement has been affirmed by the American Academy of Family Physicians [18] and the American Psychiatric Association [19].

The outcome for internationally adopted children raised by same-sex couples is essentially unknown. There are no statistics concerning the numbers of such placements. The major obstacle to any study of this special population is the identification of the sexual preference of the adopting parent(s). Most sending countries explicitly prohibit gay or lesbian persons from adopting. Others are silent on the topic but allow local agencies and courts to examine the circumstances of each adoption. It is unusual for a family study (the document detailing the characteristics of the adoptive household) to identify the prospective parent as a member of a same-sex couple. In almost all circumstances, the adopting parent is presented as a single person. Other adults in the household may be described as relatives, friends, or housemates for financial support. Even after the legal process is complete, parents and agencies are unwilling to acknowledge publicly the sexual preferences of their families or clients for fear that the sending country may exclude the individuals or the agencies from future adoptions.

A Dutch review found that being raised by a single or lesbian parent was not a risk for behavioral problems in the child but that adoption was an independent factor increasing the risk for long-term developmental issues [20]. The authors comment that, in particular, children adopted internationally presented more challenges to their families and that those risks superseded the issues of a single-parent household. Interestingly, the authors comment that these "alternative" households are often made up of "exceptionally competent parents" and thus there may be a bias toward a better outcome for their children.

The Minnesota Adoption Project, an ongoing analysis of data on almost 2300 children adopted from other countries into Minnesota, comes to some similar conclusions [21]. The study was unable to distinguish same-sex partners from heterosexual couples in an informal relationship, nor could it determine whether single parents had unidentified partners of either sex participating in the care of the children. This, however, is one of the few studies of international adoption outcome that has attempted to look at the topic in even a preliminary way without a major concern for selection bias in the type of household studied.

The single or partnered households tended to have similar educational achievement but slightly less household income and somewhat more increased financial stress than the married-couple households. More children came from China and various Latin American countries than in married-couple households. The children adopted tended to be older and to have experienced longer institutional stays and more deprivation. After adoption, the children in single-partnered households had more identified behavioral and educational issues. At the time of follow-up (when the children were an average of 7 to 8 years of age), however, there were no discernible differences in the reported behavioral or social issues of the children reared in married-couple versus alternative households. In other words, the alternative families succeeded as well as or perhaps better than the married couples in raising children with considerable preadoption stress.

In summary, almost all data currently available indicate that the children raised by same-sex parents are not fundamentally different than the children raised in heterosexual households. Nevertheless, it is not clear how the social impact of being raised by a same-sex couple may interact with a child's status as an adopted person. There are even fewer data to indicate how the special issues of international adoption may affect the children in such households. There is a desperate need for such studies for both domestic and international adoption, because there are far more children waiting for homes than there are married-couple applicants. The prospect of overcoming the barrier of accurately identifying same-sex couples without jeopardizing the few adoptions that do proceed is formidable, however.

Adoptive parents: single parents

Single-parent adoption has become increasingly more common over the past quarter century, paralleling the increase in households headed by single parents in the general population. In the United States, up to 25% of the adoptive placements of children with special needs are with single parents; single parents account for approximately 5% of all other adoptions [22,23]. Census 2000 data indicate that 17% of all adopted children in the United States live with a single parent, approximately 4% of whom report never being married and no partner present in the household [24]. Approximately 10% of intercountry adoptions are accomplished by single parents [21].

Single adoptive parent households are a heterogeneous group including unmarried adults living alone, households with same-sex or opposite sex partners sharing parenting, adult relatives (most often, sisters or a parent and grandparent) living together, combined households of two single-parent families sharing living and child care expenses, divorced parents with custody of the child previously adopted into a married household, and numerous other constellations. There have been few systematic examinations of the adult relationships existing within and around single-parent adoptive families. It may be that there are few parents truly raising a child without another significant adult presence [24–26].

In studies of domestic and international adoptions, single adopters are overwhelmingly female, 6 to 7 years older than married women adopters, and well educated but with incomes less than those of married-couple households [21,24,27]. The children placed in their homes are typically older with a higher percentage of special needs or adverse preadoption stresses [21,24,27].

Those adopting internationally are probably a selected population because many countries have different requirements for single applicants—usually a higher minimum age, minimum and maximum age gaps between the parent and the adoptive child, quotas for the number of single applicants, closer scrutiny of parental resources, and higher individual income requirements [28,29]. The more restrictive prerequisites are sometimes relaxed if the applicant is willing to adopt a child with special needs. US immigration law imposes a minimum age requirement for single applicants but not for married applicants [30].

Most studies of the outcome of single-parent adoptions are small or restricted to a geographic area or examine only certain types of adoption, such as transracial or special needs placements. Almost all studies focus on domestic adoption. The findings from many of the studies are similar, however. In general, single-parent adoptions are as successful as married parent placements [25,31–36], although single parents experience more social and economic stressors and seek postadoption services more frequently [31,37]. This is not a surprising finding, because single parents tend to adopt children who are older and more likely to have lived in foster care or to have experienced prolonged institutionalization, all of which are factors described to increase adoptive family stress [31,33,37]. In longitudinal studies of such adoptions, however, the outcome for the children has been equal to or better than that in married-couple households, and single parents report fewer problems and a more positive attitude about the effect of adoption on their lives [31,34–36]. Certain children, such as those with special needs, tend to fare better in single-parent homes [31,35]. Some experts even consider single-parent households as the "placement of choice" for the "hard to place" child.

There are no studies designed specifically to examine the outcome for internationally adopted children placed in married-couple versus single-parent homes. In large series examining such children, single-parent households account for only 2% to 10% of placements [21,39] and there is no distinction made among the various types of family constellations, which may include same-sex or opposite-sex partners or other adults living in the household. The Minnesota Adoption Project reported that despite having adopted children with higher risks for poor outcome, single parents reported outcomes for their children at least equal to those of married parents [21]. Adoption disruptions do not seem to be increased in single-parent households when other factors are held constant [31]. Large meta-analyses of the international adoption literature of the past 50 years have not identified single-parent adoption as a factor for poor mental health or behavioral outcome [21,39–41]; however, in most studies, it is not clear that the question was specifically examined.

There are considerable recent data examining the needs of parents for postadoption services and the rates of adoption disruptions. Virtually all report similar risk factors for increased stress in the household and a greater need for family supports. Child-related factors include older age at adoption; adoption from foster care; international adoption; behavioral or emotional problems; and previous neglect, abuse, or disruption. Family-related factors include a higher level of parental education, lack of previous experience as a foster or adoptive parent, fewer social supports, increased number of adopted children in the home, and younger age of parent(s) [31,33,37,41]. Because many of these risk factors for children and their parents occur at increasing rates in today's international single-parent adoptions, some experts have begun to question the wisdom of placing higher risk children with single parents. The Swedish National Board of

Intercountry Adoption, after a review of the international adoption literature worldwide, developed a policy recommendation that single or older parents should not be the placement of choice for older or higher risk children [39].

In summary, the available data seem to show that single adoptive parents are as happy with their adoption experience as married couples, despite having adopted children with more needs. Certain groups of adopted children with significant preadoption adversity, primarily from Eastern Europe and the republics of the former Soviet Union, have increased rates of behavioral problems persisting into their adoptions [40]; many of these children are adopted into single-parent homes because those countries typically do not have many restrictions on who may adopt or the characteristics of the child they choose. It is not known whether the children might be better served in different families or might have better outcomes if focused pre- or postadoption services were provided to their parents [33,37,41], however. Numerous authors have cited the need for research into the characteristics of families, single or married, that allow for increased success in international adoption [39–42].

Adoptive parents: parents with disabilities

The Americans with Disabilities Act (ADA) defines a person as disabled if he or she has now, has had in the past, or is considered to have a physical or mental impairment that may limit life's major activities [43,44]. Thus, a blind person who is self-supporting and living independently, a person with schizophrenia controlled on medication, a person who has survived cancer in the distant past, and a person who requires a personal aide for the activities of daily living are all considered to have a disability that is protected by the ADA. Homosexuality, however, is specifically excluded as a disability.

The ADA addresses adoption agencies, including private entities, stating that applicants who are disabled cannot be excluded from consideration for adoption merely on the basis of their disability [43,45]. In at least one court case, however, the judge held that an agency might consider the applicant's disability in a particular placement [46]. The court ruled that the agency's job "was not to find a child for the plaintiff's home, but the opposite: to find suitable homes for children." As a consequence, US adoption agencies cannot categorically refuse to work with prospective adoptive parents applying to adopt overseas. Currently, the working policy for most agencies is to accept applicants but to inform them of the possibility that their adoption attempt may fail as a result of overseas factors not covered by the ADA. It is suggested that the social worker should describe the abilities rather than the disabilities of the prospective parent(s) in the family study submitted to the overseas orphanage and court [47]. It is ultimately the decision of the overseas entity to accept or disapprove the parent's application, however. Clients of my own practice have reported being refused for a distant history of cancer, older age, being a single male head of a household, having a hearing impairment, being under treatment for depression, obesity, smoking, evangelical Christian religious preference, and African-American race. Nevertheless, there are parents with disabilities who succeed in adopting internationally, and there are web sites and support groups for such parents and their children [44].

There are anecdotal reports in the adoption and general popular media about the success of various adoptions by persons with disabilities [44] but no research studies on the outcome of such placements, particularly in international adoption. Because such parents tend to adopt a child with a condition similar to their own, one could hypothesize that these adoptive placements would be more successful because the parents would be better advocates, having already addressed similar special needs for themselves. Conversely, the combination of the child's needs and those of the parent could possibly be overwhelming. At least one study of disabled parents (not an adoption study) indicated that the children in households in which the parent requires aid for the activities of daily living are less likely to be immunized. The immunization status of children with parents with lesser disabilities or work limitations is equivalent to that of children living with non-disabled parents [48].

Research or even descriptive studies of this special group of adoptive parents would be useful for adoption agencies to present to courts and orphanages overseas to advocate for the placement of specific children, for prospective adoptive applicants to understand the issues in adopting and raising a particular type of child, for postadoption service providers to determine what services might be needed to improve outcome for the parents and their children, and for physicians to monitor more closely the health of the entire family unit in this possibly especially vulnerable population.

Adopted children: special needs

There is extensive literature concerning the progress of adoptions of children with special needs in the United States [31,37,38,59,60,66–80,84,86–88]. Most of the available studies have focused on parents who sought to adopt a child with special needs. Most such children are placed through the public welfare system and are eligible for a number of supports including adoption subsidy (cash for living expenses), medical subsidy or Medicaid eligibility, respite care, and mental health services.

The early studies (1970s and 1980s) concerned children with physical or developmental disabilities and found that families were generally happy with their adoption experience [68–70,73,74]. Disruption rates were low and many parents went on to adopt or foster additional children with disabilities [73]. Over time, families reported more stress as their children entered adolescence, and the children were found to have decreased school performance [69]. Behavioral and other problems did not disappear over time, but most families remained happy with their experience [67,69]. Starting in the 1990s, the children's special needs changed to include those children affected by prenatal exposure to drugs or alcohol and children with significant mental health rather than medical problems. Families reported that these adoptions were more difficult but also more re-warding than expected [71,72]. Parents who had adopted older children or those with more behavioral issues reported more stress [78]; parents with more educa-tion and higher incomes requested more services [79].

In response to these and other research findings, programs for the provision of postadoption services have been developed [77–79]. New insights into a va-riety of issues, including the cause of the children's difficult behaviors [76] and the role of children already in the home [86], have guided the development of services more responsive to adoptive parents' requests.

The outcome of international adoption of children with special needs is less clear. Parents seeking to adopt internationally a child with known special needs may be a self-selected group because they must pay large fees to process the adoption and, for the most part, the children are not eligible for the financial and medical supports available to the same children adopted within the United States. Such families may be more risk taking or more flexible in their expectations, they may have different motivations to adopt than other international adopters, or they may feel compelled to "prove" that they made a right decision in adopting such a child. Whether any of these hypotheses are true is unknown because this population has been ignored or specifically excluded in most outcome studies of intercountry adoption [39,40]. The more interesting question is not about this group at all, however.

Most applicants for international adoption are not seeking to adopt a child with special needs; yet, nearly every analysis of child characteristics, at least of children coming from institutional rather than foster care, has indicated that most children adopted internationally do have special needs. What happens to those parents who unexpectedly find themselves raising the very child they thought they were avoiding by going overseas to adopt? Do these families use their greater economic and advocacy powers to "buy" the services they need [52], or are their expectations, based their own educational and social success, too high for the expected outcomes of these children, leading to disappointment and in-creased stress [37]? Can mandated preadoption training for prospective adopters prevent unrealistic expectations of the type of the child they want to adopt? Are there ways to evaluate the skills and resources of parents to help them choose a child who best matches what the parents have (and are willing) to offer? Are there characteristics of parents or children that can predict more successful placements? Several authors have shown that the characteristics of children in foster care in the United States and children adopted from institutions overseas are similar with many medical issues, developmental delays, and mental health needs as well as past histories of prenatal substance exposure, physical abuse, and neglect [60,82]. Do the social work practices successful with the foster care population translate to good practice for internationally adopted children? Are there fundamental differences between these two groups of children or their adopting parents? The need for carefully designed research on these questions is pressing, because the numbers of international adoptions are increasing dramatically each year.

Adopted children: siblings

Should siblings always be placed together? Are there situations in which the adoption of sibling groups may be harmful to the children already in the family or to the new group of children entering? Are there settings in which siblings should be separated for safety or other reasons? These and many other questions have been examined for US adoptions [49,81,83]. Depending on the life histories and characteristics of the children and families, there are different answers to these questions for each group of children. In general, siblings should be placed together and with parents who have no other children. If placement together is not an option, some sort of contact should be maintained. Should these practices be applied to international adoption? There are some issues that are peculiar to international adoption. What happens to siblings who are adopted at different times into different families and perhaps even to different countries? What happens to siblings who are left behind in orphanages or who have remained with the birth parents? Are there long-term psychologic consequences for the children of such broken families? Are there ways in which adoptive parents can address the issue of separated siblings?

Only one large study has systematically examined issues in the placement of biologically related siblings in international adoption [84,85]. Genetic and environmental factors were found to influence the type of behavior problems noted. The study did not address any differing outcomes for related versus nonrelated siblings or children placed as singletons, however. There is a clear need for more investigation into what issues might exist for these children and how best to help families deal with them.

Adopted children: artificial twinning and instant families

In the early days of modern international adoption, after the Korean and Vietnam Wars, the process of adoption was arduous and time-consuming, even requiring special bills in Congress for the granting of individual immigrant visas. Most adoptions were accomplished through established or "traditional" child welfare agencies or through new agencies typically set up by adoptive parents specifically to place children from a particular country or region. Most agencies had strict requirements for their applicants based on the prevailing social work adoption practices (eg, parents should be married, preferably with a stay-at-home mother; the adopted child should be the youngest; there should be at least a year between adoptions; birth order should not be disturbed). In those first years, there were few agencies and parents were resigned to "following the rules" and waiting in line for the next available child. Agencies viewed their role as finding families for the children assigned to their care.

In the last decade of the century, new countries opened up to international adoption, mostly in Eastern Europe and the countries of the former Soviet Union. A new kind of adoption agency, more entrepreneurial in nature, sprang up and multiplied rapidly. With few or no restrictions placed by the sending countries and numerous children available for placement, these new agencies allowed prospective adopters much more choice in the type of child and the length of the waiting period. In other words, international adoption from some countries had become a "buyer's market." These new agencies viewed their role as finding children for the families they represent.

In such an atmosphere, where costs are far greater and children more easily available, adoptive parents began to make demands that were met by agencies anxious to keep their clientele. Thus, a new phenomenon, not seen in the domestic adoption picture, is emerging in international adoption. Applicants, anxious to save time and money, unwilling to travel more than once, and relieved at the prospect of finally accomplishing their goal of becoming parents, are asking to adopt more than one child at the same time. "Artificial twinning" is the adoption of two children closer than 8 months in age whether or not they were placed at the same time. Adoption of multiple unrelated children at the same time produces an "instant family." These practices, once extremely rare in international adoption, are increasing in prevalence. In one adoption clinic, 10% of families seeking preadoption counseling were planning to adopt more than one child at the same time [53]. Web sites and parent support groups for parents raising these children are easily available [50].

There is a small but vocal opposition to artificial twinning, at least for newborns, from the social work community [51], arguing that it is not possible to meet the needs of two unrelated close-in-age infants adequately without significant (and unnecessary) stress. Most of the available literature on this practice is expert opinion based on clinical practice [49] but none of it is supportive of the concept. There are no studies looking at the short- or long-term outcomes for unrelated adopted children raised as twins, however. One might expect that the outcome would be influenced by any special needs of the children and the parents' access to financial and other support.

Only one study has looked specifically at the outcome for multiple unrelated children adopted at the same time. Among Romanian children adopted to Canada, those families who had adopted two children at the same time reported greater parental stress and more behavioral problems in their children than families who had adopted only one child at a time [51]. An increased number of adopted children in the home, children with more special needs, and children who have experienced more preadoption adversity have been noted to increase the adoptive parent's need for counseling and other postadoption services [37,54].

Numerous studies document the increased level of preadoption adversity experienced by children adopted from Eastern European countries (see the article by Weitzman and Albers in this issue) [39–41,52,54,60]. Because these are also the countries that allow multiple-child adoptions, it seems logical to assume that families adopting more than one child can expect to face significant challenges in parenting. Anecdotal descriptions of such family life are mixed, emphasizing the most positive or most negative aspects of the experience [61,62]. Currently, most of these families are too early in their adoption experience to determine the long-term outcome. Adoption researchers have made a plea for immediate research into the issues of these adoptions for policy development and postplacement support [39].

Adoptive families: disruption and dissolution

Disruption is the removal of a child from an adoptive home before the legal process is final whereas dissolution is the removal of the child after a completed legal adoption. In practice, however, the term *disruption* is used to describe the failure of an adoptive placement at any time during or after the legal process.

There has been considerable recent media attention to the topic of "international adoption gone wrong" [55] but the actual rate of disruption in international adoption is unknown. The expected rate of failure of adoptions of children with special needs from the foster care system in the United States is approximately 10% to 15% [33,59]. The rate of failed adoptions internationally must be much lower but there does seem to be an increasing trend in the numbers of parents reporting stress severe enough to consider relinquishing the child.

One agency, specializing in the placement of US children with special needs, noted 18 unsolicited telephone calls from parents wishing to disrupt their international adoptions over the period from 1985 through 1994. The children came from a variety of countries, approximately 50% were part of a sibling group, and the mean age of the children was 9.6 years [63]. From 1994 through 2002, the same agency received 162 such calls: 70% of the children were from Eastern Europe, 10% were part of a sibling group, and the mean age of the children was 7.8 years. Most callers indicated that the reason for their dissatisfaction with the adoption was the severity and persistence of the child's behavioral and emotional problems.

In an attempt to follow up on the outcome of these telephone calls, a survey was conducted in 2003. The families who participated in the outcome study seemed to be typical of most internationally adopting parents: most were married and were experienced parents in their early 40s, and their median annual income was $90,000 [57]. The children were, on average, 5.8 years old at the time of adoption. None of the families had intended to adopt a child with special needs, and only 19% received any agency-mandated family preparation. Most parents reported receiving inadequate information about their adopted child; however, 58% did receive documents noting birth family histories of alcohol abuse, domestic violence, or extreme poverty and child histories of known abuse or neglect. The children themselves disclosed, invariably after the adoption, experiencing or witnessing homicide or suicide (20%), sexual abuse (50%), physical abuse (50%), domestic violence (30%), animal torture (4%), or separation from a twin (4%). Three quarters of the parents had concerns about their child's behavior before leaving the country of origin and, at the time of follow-up, 80% of the children were in some type of out-of-home placement ranging from adoption by a second family to foster or residential care. When queried whether the disruption could have been prevented, most felt that the relationship was doomed from the start and that if they had had adequate information about the adoption or the particular child, they would not have gone forward.

The ultimate "disruption" is death of the child. From 1996 through 2003, US newspapers have reported the deaths by the hand of their parents of 12 children adopted from Russia [56]. Detailed investigation into these cases has almost always revealed severe abuse or neglect in the child's history and poor or no adoptive parent preparation [64].

Rather than disrupt, some families have elected to continue raising the child but have sued the adoption agency for "wrongful adoption" [58]. The basis of virtually all international wrongful adoption cases has been the alleged failure of the agency to inform the parents of or to investigate the severity of the child's emotional or behavioral issues before the adoption. In those cases that were not dismissed or settled out of court, the courts have typically ruled against the parents, indicating that because the parents had the opportunity to visit the child in the orphanage, they had a responsibility to investigate for themselves the child's true condition. Most international adoption agencies also require that applicants sign a waiver absolving the agency from responsibility for information that was not transmitted from the orphanage to the agency. Although some jurisdictions have questioned the legality of such "no-fault" waivers, as yet, none have been overturned in court. Thoughtful analyses of the causes and prevention of wrongful adoption lawsuits are available [58,65].

The common theme among deaths, disruptions, and wrongful adoption lawsuits seems to be lack of preadoptive preparation for the prospective parents. There is a considerable body of information available on the factors leading to successful adoptions of children with special needs in the United States [31,66]. Whether the needs of parents and their children, and the types of supports and the way they are provided are appropriate for the parents and children of international adoption is unknown [39–41].

Summary

There is a pressing need for research into numerous social aspects of adoption. Should the lessons learned in domestic foster care adoption be applied to international adoption? Are there fundamental differences in the children or the parents that might require specially focused services? What are the characteristics of a successful adoptive family, and what kinds of parents can meet those needs? Are the "new" adoption practices of artificial twinning or multiple unrelated adoptions harmful to children or families? Are there practices from other countries that can be applied successfully in the United States? How can we accurately identify and follow the kinds of families necessary to answer these questions? The challenges are clear.

Acknowledgments

This article is dedicated to the memory of Barbara Burpee, PT.

References

[1] Kreisher K. Children's voice article: Gay adoption. January 2002. Child Welfare League of America. Available at: www.cwla.org/articles/cv0201gayadopt.htm. Accessed June 14, 2005.

[2] Connolly C. The description of gay and lesbian families in second-parent adoption cases. Behavioral Science Law 1998;16(2):225–36.

[3] National Adoption Information Clearinghouse (DHHS). 2000. Gay and lesbian adoptive parents: resources for professionals and parents. Available at: www.naic.acf.hhs.gov/pubs/f_gay/f_gayc.cfm. Accessed June 14, 2005.

[4] National Adoption Information Clearinghouse (DHHS). Legal considerations for prospective adoptive parents. 2005. Available at: www.naic.acf.hhs.gov/parents/prospective/legal/index.cfm. Accessed June 14, 2005.

[5] Craft C. About.com. 2005. Adoption by gays and lesbians. Available at: adoption.about.com/cs/gaylesbian. Accessed June 14, 2005.

[6] Martín-Ancel A. Adoption by same-sex parents. Pediatrics 2002;110(2):419–20.

[7] Perrin EC. Technical report: coparent or second-parent adoption by same-sex parents. Pediatrics 2002;109:341–4. Available at: www.pediatrics.org/cgi/content/full/109/2/341. Accessed June 14, 2005.

[8] van Nijnatten CH. Sexual orientation and Dutch family law. Med Law 1995;14(5):359–68.

[9] Anderssen N, Amlie C, Ytteroy EA. Outcomes for children with lesbian or gay parents. A review of the studies from 1978 to 2000. Scand J Psychol 2002;43(4):335–51.

[10] Ciano-Boyce C, Shelley-Sireci L. Who is Mommy tonight? Lesbian parenting issues. J Homosex 2002;43(2):1–13.

[11] Dundas S, Kaufman M. The Toronto Lesbian Family Study. J Homosex 2000;40(2):65–79.

[12] Perrin EC. A difficult adjustment to school: the importance of family constellation. Pediatrics 2004;114(5):1464–7.

[13] Brooks D, Goldberg S. Gay and lesbian adoptive and foster care placements: can they meet the needs of waiting children? Soc Work 2001;46(2):147–57.

[14] Ryan SD, Pearlmutter S, Groza V. Coming out of the closet: opening agencies to gay and lesbian adoptive parents. Soc Work 2004;49(1):85–95.

[15] Gold M, Perrin E, Futterman D, et al. Children of gay or lesbian parents. Pediatr Rev 1994;15(9):354–8.

[16] Lynch JM, Murray K. For the love of the children: the coming out process for lesbian and gay parents and stepparents. J Homosex 2000;39(1):1–24.

[17] Committee on Psychosocial Aspects of Child and Family Health, American Academy of Pediatrics. Coparent or second parent adoption by same-sex parents. Pediatrics 2002;109:339–40.

[18] Stoever J. Delegates vote for adoption policy. 2002 FP report. October 17, 2000. Available at: www.aafp.org/fpr/assembly2002/1017/7.html. Accessed June 14, 2005.

[19] American Psychiatric Association. Controversies in child custody: gay and lesbian parenting; transracial adoptions; joint versus sole custody; and custody gender issues. 1997. Available at: www.psych.org/edu/other_res/lib_archives/archives/199708.pdf. Accessed June 14, 2005.

[20] Verhulst FC, Versluis-den Bieman HO, Balmus NC. Being raised by lesbian parents or in a single-parent family is no risk factor for problem behavior, however being raised as an adopted child is. Ned Tijdschr Geneeskd 1997;141(9):414–8.

[21] Johnson D. Married vs. partnered and single parent families: is there a difference in outcome in international adoptees. Presented at the Annual Conference of the Joint Council on International Children's Services. Washington, DC, April 6, 2005.

[22] Smith DG. Single parent adoption: what you need to know. 1994. National Adoption Information Clearinghouse. Available at: library.adoption.com/Single-Parent-Adoption/Single-Parent-Adoption/article/21/1.html or naic.acf.hhs.gov/pubs/f_single/index.cfm. Accessed June 14, 2005.

[23] Marindin H. Handbook for single adoptive parents. Washington, DC: National Council for Single Adoptive Parents; 2000. p. 1–6.

[24] Kreider RM. Adopted children and stepchildren: 2000. Census 2000 special reports. US Census Bureau. October 2003. Available at: www.census.gov/prod/2003pubs/censr-6.pdf. Accessed June 14, 2005.

[25] Groze V. Adoption and single parents: a review. Child Welfare 1991;70(3):321–32.

[26] Melina LR. Adoption: an annotated bibliography and guide. New York: Garland Publishing; 1987.

[27] Marindin H. Single person adoption. In: Marshner C, Pierce WL, editors. Adoption factbook III. Waite Park, MN: National Council for Adoption; 1999. p. 489–90.

[28] China Center for Adoption Affairs. Available at: www.china-ccaa.org/english-index.htm. Accessed June 14, 2005.

[29] US Department of State. International adoption: country specific flyers. Available at: travel.state.gov/family/adoption/country/country_369.html. Accessed June 14, 2005.

[30] US Department of State. Intercountry adoption brochure. Available at: travel.state.gov/family/adoption/info/info_455.html. Accessed June 14, 2005.

[31] Shireman JF. Adoption by single parents. Marriage and Family Review 1995;20:367–88.

[32] Berry M. Adoption disruption. In: Avery RJ, editor. Adoption policy and special needs children. Westport, CT: Greenwood Publications; 1997. p. 77–106.

[33] Barth RP, Gibbs DA, Siebenaler K. Assessing the field of post-adoption services; family needs, program models, and evaluation issues. Chapel Hill, NC: Research Triangle Institute and the University of North Carolina School of Social Work; 2001.

[34] Feigelman W, Silverman AR. Single parent adoption. In: Marindin H, editor. The handbook for single adoptive parents. Chevy Chase, MD: National Council for Single Adoptive Parents; 1998. p. 123–9.

[35] Groze VK, Rosenthal JA. Single parents and their adopted children: a psychosocial analysis. Families in Society: The Journal of Contemporary Human Services 1991;72(2):130–9.

[36] Feigelman W, Silverman AR. Single parent adoptions. Soc Casework 1977;58:418–25.

[37] Bird GW, Peterson R, Miller SH. Factors associated with distress among support-seeking adoptive parents. Fam Relat 2002;51:215–20.

[38] Donley KS. Single parents as "placements of choice." In: Churchill SR, Carlson B, Nybell L, editors. No child is unadoptable: a reader on adoption of children with special needs. Beverly Hills: SAGE Publications; 1977. p. 46–7.

[39] Cederblad M. Adoption—but at what price? 2003. Swedish National Board for Intercountry Adoption (NIA). Available at: www.nia.se/english/utredneng.pdf. Accessed June 14, 2005.

[40] Juffer F, van Ijzendoorn MH. Behavioral problems and mental health referrals of international adoptees: a meta-analysis. JAMA 2005;293:2501–15.

[41] Miller LC. International adoption, behavior and mental health. JAMA 2005;293:2533–5.

[42] Barth RP, Miller JM. Building effective post-adoption services: what is the empirical foundation? Fam Relat 2000;49:447–55.

[43] US Department of Justice. ADA home page. Available at: www.usdoj.gov/crt/ada/adahom1.htm. Accessed June 14, 2005.

[44] Adoptioninformation.com. Disabled persons can adopt. It's the law. Available at: www.adoptioninformation.com/resources/article/081099.htm. Accessed June 14, 2005.

[45] Freundlich M. The Americans with Disabilities Act: what adoption agencies need to know. Evan B Donaldson Adoption Institute. Available at: www.adoptioninstitute.org/policy/ada/html. Accessed June 14, 2005.

[46] Peterson L. Court rules agencies may deny placement based on prospective parent's disability. Child Welfare League of America. Available at: www.cwla.org/programs/adoption/americans_with_diasabilites2.htm. Accessed June 14, 2005.

[47] Jenista JA. Parents with disabilities. Presented at the Annual Meeting of the Joint Council on International Children's Services. Washington, DC, April 6, 2005.

[48] Hyatt Jr RR, Allen SM. Disability as a "family affair": parental disability and childhood immunization. Med Care 2005;43(6):600–6.

[49] Kockeritz N. The effects of adoptive family composition on outcomes for children. 2004. Intercountry Adoption Services. Social Development Canada. Available at: www.adoption.ca/pdfs/artifical_twinning_e.pdf. Accessed June 14, 2005.

[50] Adoptioninformatin.com. Artificial twinning. Available at: www.adoptioninformation.com/directory/twinning.htm. Accessed June 14, 2005.

[51] Johnson PI. Instant family? A case against artificial twinning. Available at: library.adoption.com/Parenting-and-Families/Instant-Familiy-A-Case-Against_Artificial_Twinning.html. Accessed June 14, 2005.

[52] Ames E. The development of Romanian children adopted into Canada: final report. Burnaby (BC): Simon Fraser University; 1997.

[53] Jenista JA. Preadoption review of medical records. Pediatr Ann 2000;29(4):212–5.

[54] Judge S. Determinants of parental stress in families adopting children from Eastern Europe. Fam Relat 2003;52(30):241–8.

[55] Working R, Madhani A. Parents often not ready for needy foreign kids: adoptions from Eastern Europe put added stress on parents as children often suffer a range of emotional or physical problems, experts say. Chicago Tribune December 28, 2003.

[56] Working R. Adoptee deaths rare, experts say: 12 Russian cases troubling, puzzling. Chicago Tribune May 21, 2004.

[57] McNamara J, McNamara B, Holtan B. Preparation for international adoption. Presented at the 30th North American Council on Adoptable Children Training Conference. Minneapolis, MN, August 9, 2004.

[58] Freundlich M, Peterson L. Wrongful adoption: law, policy and practice. Washington, DC: Child Welfare League of America; 1998.

[59] Berry M, Barth RP. A study of disrupted adoptive placements of adolescents. Child Welfare 1990;69(3):209–25.

[60] Groza V, Ryan SD. Pre-adoption stress and its association with child behavior in domestic special needs and international adoptions. Psychoneuroendocrinology 2002;27(1–2):181–97.

[61] Ciccarelli D. Steppe children: gifts from mother Russia. FACE Facts 1996;19(4):8–14.

[62] Galbraith L. Romanian orphans, adopted daughters. Harrowsmith, Ontario: Stoneridge Publishing; 1998.

[63] Holtan B, Jenista JA, Tepper T. Troubled Eastern European adoptions. Presented at the Annual North American Council for Adoptable Children Training Conference. Baltimore, MD, August 2002.

[64] Working R, Rodriguez A. Rescue of boy ends in tragedy. Chicago Tribune May 21, 2004.

[65] National Adoption Information Clearinghouse. Providing background information to adoptive parents: a bulletin for professionals. 2003. Available at: naic.acf.hhs.gov/pubs/f_background bulletin.cfm. Accessed June 14, 2005.

[66] Groze V. Successful adoptive families: a longitudinal study of special needs adoption. Westport, CT: Praeger Publications; 1996.

[67] Rosenthal JA, Groze VK. A longitudinal study of special-needs adoptive families. Child Welfare 1994;73(6):689–706.

[68] Lewis RG. Adoption and mental retardation. Pediatr Ann 1989;18(10):637–44.

[69] Glidden LM, Johnson VE. Twelve years later: adjustment in families who adopted children with developmental disabilities. Ment Retard 1999;37(1):16–24.

[70] Hockey A. Evaluation of adoption of the intellectually handicapped: a retrospective analysis of 137 cases. J Ment Defic Res 1980;24(3):187–202.

[71] McCarty C, Waterman J, Burge D, et al. Experiences, concerns, and service needs of families adopting children with prenatal substance exposure: summary and recommendations. Child Welfare 1999;78(5):561–77.

[72] McClone K, Santos L, Kazama L, et al. Psychological stress in adoptive parents of special-needs children. Child Welfare 2002;81(2):151–71.

[73] Glidden LM, Pursley JT. Longitudinal comparisons of families who have adopted children with mental retardation. Am J Ment Retard 1989;94(3):272–7.

[74] Coyne A, Brown ME. Developmentally disabled children can be adopted. Child Welfare 1985; 64(6):607–15.

[75] Rosenthal JA, Groze V, Aguilar GD. Adoption outcomes for children with handicaps. Child Welfare 1991;70(6):623–36.

[76] Henry DL. Resilience in maltreated children: implications for special needs adoption. Child Welfare 1999;78(5):519–40.

[77] Kramer L, Houston D. Hope for the children: a community-based approach to supporting families who adopt children with special needs. Child Welfare 1999;78(5):611–35.

[78] McDonald TP, Propp JR, Murphy KC. The postadoption experience: child, parent and family predictors of family adjustment to adoption. Child Welfare 2001;80(1):71–94.

[79] Kramer L, Houston D. Supporting families as they adopt children with special needs. Fam Relat 1998;47:423–32.

[80] Groze V. Clinical and non-clinical adoptive families of special needs children. Fam Soc 1994; 75:90.

[81] Erich S, Leung P. The impact of previous type of abuse and sibling adoption upon adoptive families. Child Abuse Negl 2002;26(10):1045–58.

[82] Jenista JA. Medical issues in adoption. In: Marshner C, Pierce WL, editors. Adoption factbook III. Waite Park, MN: National Council for Adoption; 1999. p. 417–22.

[83] Boer F, Versluis-den Bieman HJM, Verhulst FC. International adoption of children with siblings: behavioural outcomes. Am J Orthopsychiatry 1994;64:252–62.

[84] van den Oord EJ, Boomsma DI, Verhulst FC. A study of problem behaviors in 10- to 15-year-old biologically related and unrelated international adoptees. Behav Genet 1994;24(3):193–205.

[85] van der Valk JC, Verhulst FC, Neale MC, et al. Longitudinal genetic analysis of problem behaviors in biologically related and unrelated adoptees. Behav Genet 1998;28(5):365–80.

[86] Mullin ES, Johnson L. The role of birth/previously adopted children in families choosing to adopt children with special needs. Child Welfare 1999;78(5):579–91.

[87] Grover S. Did I make the grade? Ethical issues in psychosocial screening of children for adoptive placement. Ethical Human Psychological Psychiatry 2004;6(2):125–33.

[88] Edelstein SB. Children with prenatal alcohol and/or other drug exposure: weighing the risks of adoption. Washington, DC: Child Welfare League of America; 1995.

ELSEVIER
SAUNDERS

PEDIATRIC CLINICS
OF NORTH AMERICA

Pediatr Clin N Am 52 (2005) 1495–1506

Intercountry Adoption: Young Adult Issues and Transition to Adulthood

Susan Soon-keum Cox[a,*], Joy Lieberthal, LMSW[b]

[a]Holt International Children's Services, PO Box 2880, Eugene, OR 97402, USA
[b]Also-Known-As, New York, NY, USA

For literally thousands of children in countries throughout the world, intercountry adoption is the only viable possibility for them to have a permanent loving family. Whenever there is a disaster, whether by natural causes or resulting from armed conflict or human atrocities, the predictable consequence is that children are the most vulnerable. Children's immediate and long-term survival is the most fragile.

Intercountry adoption is an extremely sensitive and emotional issue for the citizens of the sending countries as well as for those in other, often more affluent, countries who adopt these children. It must be a priority to respect the dignity of the child's birth country as well as the dignity of the child.

More than 20,000 children are adopted internationally each year by US families. Five decades of intercountry adoption to the United States translates into more than 200,000 children in this country who are international adoptees. Beyond the adoptees themselves, those affected by adoption expand to include adoptive parents, siblings, grandparents, aunts, uncles, cousins, and wide extended family as well as normal close attachments through friends, neighbors, church, and school. This represents a significant community of lives that are touched by the experience of international adoption.

Most individuals living the United States are aware of intercountry adoption, even if only from reading an article or seeing news reports. In spite of the scope of intercountry adoption in the United States, outside the immediate adoptive circle, there is minimal understanding of more than superficial issues. For the most part, intercountry adoption is accepted and acknowledged as

* Corresponding author.
E-mail address: ssoonkeum@aol.com (S.S.-K. Cox).

beneficial for the child and the family. The volume of awkward and sometimes intrusive inquiries that international adoptees and their families are often required to endure provides evidence that a deeper public sensitivity to the unique situations of these families and children has not developed. Another perspective is that these children and families are considered the same as any other and that no special consideration is needed or required.

A "social experiment"

The modern era of intercountry adoption began in 1956 when children from Korea, many fathered by United Nations soldier fathers and orphaned by the Korean War, were adopted by families in the United States. In the beginning, the concept of intercountry adoption was not universally embraced. Although American families had adopted children from Europe, these adoptions from Korea had the added complication of distinct racial differences between parents and children. Some critics considered it a crazy social experiment, and others acknowledged that these were cute babies and delightful toddlers but worried about what would happen to them when they grew up. Who would give them jobs? Who would marry them?

In spite of the skeptics, hundreds of American families adopted children from Korea, and within a few years, thousands of Korean children with Asian faces who arrived in the United States with names like Kim or Lee became Jones or Smith. They lived in communities across the United States, became American citizens, and became "Americanized" in every way possible.

Families who were pioneers in this process were encouraged to "love these children as your own." They were also advised to help their adopted children learn the language, food, customs, and culture as quickly as possible. "Fitting in" to American society was considered a necessary priority. Nearly all the children first adopted from Korea were Amerasian, and their appearance often varied greatly from one another. Some children were light skinned with blond hair and limited visible evidence of their Korean heritage. Children with black fathers appeared less Korean and more black biracial like their fathers. Many children looked distinctly Korean. The primary emphasis for Korean adoptees was to absorb them into the culture of their new adoptive families as quickly and completely as possible.

There was widespread concern that for these adoptions to be considered successful, it was necessary to demonstrate that children from another country and culture could effectively assimilate into their new family and American society. Children adopted from Korea, then from Vietnam, and later from other Asian and Latin American countries were convincing evidence of children's typical ability to be successfully transplanted from one culture to another. These adopted children are considered to be more American by culture than defined by their birth heritage and physical appearance. Simply by osmosis, it is their primary nationality.

As intercountry adoption has evolved and matured, there is less fearfulness and anxiety surrounding the necessity of proving its appropriateness. More attention and concern are focused on embracing the child's birth country and ethnicity as valued and important for the adopted child while supporting his or her healthy sense of self.

Race and identity

Being an international adoptee is a unique experience. A significant number of international adoptions are interracial adoptions, with clear racial differences between adoptees, their parents, other family members, and, in general, the community in which they live. These obvious physical differences generate intense speculation and curiosity from a variety of sources, including other family members, complete strangers, and casual observers. Dissimilarities of race and culture between adoptees and their adoptive families typically characterize intercountry adoption.

> More often than not, we grew up as the only Koreans in our community. We looked different from everyone around us—including our mothers and fathers. How we fit into our families was a curiosity to others who saw how we looked but did not understand how we felt. Repeatedly we were asked, 'Who are your real mom and dad?' [1]

International adoptees and their families do see themselves as comparable to any other family—with all the usual complexities. The issues that typically delineate distinctions between birth and adoptive families are more obvious for intercountry adoption, because the physical differences may be so obvious and public. As a normal part of child development, all adopted children experience the realization that they are not their parents' biologic children. It is not unusual for them to wonder about their birth parents, especially how they looked.

The differences are real. No one understands that with greater clarity than the adoptive family and, ultimately, the adoptee. Early in the adoption process, prospective adoptive parents must explore their feelings about these issues with their extended family, social worker, or adoption facilitator. Most importantly, they must explore and come to peace with these issues deep within themselves.

Beginning with the first social introduction outside the home as a toddler and throughout the lifetime of an international adoptee, individuals may be questioned about their adoption because of how they look. Strangers in supermarkets inquire why the child "looks different," "couldn't you have children of your own," and "how lucky that little child is."

Adoptive parents give voice to the necessary explanations until the children are old enough to take on the responsibility to articulate the answers for themselves. It is beneficial when adoptive families consider this challenge thoughtfully. The answers provided by parents are later echoed by the adoptee when he or she can speak on his or her own behalf. Parents and other significant adults can guide the adoptee in learning the appropriate boundaries of what should be shared about their adoption experience. In respecting the normal relations of communication, adoptees should also learn to respect and honor their own right to privacy. Their adoption experience belongs to them, and they should share their information only when they think it is appropriate. During childhood and adolescence, whenever questions are asked, it is an opportunity for adoptive families to encourage the use of appropriate adoption language.

At some time in an adoptee's development, he or she may find this public curiosity about himself or herself confusing. Sometimes it is annoying and intrusive. Adoptees have various tolerance levels of these situations determined by their own personalities. Confronting the normal issues of adolescence at the same time that an adoptee is confronting his or her racial and cultural identity can be a confusing, difficult, and overwhelming experience. For some adoptees, these issues are deeply uncomfortable and troubling. It is essential that they feel confident they can share these concerns with others and be supported by their adoptive families, who sometimes find these issues to be difficult for them as well.

Family relationships are defined by emotions, feelings, characteristics, and personalities of individual family members. What is felt, more than what is reflected on individual faces, establishes and binds families together. This is the true essence of adoption. Those feelings evolve from being with one another and creating a shared history. This commitment is understood by adoptive families but often seems mysterious to others beyond the extended family.

Culture and heritage

Acknowledging and demonstrating respect for an adoptee's cultural and racial heritage are critical responsibilities of adoptive parents and family, including extended family members who are a part of the child's life. Other adults who have regular contact with adoptees through school, church, sports, and other social activities may have a tremendous impact on how international adoptees view themselves.

An adoptive family may ignore or make little effort to include the cultural heritage of the adopted child as a part of their parenting. That decision does not necessarily indicate that the child is not accepted, loved, or cherished as their own son or daughter. When the adoptive family also accepts and honors the cultural identity of the child's birth heritage, however, it enriches not only the adoptee but the entire family and extended family as well.

The challenge is to achieve a competent level of understanding that ensures sensitivity to important and relevant concerns without overcompensating. It is a critical and necessary objective for adoptive parents to reach a comfortable balance between heritage and ethnicity for their adopted child. Each child reacts in a manner that is consistent with his or her personality. Adopted children also respond differently to adoption issues at various times as part of normal child development.

How comfortable an adoptee is with these issues is influenced by his or her general temperament, family dynamics, social environment, and other circumstances. The manner in which these issues are addressed during the early developmental years has tremendous influence in determining how an adoptee acknowledges and embraces his or her race, ethnicity and birth heritage in the context of who he or she is within the adopted family and adopted nationality, however. Internationally adopted children who have been exposed with openness and regularity to their birth culture and heritage are generally more comfortable and grounded than adoptees entering adolescence with no previous exposure to those issues or experiences.

> The non-adopted person is surrounded by genetic heritage and has easy access to family history. In families formed biologically, answers abound and are absorbed before the need for a question arises. Feelings of belonging and relatedness are taken for granted as they develop gradually and become a part of the person's identity. Shared ancestry, family resemblances, and, in some cases, cultural heritage are denied the adopted person who grows up separated from blood relations. As the adopted person matures, the need for information about his birth family may grow. Both external life events and internal processes may trigger the desire for additional knowledge or bring to the surface the need to know one's roots [2].

What is important are the efforts of adoptive parents to demonstrate to the adoptee and other family members their willingness to absorb the child's ethnicity into the family. These attempts to highlight and celebrate a child's birth culture should include the entire family and be in harmony with other family activities. If limited to the adoptee, it underscores differences rather than becoming an opportunity to share what the child brings to the family. Extreme efforts to provide cultural sensitivity and awareness to adoptees may meet with resistance, however, because such efforts glaringly articulate that an adoptee is unique from other family members.

Adoptive families who pursue relationships and friendships with individuals of the same ethnic heritage as their adopted family member in their communities help the adoptee to experience other children and adults who look similar to them. The clear message to the child and ethnic community is that the family is comfortable with and values the ethnicity of the child.

Across the United States, there are increasing numbers of culture and heritage camps for children adopted internationally. There are a variety of camps to choose from, including day camps for elementary school–aged children to week-long camps for adolescents. Particularly for adoptees living in communities in which they have little opportunity to be with other adoptees or children of color, camps are a valuable learning experience. A critical outcome of these activities is for the adoptee to be with others who are "just like me." The longing to not be the only person who looks and feels different can be deeply felt, and the shared time and friendship with other adoptees provide powerful support.

Tours for adoptees and their families to visit a child's birth country represent an extension of the concept of heritage and culture camps. These trips back with other adoptees are often considered a positive but dramatic life experience for young adult adoptees. When an internationally adopted child's experience includes his or her heritage and culture in an ongoing manner, adoption books, camps, tours, and adoptee groups are simply a normal progression of their adoption experience.

In the early 1990s, adoptions from China and Eastern Europe began to dominate the number of children adopted internationally. These countries required adoptive families to travel to the country to bring home their adopted children, promoting a greater understanding and connection of adoptive parents to the child's culture and heritage. This has provided a network of support and community among adoptive families and adoptees that ensures children adopted today do not have to grow up feeling isolated and different from everyone else around them.

Search and identity

> Every adoptee has his or her own very personal and unique adoption story. That history is a part of who they are as they move from childhood through adolescence to adulthood. It is important for adoptees to come to their own peace with how adoption fits into their life and achieve a comfortable balance. For international adoptees, their story began in another country and culture and includes issues of race, ethnicity and heritage [3].

It is normal that adoptive parents consider the birth parents, primarily the birth mother, of their adopted child. It is natural that some parents feel a certain amount of anxiety about the birth mother coming back well into the future, changing her mind, and wanting to retrieve the child who is now "theirs." Some adoptive parents fear the existence of and possible intrusion by the birth mother into the life of the adoptee and adoptive family. These adoptive parents may seek intercountry adoption believing foreign adoption reduces the risks and provides assurances and a sense of security from the possibility of being "found" by the birth mother.

It is true that the possibility of an international adoptee being discovered by a birth mother in another country is greatly reduced by barriers of geographic distance, resources, and language. The greatest separation and difference are cultural, however. Similar to US adoptions, which were once shrouded in whispers, shame, and secrecy, birth mothers overseas commonly relinquish their children for adoption in secrecy. Privacy allows them to melt back into society after the birth of the child. The unfortunate consequence is that there is seldom accurate information available should the adoptee desire to initiate a search for immediate extended birth family as an adult.

This commitment to secrecy also affects information regarding the child who is to be relinquished for adoption. Concern about protecting the confidentiality of the birth mother and the possibility that she might someday be identified without her consent has the unintended and undesired effect of false identifying information being presented at the time of relinquishment. This information includes medical history, personal history and other pertinent data that are critical for a family considering adopting, and possibly for the adoptee in the future.

This is changing steadily. More frequently, international searches have been completed successfully by adoptees and birth parents. These occurrences are still rare but are likely to increase similar to the trend in the United States regarding domestic adoptions. It is imperative to continue to advocate for truthful and open dialogue between birth mothers and social workers during the relinquishment and adoption process. The necessary commitment to educate and reassure birth mothers, social workers, and others who are part of the adoption process worldwide should include a responsible tone of caution and not preclude the importance of understanding the diverse and profound cultural sensitivities these issues present.

> I went back to Vietnam because I wanted to try to find my birth family. I was four years old when I was adopted and so I could remember them. I did find them and it has been good. I was able to introduce my birth mother and my adopted mother to each other. But since then, it has been hard. I feel torn sometimes between two places and responsibilities. If you are going to search, you better be prepared for what you may find. Search is not easy. I'm glad I did it, but it makes relationships more difficult [4].

Clinical issues in adoption

> Young adulthood is a period of many changes. It is during this time that a young adult evolves into a member of a couple, a person with a career, eventually, maybe, a parent. Each of these changes can rock any prior sense of stability or inviolability as the young adult struggles with a changing definition of him/ herself [5].

Physicians and other medical personnel are privy to private information that can blur the boundaries at times, because some families may choose information to be private or secret. In adoption, there are times when families choose not to reveal to others the adoption status of the child; thus, it is important for physicians to be clear on how openly they may be able to speak with their patient about his or her adoption experience. When approaching the subject of adoption, it is also essential for practitioners to be self-aware of their own biases on adoption and what it means to be adopted. Some pitfalls to keep in mind include the following [6]:

- The problem is all about adoption, or adoption is unrelated to the problem.
- Beliefs about adoption include that it is the cause of a primal wound and thus the cause of extreme distress, that a person who is adopted is not complete, and that an adoptive family is dysfunctional.

- Adoption work is short-term.
- Like any significant issues a person has, adoption issues are revisited at every developmental stage and milestone.

Although international adoptions may be on the rise and becoming increasingly more visible, adoption myths and beliefs still remain in the mainstream that leave adoptive families feeling marginalized. Specific to adoptees, the first myth is that "being adopted is the same as staying with the family one is born to." This belief that an adoptive family can make up for the loss of being with a birth family and that differences between adoptive and birth families should be eliminated fails to acknowledge truth and leaves the adopted person vulnerable if he or she is asking questions about his or her past.

Another myth is that "all the child's needs can be met by the adoptive family." Not only is this a huge disservice to the child, but the reality is that this statement is false. To disregard a child's beginnings and the genetic connection that he or she has to another family is to disregard the essence of who a child is and can sometimes be dangerous to the health of the child. Another myth is that "triad members need to be protected so that birth mothers are not judged, adoptive parents do not feel stigmatized, and the adoptee is protected from the reality of why he or she was placed for adoption." This presumes that there is an inherent shame or guilt involved with adoption.

There are those who still consider "adoption as an event." It is important to appreciate that the understanding of being adopted evolves at every life stage of a human being. Lastly, "adoption is a win-win-win situation." This statement is incomplete; to have a winning situation, there must have been a loss somewhere else [6].

As young adoptees enter the world of adulthood, their adoption story evolves along with their bodies and minds. As Joyce Maguire Pavao shares [7], "adoption issues do not end at the threshold of adulthood—far from it. They continue throughout the life of the adopted person and into the next generation, for all parties connected to adoption."

The key aspect of young adulthood is the search for the individual. It is a time in which most young adults seek independence more literally—by going to college or moving out of the home—and figuratively in their attempts to try and create a community, family, or niche of their own. As Maguire Pavao [7] continues, this journey of self-discovery "for an adopted person...are times of distinct normative crisis."

If we look at the core clinical issues in adoption mapped out by Roszia and Silverstein [8], these are issues that transcend age and stage. Their article has served as a cornerstone for many professionals working with families formed through adoption. "Regardless of the circumstances of the participants, [all deal with various aspects of the following]: loss, rejection, guilt and shame, grief, identity, intimacy, and mastery/control" [8].

From this basis, Taddonio and Lieberthal [6] have expanded on these issues to include issues of attachment and bonding, loyalty, and entitlement.

Most relevant to pediatricians who are terminating their association with their young adult patients are the following issues.

Loss

For the adopted person, to become an adoptee, one must have lost the family to whom he or she was born. Fundamentally, this is the most profound of all the issues. "This fact is particularly evident during the adoptee's adolescence when the issues of...impending emancipation may rekindle the loss issue" [8].

The permanent severing of birth ties through adoption can make "any subsequent loss, or perceived threat of separation, become more formidable for the adoptees than for their non-adopted peers" [8].

Furthermore, as the young adult is embarking on adulthood, the thought of losing his or her adoptive family can cause great anxiety. Because so much of being identified as an adopted person is equated to being part of the adoptive family, to separate from that family may cause inner conflict and reason to take the next steps to adulthood eagerly. This concept is further substantiated by Pavao [7] when she writes, "An idea that many adopted people carry around is that at age eighteen, they will no longer be adopted, that they will no longer belong to their adoptive family."

For transracially adopted youth, this is further complicated by the realization that they now have to learn to identify as a person of color separate and apart from their adoptive identity, which has been so obvious when they are in the company of their parents. For practitioners, it is essential to acknowledge the profound effect that such a loss as family (adoptive and birth) may have on the decision-making process of young adults. It is often noted that adoptees tend to stay connected physically and financially to their adoptive parents long after their peers are emancipated from their families.

As part of the developmental stage of young adulthood, the question of "Who am I?" evolves into a more focused inquiry of "self in relationship to others and in the broader society" [5]. It is in this search for self that "the loss of part of themselves is felt intensely, almost physically, as they become self-reflective adults" [5].

Thus, the search for identity through seeking out birth relatives, becoming a member of an adoption community, and trying on various perceived aspects of one's birth story is prevalent for this group. An example of this would be if a young woman, who was adopted from Latin America into an upper middle class white Jewish family, begins dating boys who are from a poor socioeconomic status. Her perception of her adoption was that her birth family was too poor and uneducated to keep her. As she seeks out partners for herself, it seems that she is perpetuating the "fantasy" she has of her beginnings and seeks out those who she thinks she is "supposed to be with."

Loyalty

Young adulthood is a time for searching for self. For adopted youth, this may become complicated as they seek to learn more about themselves in relation to their birth family or birth culture. The adoptee may feel torn between his or her birth parents and adoptive parents and think that a choice needs to be made. To ask to connect with birth family or seek a better understanding of birth culture may feel disloyal to the adoptive family. As Deann Borshay, a Korean adoptee, shared in her documentary, "First Person Plural" [9], "I can't talk to my (adoptive) mother about my (birth) mother," [because] "it feels like I am putting dirt in my mouth." It is not uncommon for adopted people to feel that they must be grateful to be adopted; thus, to inquire about birth family would mean they have squandered this gift of family.

Another aspect of loyalty is in whom the adopted person thinks he or she should identify with. For some, their loyalty is to their birth family; these individuals emulate the life that should have been. Others overidentify with their adoptive family, rejecting any knowledge they have about their birth family. For some, their loyalty is to their birth culture; they reclaim their birth names and seek out others who reflect their birth community.

Identity

For all young adults, the seeking of identity is key to becoming a self-actualized person. For the adoptee, this process is complicated in that there are more labels and identities to absorb and process [6]. There is the identity of the birth family, the birth culture, the adoptive family, and the adoptive culture.

For those who have grown up within their birth family, there are clear "identity markers" that help to form who they are. For example, a person would know where he or she got a particular body feature, what he or she might look like at the age of 65 years, and from whom he or she inherited a particular affinity to art or music. For the adopted person, the absence of such identity markers for the future leads to a lack of emotional preparedness, to experimentation with stereotypes, to filling in the gaps with fantasy, or to self-education on how to be "Black, Asian, low-class, etc." [6]. This then further complicates an adoptee's perception of body and sexuality, which, in turn, affects relationships and intimacy. "True intimacy requires a strong sense of identity. And to the extent that identity is compromised for adoptees—or, for that matter, for any adult—the ability to find intimacy is compromised as well" [5]. Pavao adds, "It takes knowing who you are to know who you can be with" [7].

Control

Because of the significant defining moment when adoptees had no control (ie, no part in the decision-making process of becoming an adoptee), control is an important issue for many adoptees to resolve. For some, the adoption experience has led them to always be in control of every aspect of their lives and those who are close to them. For others, they become victimized and feel they have no power over any aspect of their life. For still others, there is an absence of acknowledgment of one's own responsibility, blaming adoption as the cause of lack of decision-making skills.

Entitlement and gratitude

Feeling grateful and entitled to let that go culminates all the previously discussed issues in adoption. For adoptees, it is important to feel entitled to be a legitimate member of a family. This entitlement then absolves the adoptee of the fear to show negative traits or behaviors and not to feel compelled to try to be "perfect" and full of gratitude [6]. It is that sense of entitlement that frees adoptees to make sense of the losses in their life, to explore their identity, to be a part of their birth and adoptive families, and to engage in healthy and mutually beneficial relationships.

How the professional community can help

As increasing numbers of children are adopted from other countries, educators, physicians, public policy leaders, clergy, and others should consider the profile of these children and families. These families, who are routinely called on to validate that they are a "real" family, would benefit from the combined support base of a fundamental understanding of international adoption issues.

Parent support groups are a critical resource before and after adoptive placement. These groups are an important source of information as well as support and encouragement during the sometimes long and difficult adoption process. Parent groups can alert those in the process of adopting to issues of irregularity and concern. The network of information gathering that is accumulated and shared by adoptive families through support groups is amazingly swift and sophisticated. They share the commonality of wanting to protect and secure the adoption process and the children who are to be adopted. Those interested in adopting a child should connect with a parent group. Joining with other parents and adoptive families is powerful support. The relationships can be richly rewarding long after the adoption is complete.

As adoption has expanded, so has an adoption-related consumer industry. There is a growing inventory of books, magazines, newsletters, and videotapes available. Some of these resources attempt to address the specific issues regarding intercountry adoption. There are excellent books about more general adoption issues that are appropriate for any adopted child.

Lifelong experience of adoption

As would be expected, the global community of international adoptees represents a wide range of life experiences, education, vocations, and family life as adults. They also represent diverse perspectives on how they view politics, religion, and social issues in general. A growing number of adult adoptee organizations have been established. Some groups are primarily social organizations, but others have a more political or ideologic agenda and focus that often relates directly to adoption.

As increasing numbers of adult adoptees are meeting and marrying other adoptees, an emerging number of adoptees are also adopting children. As international adoptees have their own families, the generational and lifelong implications of adoption become clear. Adoptees who grew up looking different from their adoptive parents are often raising children, not adopted but born to them, who are continuing the profile of interracial families.

If you are adopted, you are an adopted person forever. This includes international adoptees. The issues of adoption, race, and ethnicity change with individual life experiences. International adoptees grow up. They get married, become parents, and some have already become grandparents.

International adoptees are living ordinary lives in communities throughout the world. Their individual experiences are as varied and rich as the individual families that adopted them. Collectively, they represent the enormous capacity of human resilience that children are capable of. Families are the most enduring and important of relationships.

Intercountry adoption transcends the boundaries of race, nationality, and culture. It gives a child a family that is as "real" as any family. International adoptive families illustrate what is possible when people are willing to recognize and honor differences while discovering and making commitments to the common need for "family" that exists in each of us.

References

[1] Cox SS-K. Voices from another place. St. Paul (MN): Yeong & Yeong Book Company; 1999.
[2] Demuth CL. Biological clock: key times in an adopted person's life. Adoptalk 1991;Fall.
[3] Cox SS-K. Joint Council on International Children's Services. The Bulletin 1999;Summer.
[4] Tuy, from Vietnam. Joint Council on International Children's Services. The Bulletin 1999;Summer.
[5] Brodzinsky DM, Schecter MD, Henig RM. Being adopted: the lifelong search for self. New York: Doubleday; 1992.
[6] Taddonio R, Lieberthal J. Clinical issues in adoption. Presented at Yale Child Study Center, New Haven, CT, October 1, 2003.
[7] Pavao JM. The family of adoption. Boston (MA): Beacon Press; 1998.
[8] Silverstein D, Kaplan S. Lifelong issues in adoption. Adoptive Families Magazine 1999.
[9] Borshay D. First person plural. POV 2000.

ELSEVIER
SAUNDERS

PEDIATRIC CLINICS
OF NORTH AMERICA

Pediatr Clin N Am 52 (2005) 1507–1515

International Adoption: A Personal Perspective

Judith Eckerle Kang, MD

Department of Pediatrics, New York Presbyterian Hospital, Weill Cornell Medical Center,
525 East 68th Street, New York, NY 10021, USA

I am an international adoptee from Korea and a first-year resident in pediatrics. At this point in my life, I am finally able to talk frankly about my feelings and my journey as an adopted person. My intent is to share my personal perspective based on my experiences, but I must acknowledge that my own views have been colored by stories shared with me by other adoptees and their parents. We are a diverse group, and each adoptee's story is different. This is mine.

Beginnings

The story in my adoption papers told that I was born in Sungdong-gu, a section of Seoul, South Korea, near what is now Olympic Park and was found at a police station at approximately 1 week of age. When I take care of neonates, I often wonder if the authorities guessed my age by the state of my umbilical cord stump, but my birth date was probably arbitrarily assigned. I stayed in a hospital for a few weeks until social workers found a foster home in a poor part of the city with a single mother who was raising six other children on her own. My paperwork stated that my foster home consisted of two parents in the countryside, "where the air is clean and pretty," with two teenaged children to help care for my every need. I only discovered the discrepancy when I was reunited with my foster mother 2 years ago. Although reality was not as rosy as the picture painted in my adoption records, I do believe that I was loved and

E-mail address: jue9004@nyp.org

well cared for because I was a fat and happy baby when I arrived in the United States 4 months later.

Family

My adoptive father was stationed in Seoul in 1970. Newly wed, my adoptive mother joined him in Korea and taught English to businessmen and children in the community. They decided that they would someday adopt a Korean child. After returning to the United States in 1972, they had two biologic children, Jenn and Jeff, and then started the adoption process in 1975. They began to receive letters and photographs of the child who would soon join their family, but approximately 1 month before the expected arrival, the photographs and name unexpectedly changed to mine. I have wondered what happened to that other child, but I consider it luck or fate that I came to my family instead. A little over a year after I arrived, my little brother Joey was born, my parents' third birth child.

Arrival

I arrived February 4, 1977. Consistent with the uncertainty of the rest of my history, one passenger from the airplane told my parents that I slept the entire way from Korea and another told them that I cried the whole trip. The photographs documenting my arrival are few—my older sister and brother watching for my plane with their noses pressed against the terminal window, a few pictures of my parents' friends, and, finally, me, incredibly overbundled and looking guarded and confused in some and outright crying in others. The pictures taken during my first few days in the United States show me asleep in my high chair, chubby cheek down in my food. Within a short time, the pictures of me were all smiles— I was home.

Childhood

I do not remember ever feeling that different from my siblings or my peers. I started out in a city school with incredible racial diversity, so I did not think twice about being a minority. In the third grade, I moved to a suburb of Minneapolis, the unofficial Korean adoptee capitol of the world. There were four Korean adoptees in my grade alone. Although I was teased about having a "flat face" and occasionally called a "chink," my classmates teased me more about the fact that I was so thin. My sibling relationships were pretty typical—I adored my older sister, was protective of my little brother, and fought constantly with my older brother. One day after one of countless fights with him, my mother sat us down and asked Jeff if our fighting had anything to do with me being adopted. His emphatic reply was, "No! She's just a jerk!" We outgrew the fighting as we matured, and I do not think any of us thought a great deal about me being adopted. Although most international adoptees grow up with white parents, people often ask me if it was especially hard to grow up as the only minority member of the family surrounded by biologic children. We never thought about it, and I was celebrated for being different. With that encouragement, I eventually grew to appreciate being unique.

Looking back, I realize that my parents were progressive for the times. They did a lot that adoptive parents are doing now. They talked about Korea. We have celebrated my adoption day every year that I can remember, something that always made adoption seem special. My mother and I would occasionally give demonstrations at local high schools about aspects of Korean culture. I owned a *hanbok*, a traditional Korean dress, but seldom ever wore it. One of my birthday parties had a Korean theme. I also have a poem that my parents put by my bedside. It is an anonymous adoptive author telling a child, "You did not grow under my heart, but in it."

All these things made me more secure in my adoptive identity. There were never any secrets and never any shame in being adopted or different. There were even times when my parents would "forget" that I was adopted, such as the time my mother was filling out a family medical history form for me in high school. She began writing "grandmother had diabetes and glaucoma...," and I had to remind her that I am adopted. So although they provided links to my Korean heritage, my family never pushed or forced me to seek a Korean identity. I was and am just one of their kids.

I also do not remember that my doctor ever talked about my being adopted, although I think it might have been a good thing to talk about every now and then. I believe there may be a role for pediatricians to ask basic screening questions for problems related to identity or attachment. I am glad that he did not make a big issue about me being adopted, however, because his choice allowed me to address things naturally and at my own pace.

Adolescence

I believe it was my awkwardness and thin stature that contributed to my feelings of inadequacy during adolescence, but I have many Korean adoptee friends who felt unattractive solely because they were not blond-haired and blue-eyed like the teens with whom they attended school. As noted in many adoptee texts, my friends were often "surprised" when they looked in the mirror and saw a dark-haired and almond-eyed person instead of the white daughter they believed they were. I remember pinching the end of my nose, night after night, trying to mold it into a "ski-jump" nose like my sister's. It was hard to grow up in a time when there were few Asian role models to look up to. Even today, there are few ethnic role models for minority kids growing up in predominantly white communities.

Environment Versus Genetics

I had quirks growing up, as everyone does, but I did not think twice about them until I got to Korea and learned more about Korean culture. The first is that I never adapted to the time change in the United States. My family always joked that I was on perpetual "Korean time," because I would stay up all night and sleep all day. I was in professional theater as a child and thrived on the schedule of night performances, when my bedtime was extended until midnight. I happily worked the graveyard shift as a waitress all through high school and college. During medical school, I would study from 10:00 PM to 6:00 AM, and I now take all the night shifts I can in the pediatric emergency room. Conversely, when I travel to Korea, I am tired by 10:00 PM and wide awake at 7:00 or 8:00 AM, even after being there for months. It seems that my body really did stay on Korean time.

In grade school, my mother would find me on the floor some mornings, having laid out some blankets and pillows from my bed on which to sleep. I could not explain why I felt more comfortable there, but my first trip to Korea was spent on padded blankets called *yiboo* that are put on the floor and then folded up and put away during the day. Maybe I was remembering an earlier sleeping arrangement when I took to the floor as a child.

Starting in grade school, I requested soup at every meal. My mother made me soup for breakfast and put soup in my thermos to take to school for lunch. This craving has continued throughout my life—my college roommates could tell stories of my nightly soup being cooked in the electric hotpot. I was stunned when I went to Korea for the first time and saw that they ate soup for breakfast, lunch, and dinner. Koreans did not think I was "weird" for having soup for every meal, as I had felt my whole life in the United States, where I grew up on meat and potatoes in a traditional midwestern household—absolutely no spicy food. But when I was introduced to Korean food, I came to crave it, and I now eat it all the time. I thought that if it were just a phase or an attempt to connect with my newfound Korean heritage, I would grow out of it, but 6 years later, I still crave Korean food as much as ever. A recent article in *Pediatrics* theorized that infants could be influenced by the flavors of the mother's food that permeate into the amniotic fluid and breast milk [1]. Although I was not breastfed for long, I do wonder if my in utero exposures contributed to my current and childhood food preferences, especially because my adoptive family did not introduce me to most of the Korean flavors that I currently enjoy.

Attachment

People frequently comment on attachment disorders when it comes to international adoptees. From my perspective, most adoptees are firmly and securely attached in their relationships, but I do believe that adoption poses some attachment issues. When I was young, I always had a hard time with my father going on business trips. The John Denver song "Leaving on a Jet Plane" brought me to tears every time I heard it, to the point where my brothers and sisters would play the record as a joke because everyone knew it would make me cry instantly. At the time, I did not know why it made me so sad, but I think that the prospect of my dad leaving was especially scary for me. No matter how many times he went on short business trips, I was never sure that he would come back.

When forming close relationships in college, including my first serious romantic relationship, I always had a fear of being abandoned. It took me a long time to trust the people I was close to, and I held back to an extreme that I openly attribute to my fear of abandonment. I also had problems when loved ones moved away or were physically far from me. A psychiatry resident once told me she thought that my "object permanence" was underdeveloped, which made sense to me. I had been born to a birth mother with whom I spent only a few days or weeks and was then taken care of by numerous hospital personnel. I was loved by a foster mother and was able to bond with her for a few months but then left once again to fly across the world to a new home in Minnesota. During my first 6 months of life, the few relationships I did form were repeatedly broken. In high school and college, I believed that babies had little awareness of their surroundings and that it was unlikely I was affected by all the changes that took place during those first 6 months. As a medical student and new doctor, however, I witness the depth to which babies know their parents and caretakers. It now seems plausible that so much change and disruption could have a long-term effect on my feelings of security.

That said, I believe that I grew up in the healthiest environment possible, with love and support from all sides. Nevertheless, the fact remains that I grew up with the knowledge that for whatever reason, I had been abandoned at birth by the one person who was supposed to love me the most. Some adoptees with whom I have spoken report that they never really thought about their birth parents while growing up, but I have always wondered about the circumstances surrounding the decision to give me up for adoption.

Searching

Because of the scant information contained in my poorly documented adoption records, I thought I would never have enough information to conduct a birth parent search. My world was shaken on my second trip to Korea when another adoptee told me she had similarly poor birth records but had made an appearance on television and been reunited with her birth parents. I contemplated this idea for an entire year, the first small steps toward actually doing my own search. I am grateful that my parents and friends neither pushed nor discouraged me during that time.

I learned that friends who had found their birth parents often had traumatic reunions. One found his birth mother only to discover that she was schizophrenic. Another friend's birth mother would meet him only in secret and would not introduce him to his brothers or sisters because she had never told them that he had been given up. He felt abandoned and rejected for a second time. A few who found their birth parents had positive experiences, but many were reunited only to be chastised for not speaking Korean or for not understanding Korean culture. I told myself that maybe it would be better if I never found my birth parents, but I decided that the stories of my abandonment I had invented over the years had to be worse than whatever truth I might find. I longed just to look like someone, to "have" someone's eyes, or to hear the story about my birth, things I believe other people take for granted.

I laid some groundwork for a birth parent search during my third trip to Korea, and on the fourth trip, I felt ready to conduct a serious search. With the help of a volunteer-run adoptee organization in Seoul, I contacted national newspapers that ran human interest stories about my search. I told my story on the Korean television equivalent of *Oprah*. A major network television station and a police officer went to my adoption agency to search through old records for previously concealed facts about my birth parents. A cable television network made an hour-long special about my search and life story. After this, I felt like I had exhausted all possible options.

The hour-long special aired four times during prime time. The other talk show aired to a viewing audience of nearly 5 million people, which is a huge audience considering that Korea is approximately the size of Indiana. Three major newspapers ran my story in print and on the Internet. During my third year of medical school, in one last-ditch effort for publicity, I entered and won the title Miss Wisconsin USA, going on to compete in the 2003 Miss USA competition. Again, Korean national newspapers, Internet publications, and a few Korean-American publications covered my story. To date, no one has responded.

Reflection

In my third year of medical school, in the midst of my birth parent search, I helped to lead an art therapy session for an inpatient group of adult psychiatric patients. The task assigned by the therapist was to draw a bridge going from "somewhere to anywhere" (Fig. 1). In the 10 minutes we had to work, I drew what I thought was a happy picture of me on a bridge that stretched from the United States to Korea. On the American side, I drew stick figures of my immediate family standing in front of my parents' house. The bridge was a single lane that arched across the two bodies of land, separated by a blue ocean, with me standing in the middle of it, smiling and waving. On the Korean side, I drew the Korean flag and large buildings as I remembered them from Seoul. I placed a sun and fluffy clouds on the US side and stars and the moon on the Korea side. During our reflection on the drawings, the therapist commented to the group that the sturdier the bridge we had drawn, the more secure was the path we thought we were on. I had drawn no supports and no railings for my spindly little bridge that stretched across the ocean. Although I had a serious boyfriend at the time, I

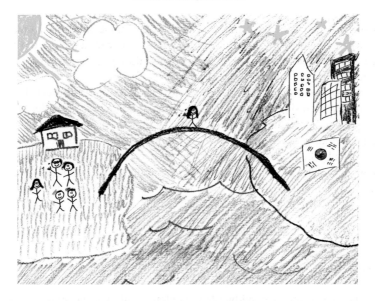

Fig. 1. Art therapy session assignment to draw a bridge going from "somewhere to anywhere."

had not depicted him or any of my roommates or friends in my drawing. I realized that I have often felt alone in my birth parent and cultural identity search, because it is nearly impossible for nonadoptees to understand the complexities that adoptees experience during this kind of search. It makes sense that I had also drawn myself standing alone in the middle of the bridge. I had drawn my family, and I knew that they were there if I needed them, but they were not on this journey with me. I had drawn no faces and no people in Korea, just buildings and a flag, representing the fact that I had no deep connections to family or people there at the time.

Where I Am Now

Approximately 1 year ago, I married a Korean-American man. I finally gave up my birth parent search, and I think it ended for a reason. My Korean in-laws wholeheartedly accepted me as a daughter. In a way, it felt like I had been readopted and that I had come full circle. Sometimes, when I am in a car with Korean adopted friends or with my in-laws, I think about how different my life might have been if I had been reared in Korea, and I am wistful for what might have been. I used to get quite emotional when talking about adoption, but I now feel like I have come to terms with my abandonment, my adoption, and my role as a Korean adoptee in the United States. I still sometimes cry when I see adoptive "reunions" on cheesy talk shows or watch television dramatizations of such events. I have not watched the videotape from the Korean talk show, where I poured my heart out to the viewers. It would still be too painful to see the raw emotions I was experiencing during those stressful months of searching.

I am now a proud aunt many times over. I also love the work that I do with kids through my residency program. Kids often do not notice the differences that adults notice. For example, our wedding festivities ended with a traditional Korean ceremony, and when my sister's daughter saw the pictures, she turned to my sister and asked, "Where are the pictures of your Korean ceremony, Mom?" Through my young niece's eyes, I was reminded that I am not an "adoptee," just one of the family like everyone else. This is how my siblings and I grew up: knowing that I was adopted but not really seeing any difference in that.

Future

I grew up in a suburban, midwestern, predominantly white community; thus, it just did not occur to me to date within my ethnicity. It was not until I had traveled to Korea that it became important to me to someday marry a Korean-American man. I realized there were many things about the Korean culture that I had not had the chance to learn, and I realized, too, that I would never know enough to be fully able to teach my children the things that are now important to me. My husband and I plan to adopt from Korea. I wonder how my adopted child's experiences are going to differ from mine, because she or he is going to grow up with a strong connection (through my in-laws) to Korean heritage and without racial differences in the immediate household. After residency, I plan to be involved in adoption medicine and, hopefully, to build a practice in which I can advise prospective and new adoptive parents and work with kids as they come to the United States. I believe that my adoption journey has helped to prepare me for this career choice, and I hope that I can contribute positively to the lives of future parents and adoptees. Based on my experiences, I would offer the following suggestions to parents and health care professionals.

1. Celebrate your child in as many ways as possible. In particular, have a special day each year when you celebrate your child's adoption.
2. Some kids and teenagers have unresolved issues surrounding their adoption. Do not be afraid to seek out and offer them support aided by therapists or psychiatrists.
3. If your child is interested, there are also a number of adoptee organizations that are wonderful resources in the United States and abroad. They can provide links to other adoptees, assist with travel, provide translation services, and assist in birth parent searches.
4. Let your child choose the timing and direction that he or she takes in exploring his or her heritage. Some adoptees never want to start down that

path, whereas others are willing to fly across oceans to search for answers. Whatever their choice, support them at their own pace.

5. Although I am proud to be an adoptee, I believe that kids do not usually want to be known as "the adopted child," lest they be defined by that fact alone. Kids just want to be kids like everyone else around them.

Reference

[1] Lederman SA, Akabas SR, Moore BJ. Overview of the conference on preventing childhood obesity. Pediatrics 2004;114:1139–45.

ELSEVIER
SAUNDERS

PEDIATRIC CLINICS
OF NORTH AMERICA

Pediatr Clin N Am 52 (2005) 1517–1523

Appendix

Adoption Bibliography

Kay Seligsohn, PhD*, Lisa Albers, MD, MPH

Adoption Program, Children's Hospital Boston, 300 Longwood Avenue, Boston, MA 02115, USA

General adoption issues

Gray, Deborah. *Attaching in Adoption: Practical Tools for Today's Parents.* Indianapolis, IN: Perspectives Press, 2002.

The author provides readers with a comprehensive understanding of the range of child and parent factors that support or prevent parents and children from fostering a healthy attachment after adoption. Through the use of case examples, she discusses how previous trauma, normal grief expected during the adoption process, and several neurologically based conditions—including attention and learning problems—may impact a child's and family's capacity for and quality of interpersonal attachment. After acknowledging the myriad factors that must be considered when supporting the attachment process between adoptive children and their parents, she clarifies when families need to seek further support for their child or for themselves and outlines key questions to ask of potential therapists.

Audience: Strongly recommended reading for parents considering adoption, those who have adopted children, and those who work with adopted children.

Caveats: Some of the parent checklists, although useful as guidelines, must not be used for diagnostic purposes but rather are helpful in identifying a child's need for further evaluation.

Hopkins-Best, Mary. *Toddler Adoption: The Weaver's Craft.* Indianapolis, IN: Perspectives Press, Inc., 1997.

This is a thorough guide to adjustment, attachment, learning, and parenting for parents of children who arrive home between 1 and 4 years of age. The author

---

* Corresponding author.
E-mail address: kay.seligsohn@childrens.harvard.edu (K. Seligsohn).

0031-3955/05/$ – see front matter © 2005 Elsevier Inc. All rights reserved.
doi:10.1016/j.pcl.2005.06.001

pediatric.theclinics.com

provides information that helps parents make informed decisions about the unique aspects of adopting a toddler. Specific recommendations are provided to foster attachment and to manage behaviors of concern.

Audience: Parents who are considering or have adopted a toddler.

Caveats: Although solidly based in clinical experience, this book does not adequately address challenges that may arise with developmental or learning concerns.

Meese, Ruth Lyn. *Children of Intercountry Adoptions in School: A Primer for Parents and Professionals.* Westport, CT: Bergin and Garvey, 2002.

This is a thorough and practical guide for working with schools, with an emphasis on special considerations for children and their families after international adoption. Written by a special educator who is also an adoptive parent, this book provides both background information about factors that may impact children after international adoption and strategies to address concerns children may have in school. Separate chapters address practical topics such as classroom strategies and the importance of potential language impairments on learning after international adoption. This primer also describes legal rights as well as practical approaches to obtaining appropriate educational services from a child's school system.

Audience: Parents, educators, and other professionals who work with children after international adoption.

Caveats: Although it provides a thorough approach to supporting children within the educational system, this book minimally addresses the long-term emotional issues that may impact children after international adoption, both at home and at school.

Miller, Laurie. *The Handbook of International Adoption Medicine: A Guide for Physicians, Parents and Providers.* Oxford, UK: Oxford University Press, 2005.

An extremely helpful reference describing current research pertinent to parents and professionals working with children and their families before, during, and after international adoption. Cases and available research data are used to highlight clinical points.

Audience: Parents, health care providers, and allied health professionals who work with international adoptees.

Caveats: Intended as a reference for the reader rather than a comprehensive approach to many postadoptive developmental, learning, or emotional concerns.

Adoption and identity development

Brodzinsky, David M.; Schechter, Marshall D.; Henig, Robin M. *Being Adopted: The Lifelong Search for Self,* New York: Vintage & Anchor Books, 1992.

This book places adoption within the context of the developmental continuum from birth through adolescence. It focuses on the adjustments adopted children make at the time of adoption, as well as their progress through different developmental stages with reference to Erikson's and Piaget's stages of identity and cognitive development as a framework for understanding specific issues adopted children may face.

Suggested audience: Parents and professionals involved with children who have a history of adoption.

Caveats: Although it provides a basic developmental framework, this book does not incorporate more recent research regarding adoption, attachment, or development.

O'Malley, Beth. *Lifebooks: Creating a Treasure for the Adopted Child.* Winthrop, MA: Adoption-Works, 2000.

A lifebook tells the child's life story though words, artwork, photos, graphics, and memorabilia. This book provides a thoughtful and highly practical guide for adoptive parents to make a lifebook for their child. It gives wonderful illustrations, examples, and explanations.

Audience: All.

Focus on children with developmental and behavioral challenges after international adoption

Federici, Ronald. *Help for the Hopeless Child: A Guide for Families (with Special Discussion for Assessing and Treating the Post-Institutionalized Child).* 2nd edition. Alexandria, VA: Ronald S. Federici and Associates, 2003.

Written by a pediatric neuropsychologist with extensive clinical experience working with school-aged children and adolescents impacted by trauma, institutionalization, and medical concerns, this book provides families with a guide to identifying the appropriate assessments and treatment for children with complex developmental disorders. The author also describes an intensive family treatment program and multidisciplinary intervention to address significant behavioral concerns. For children with prenatal substance exposure, significant neurologically based disorders, and other severe behavioral concerns, the author outlines important considerations when seeking appropriate treatment and interventions.

Audience: Professionals working with postinstitutionalized children; parents considering adoption of an older child; and parents who have adopted older children after institutionalization and may have exhausted routine emotional, psychiatric, and school-based interventions.

Caveats: Controversial techniques are described for addressing severe behavioral concerns. This is not a "do it yourself" manual to identify neuropsychologic or psychiatric concerns for children. The straightforward approach to diagnosis described in this manual for any child requires collaboration with knowledgeable psychologic, medical, and mental health providers. The family-based interventions require intense dedication of time and emotional resources and are best performed in collaboration with an experienced and sophisticated local mental health provider.

Keck, Greg; Kupeckny, Regina. *Adopting the Hurt Child.* Harrisburg, PA: Nav Press, 1998.

Keck, Greg; Kupeckny, Regina. *Parenting the Hurt Child.* Harrisburg, PA: NAV Press, 2002.

The authors of these books explore how parents can help adopted or foster children who have suffered neglect or abuse. They discuss control issues as well as parenting techniques that work (praise, consistency, flexibility, anger management) and those that do not (punishment, withholding parental love, grounding, time-outs, deprivation). The authors advise foster or adoptive parents to claim the role of parent and suggest ways to deal with teachers and other authority figures in the child's life.

Audience: Parents and professionals.

Caveats: Controversial and unproven techniques are described.

Tepper, Thais; Hannon, Lois; Sandstrom, Dorothy. *International Adoption: Challenges and Opportunities.* 2nd edition. Meadowlands, PA: Parent Network for the Post-Institutionalized Child, 2000.

Assembled by parents of children adopted from institutions primarily in Eastern Europe, this manual provides some of the best research-based recommendations to address postadoptive concerns for children. Topics include the impact of institutions and alcohol on a child's developing nervous system, as well as specific chapters addressing speech and language difficulties, learning challenges, and complex neurobehavioral disorders.

Audience: Professionals and parents with an interest in evidence-based recommendations.

Caveats: Although this book provides a solid research basis when available, many chapters are not current with respect to available evidence or resources.

Prenatal substance exposure

Barth, Richard; Freundlich, Marilyn; Brodzinsky, David. *Adoption and Prenatal Alcohol and Drug Exposure: Research, Policy, and Practice.* Washington, DC: Child Welfare League of America, 2000.

This is an outstanding summary of a 1997 conference highlighting the implications of prenatal substance exposure for adoptive families. While focusing on the different outcomes that may be pertinent for families, this book describes the remedial effects of a positive postnatal environment and suggests services and supports to maximize positive outcomes.

Audience: Parents of children with prenatal alcohol exposure and professionals working with such children in home and school settings.

Caveat: Although the book highlights successes, it may be overwhelming to families.

Kleinfeld, Judith; Wescott, Siobhan. *Fantastic Antoine Succeeds! Experiences in Educating Children with Fetal Alcohol Syndrome.* Fairbanks, AK: University of Alaska Press, 1993.

This is a summary of a 1991 conference on educating children with fetal alcohol syndrome that discusses the importance of early interventions and educational strategies for children affected by prenatal exposure to alcohol.

Audience: Parents of children with prenatal alcohol exposure and professionals working with these children in home and school settings.

Caveat: Although the book highlights successes, it may be overwhelming to families.

Kleinfeld, Judith; Morse, Barbara; Wescott, Siobhan. *Fantastic Antoine Grows Up: Adolescents and Adults with Fetal Alcohol Syndrome.* Fairbanks, AK: University of Alaska Press, 1993.

Written from the perspective of and with input from individuals with prenatal alcohol exposure, their parents, educators, and the professionals who work with them, this book shares practical lessons learned through experience. The authors demonstrate why the methods used on young children with prenatal alcohol exposure do not necessarily work when they are older. Specifically, the authors discuss why methods often used successfully with other special-needs children often fail with children who have prenatal alcohol exposure.

Audience: Parents of children with prenatal alcohol exposure and professionals working with these children in home and school settings.

Caveat: Although the book highlights successes, it may be overwhelming to families.

Streissguth, Ann. *Fetal Alcohol Syndrome: A Guide for Families and Communities.* Baltimore, MD: Brookes, 1997.

Streissguth, Ann; Kanter, Jonathan. *The Challenge of Fetal Alcohol Syndrome: Overcoming Secondary Disabilities.* Seattle, WA: University of Washington Press, 1997.

Both of these books provide an overview of the clinical condition of fetal alcohol syndrome (FAS) and fetal alcohol effects (FAE) and discuss the diagnostic process, research conducted since the syndrome was first recognized in 1973, and strategies for prevention of primary and secondary disabilities. Her suggestions for helping those with FAS/FAE focus on needs across the lifespan and on advocacy for children and their families.

Audience: Adoptive parents and professionals who work to help children with a range of developmental and behavioral concerns for children prenatally exposed to alcohol.

Caveat: Although the book highlights successes, it may be overwhelming to families.

Books for children

Koehler, Phoebe. *The Day We Met You.* New York, NY: Aladdin Paperbacks, 1990.

A description of adoption in the simplest terms, geared toward very young children.

Audience: Toddlers and preschool ages.

McCutcheon, John. *Happy Adoption Day.* Boston, MA; New York, NY: Little, Brown and Company, 1996.

This book and its accompanying music (found on *Family Garden*, Rounder Records) celebrates the adoption day—the day the family is formed through beautiful verse and wonderful illustrations.

Audience: Toddlers and preschool ages.

Jeram, Anita. *All Together Now.* Cambridge, MA: Candlewick Press, 1999.

Little Duckling and Miss Mouse come to live with Mommy Rabbit and her bunny. This story explores similarities and differences between members of the same family.

Audience: Toddlers and preschool ages.

Hichks, Randall B. *Adoption Stories for Young Children.* Sun City, CA: Wordslinger Press, 1995.

Through a personal story, this book provides a good description of domestic open adoption. In simple terms, it describes why the birth mother made an adoption plan for her child and what motivated the adoptive parents to choose to adopt.

Audience: Late preschool and early elementary school ages.

Thomas, Pat. *My New Family: A First Look at Adoption.* Hauppauge, NY: Barron's Educational Services, Inc., 2003.

Gives clear, concrete, and concise definitions to terms such as *birth parent*, *foster family*, and *adoption*. Describes the different ways in which families are formed and explains differences in families. Also includes a discussion guide for parents at the end to facilitate use of this book, as well as conversations about adoption.

Audience: Preschool and early elementary school ages.

Cole, Joanna. *How I Was Adopted.* New York, NY: Morrow Jr. Books, 1995.

Told from the child's perspective, this book explains adoption well. It includes information about the child growing as a fetus, her birth mother's uterus, and the birth—a fact that is often neglected in books and discussions of adoption yet is crucial to a child's understanding of adoption. This book also contains a forward for parents that discusses talking to children about adoption and ways to make use of the book.

Mandelbaum, Pili. *You Be Me I'll Be You.* Brooklyn, NY: Kane Miller Book Publishers, 1993.

A brown-skinned daughter and her white father experiment to see what it would be like to have each other's skin in this beautifully written and illustrated story. Concepts about racial identity, societal definitions of beauty, and transracial families are illustrated in children's terms.

Audience: Preschool and early elementary school ages.

Walvoord Girard, Linda. *We Adopted You, Benjamin Koo.* Morton Grove, IL: Albert Whitman & Company, 1989.

Benjamin Koo narrates his international, transracial adoption story. Benjamin eloquently describes his emerging awareness of the physical differences between himself and his parents as well as his deeper understanding of the loss that adoption entails. It nicely describes how adopted children often become aware of and grieve the loss of their birth family during the elementary school years. It also illustrates how therapy can help children come to a better understanding of adoption and manage unresolved grief.

Audience: Elementary school ages.

Peacock, Carol Antoinette. *Mommy Far, Mommy Near.* Morton Grove, IL: Albert Whitman & Company, 2000.

Elizabeth, who was born in China, describes the family who has adopted her and the complex feelings she has about being adopted. The story depicts her increasing understanding of adoption as she develops.

Audience: Elementary school ages.

Kroll, Virginia. *Beginnings: How Families Come to Be.* Morton Grove, IL: Albert Whitman & Company, 1994.

Six vignettes tell how families are formed. Each vignette is a conversation between a parent and child telling the story of how that child joined the family. The vignettes include birth, international adoption, kinship adoption, single parent adoption, domestic adoption, and adoption through the foster care system.

Audience: Preschool and early elementary school ages.

Tax, Meredith. *Families.* New York, NY: Feminist Press of the City University of New York, 1981.

Angie, age 6, describes her family structure and the families of her friends and extended family. This book nicely describes the differences that can exist within modern step, blended, multigenerational, and multiethnic families.

Audience: Preschool and early elementary school ages.

Braff Brodzinsky, Anne. *The Mulberry Bird.* Indianapolis, IN: Perspectives Press, Inc, revised 1996.

Using personified birds, this book provides a compassionate view of the issues and events that may lead a birthmother to make an adoption plan for her child. This book is especially helpful for children with a history of poor care before adoption and provides the perspective of the birth mother, adoptive families, and adopted children.

Audience: Elementary school ages.

ELSEVIER
SAUNDERS

PEDIATRIC CLINICS

OF NORTH AMERICA

Pediatr Clin N Am 52 (2005) 1525–1531

Index

Note: Page numbers of article titles are in **boldface** type.

pediatric.theclinics.com